Recent Advances in Veterinary Surgery

Recent Advances in Veterinary Surgery

Editor: Orla O'Connell

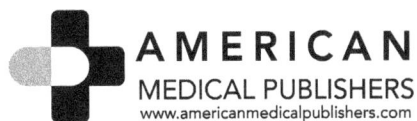

AMERICAN
MEDICAL PUBLISHERS
www.americanmedicalpublishers.com

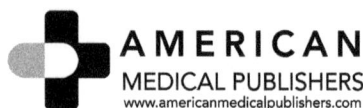

AMERICAN
MEDICAL PUBLISHERS
www.americanmedicalpublishers.com

Cataloging-in-Publication Data

Recent advances in veterinary surgery / edited by Orla O'Connell.
      p. cm.
Includes bibliographical references and index.
ISBN 978-1-63927-523-6
1. Veterinary surgery. 2. Veterinary medicine. 3. Animals--Diseases. 4. Surgery. I. O'Connell, Orla.
SF911 .R43 2022
636.089 7--dc23

American Medical Publishers,
41 Flatbush Avenue,
1st Floor, New York,
NY 11217, USA

ISBN 978-1-63927-523-6 (Hardback)

Contents

Preface IX

Chapter 1 **Kinetic, kinematic, magnetic resonance and owner evaluation of dogs before
and after the amputation of a hind limb** 1
Vladimir Galindo-Zamora, Verena von Babo, Nina Eberle, Daniela Betz,
Ingo Nolte and Patrick Wefstaedt

Chapter 2 **Regeneration of dermal patterns from the remaining pigments after surgery
in *Eublepharis macularius*** 15
Noriyuki Nakashima

Chapter 3 **Prognostic indicators for perioperative survival after diaphragmatic
herniorrhaphy in cats and dogs: 96 cases (2001-2013)** 19
Claire Legallet, Kelley Thieman Mankin and Laura E. Selmic

Chapter 4 **Course of serum amyloid A (SAA) plasma concentrations in horses
undergoing surgery for injuries penetrating synovial structures** 26
Eva Haltmayer, Ilse Schwendenwein and Theresia F. Licka

Chapter 5 **Biomechanical evaluation of monosegmental pedicle instrumentation in a
calf spine model and the role of fractured vertebrae in screw stability** 37
Fuxin Wei, Zhiyu Zhou, Le Wang, Shaoyu Liu, Rui Zhong, Xizhe Liu,
Shangbin Cui, Ximin Pan, Manman Gao and Yajing Zhao

Chapter 6 **Ultrasonographic findings in cows with left displacement of abomasum,
before and after reposition surgery** 47
Xin-Wei Li, Qiu-Shi Xu, Ren-He Zhang, Wei Yang, Yu Li, Yu-Ming Zhang,
Yu Tian, Min Zhang, Zhe Wang, Guo-wen Liu, Cheng Xia and Xiao-Bing Li

Chapter 7 **Comparative measurements of bone mineral density and bone contrast values
in canine femora using dual-energy X-ray absorptiometry and conventional
digital radiography** 54
K. Lucas, I. Nolte, V. Galindo-Zamora, M. Lerch, C. Stukenborg-Colsman,
B. A. Behrens, A. Bouguecha, S. Betancur, A. Almohallami and P. Wefstaedt

Chapter 8 **Skin asepsis protocols as a preventive measure of surgical site infections in
dogs: chlorhexidine–alcohol versus povidone–iodine** 63
Luís Belo, Isa Serrano, Eva Cunha, Carla Carneiro, Luis Tavares,
L. Miguel Carreira and Manuela Oliveira

Chapter 9 **Diagnosis and surgical management of malignant ovarian teratoma in a green
iguana (*Iguana iguana*)** 69
Lucia Bel, Marco Tecilla, Gabriel Borza, Cosmin Pestean, Robert Purdoiu,
Ciprian Ober, Liviu Oana and Marian Taulescu

Chapter 10   **Evaluation of chemical castration with calcium chloride versus surgical castration in donkeys: testosterone as an endpoint marker** 74
Ahmed Ibrahim, Magda M. Ali, Nasser S. Abou-Khalil and Marwa F. Ali

Chapter 11   **Prospective clinical study to evaluate an oscillometric blood pressure monitor in pet rabbits** 83
Luca Bellini, Irene A. Veladiano, Magdalena Schrank, Matteo Candaten and Antonio Mollo

Chapter 12   **A comparison of microRNA expression profiles from splenic hemangiosarcoma, splenic nodular hyperplasia, and normal spleens of dogs** 91
Janet A. Grimes, Nripesh Prasad, Shawn Levy, Russell Cattley, Stephanie Lindley, Harry W. Boothe, Ralph A. Henderson and Bruce F. Smith

Chapter 13   **Surgical treatment of traumatic eventration with polyester button and polypropylene mesh to strengthen the suture technique in equine** 103
Carla Faria Orlandini, Denis Steiner, André Giarola Boscarato, Gabriel Coelho Gimenes and Luiz Romulo Alberton

Chapter 14   **Faecal transplantation for the treatment of *Clostridium difficile* infection in a marmoset** 109
Yumiko Yamazaki, Shinpei Kawarai, Hidetoshi Morita, Takefumi Kikusui and Atsushi Iriki

Chapter 15   **Efficacy of oral meloxicam suspension for prevention of pain and inflammation following band and surgical castration in calves** 114
M. E. Olson, Brenda Ralston, Les Burwash, Heather Matheson-Bird and Nick D. Allan

Chapter 16   **Investigation of short-term surgical complications in a low-resource, high-volume dog sterilisation clinic in India** 125
I. Airikkala-Otter, L. Gamble, S. Mazeri, I. G. Handel, B. M. de C. Bronsvoort, R. J. Mellanby and N. V. Meunier

Chapter 17   **A large animal model for standardized testing of bone regeneration strategies** 133
James C. Ferguson, Stefan Tangl, Dirk Barnewitz, Antje Genzel, Patrick Heimel, Veronika Hruschka, Heinz Redl and Thomas Nau

Chapter 18   **Tiludronate and clodronate do not affect bone structure or remodeling kinetics over a 60 day randomized trial** 143
Heather A. Richbourg, Colin F. Mitchell, Ashley N. Gillett and Margaret A. McNulty

Chapter 19   **Comparison of three imaging modalities used to evaluate bone healing after tibial tuberosity advancement in cranial cruciate ligament-deficient dogs and comparison of the effect of a gelatinous matrix and a demineralized bone matrix mix on bone healing** 153
Marije Risselada, Matthew D. Winter, Daniel D. Lewis, Emily Griffith and Antonio Pozzi

Chapter 20   **Exploring the behavioural drivers of veterinary surgeon antibiotic prescribing: a qualitative study of companion animal veterinary surgeons**...................................165
C. King, M. Smith, K. Currie, A. Dickson, F. Smith, M. Davis and P. Flowers

Chapter 21   **Factors contributing to the decision to perform a cesarean section in Labrador retrievers** 174
Gaudenz Dolf, Claude Gaillard, Jane Russenberger, Lou Moseley and Claude Schelling

Chapter 22   **Postoperative pain and short-term complications after two elective sterilization techniques: ovariohysterectomy or ovariectomy in cats** 183
Marco Aurélio A. Pereira, Lucas A. Gonçalves, Marina C. Evangelista, Rosana S. Thurler, Karina D. Campos, Maira R. Formenton, Geni C. F. Patricio, Julia M. Matera, Aline M. Ambrósio and Denise T. Fantoni

Chapter 23   **Treatment of calvarial defects by resorbable and non-resorbable sonic activated polymer pins and mouldable titanium mesh in two dogs** 190
Pierre Langer, Cameron Black, Padraig Egan and Noel Fitzpatrick

Chapter 24   **Evaluation of P16 expression in canine appendicular osteosarcoma** 199
B. G. Murphy, M. Y. Mok, D. York, R. Rebhun, K. D. Woolard, C. Hillman, P. Dickinson and K. Skorupski

Permissions

List of Contributors

Index

Preface

This book has been a concerted effort by a group of academicians, researchers and scientists, who have contributed their research works for the realization of the book. This book has materialized in the wake of emerging advancements and innovations in this field. Therefore, the need of the hour was to compile all the required researches and disseminate the knowledge to a broad spectrum of people comprising of students, researchers and specialists of the field.

The surgery that is performed by veterinarians on animals is known as veterinary surgery. It has been divided into three broad categories, namely, orthopedics, soft tissue surgery and neurosurgery. Orthopedics surgery is the surgery of joints, bones and muscles. A few examples of orthopedic surgery are bone fracture repair, hip dysplasia and arthroscopy. Soft tissue surgery includes the surgery related to body cavities, skin, cardiovascular system and respiratory tracts. Some of the other surgical procedures which are used in modern veterinary surgery are joint replacement, skin grafts and urogenital procedures. The surgical procedures which do not involve life-threatening conditions are known as elective procedures. A few examples of these surgeries are sterilization surgery, dental surgery, ophthalmic surgery and cardiology surgery. This book contains some path-breaking studies in the field of veterinary surgery and its advances. It also traces the progress of this field and highlights some of its key concepts and applications. This book is appropriate for students seeking detailed information in this area as well as for experts.

At the end of the preface, I would like to thank the authors for their brilliant chapters and the publisher for guiding us all-through the making of the book till its final stage. Also, I would like to thank my family for providing the support and encouragement throughout my academic career and research projects.

Editor

Kinetic, kinematic, magnetic resonance and owner evaluation of dogs before and after the amputation of a hind limb

Vladimir Galindo-Zamora[1,2], Verena von Babo[1], Nina Eberle[1], Daniela Betz[1], Ingo Nolte[1*] and Patrick Wefstaedt[1]

Abstract

Background: The amputation of a limb is a surgical procedure that is regularly performed in small animal practice. In spite of several clinical reports indicating high owner satisfaction after limb amputation in dogs, an amputation is still very critically seen by the owners, and even by some veterinarians, due to the lack of accurate information about the recovery of amputee patients. Thus, the objective of this study was to prospectively evaluate, both objectively and subjectively, the recovery outcome of dogs undergoing a hind limb amputation. Twelve patients in which a hind limb amputation was scheduled were studied. Kinetic and kinematic gait analyses were performed before the amputation, and 10, 30, 90 and 120 days after surgery. Magnetic resonance (MR) examination of the contralateral stifle joint was performed before and 120 days after amputation. The subjective impressions of the owners were gathered at the same examination times of the gait analyses.

Results: Kinetic data showed a redistribution of the load to all remaining limbs after the amputation; ten days after the procedure patients had already established their new locomotory pattern. Kinematic data showed significant differences between sessions in the mean angle progression curves of almost all analyzed joints; however, the ranges of motion were very similar before and after the amputation, and remained constant in the subsequent sessions after the amputation. No changes in the signal intensity of the soft tissues evaluated, and no evidence of cartilage damage or osteoarthritis was seen on the MR examination of the contralateral stifle. Owners evaluated the results of the amputation very positively, both during and at the end of the study.

Conclusions: Dogs had a quick adaptation after a hind limb amputation, and the adaptation process began before the amputation was performed. This happened without evidence of morphologic changes in the contralateral stifle joint, and with a very positive evaluation from the owner.

Keywords: Hind limb amputation, Kinetic and kinematic analyses, Magnetic resonance imaging, Owner evaluation

Background

The amputation of a limb is a surgical procedure that is regularly performed in small animal practice. Severe trauma and limb tumors are the most common reasons for performing an amputation; other indications include chronic osteomyelitis, neurological dysfunctions such as sciatic neuropathy and brachial plexus paralysis, congenital limb deformities, vascular disease and arteriovenous fistulas [1–3].

In spite of several clinical reports indicating high owner satisfaction after limb amputation in dogs [4–7], an amputation is still very critically seen by the owners, and even by some veterinarians. Particularly, owners have the tendency to think that the procedure may affect the animals emotionally, as it indeed happens in people [8], or that it will be disabling for them. Besides, owners are often worried about the possibility of overload of the remaining limbs, leading to hypothetical secondary joint pathologies. Thus, many owners are reluctant to have their dog amputated and reject the amputation as an alternative to euthanasia or take the decision only after

* Correspondence: ingo.nolte@tiho-hannover.de

The preliminary results of this study were presented at the 56. Jahreskongress der Deutsche Gesellschaft für Kleintiermedizin on October 22, 2010 in Düsseldorf (Germany).

[1]Small Animal Hospital, University of Veterinary Medicine Hannover, Foundation, Bünteweg 9, D-30559 Hannover, Germany
Full list of author information is available at the end of the article

the patient has gone through a painful surgical and/or medical treatment process.

The lack of objective information prevents the veterinarian from providing the owners with accurate information about these concerns. A hesitant veterinarian might then play a role in the owner deciding against the amputation. There is only one previously published report objectively evaluating the gait of amputated dogs [9]. In that study, force plate analyses were carried out to measure ground reaction forces (GRF) and contact times in a population of 10 large-breed dogs which had a limb amputation (five forelimbs and five hind limbs). Additionally, the center of gravity was calculated in those patients. It was found that the absence of a limb caused statistically significant changes in the GRF, impulses and contact times of the remaining limbs and the location of the animal's centre of gravity, in comparison to a control group of 22 healthy dogs. However, there are no prospective studies with animals which are planned to be amputated, and no study has been performed objectively evaluating kinematics (joint movement) or possible joint changes after a hind limb amputation in dogs.

The general objective of the present study was therefore to prospectively characterize the recovery outcome of dogs undergoing a hind limb amputation. In order to evaluate the motion and weight bearing characteristics, as well as the duration of adaptation to the three-legged gait, kinematic and kinetic analyses were carried out. Furthermore, MR images of the remaining contralateral femorotibial (stifle) joint were made before and 4 months after the amputation, in order to investigate possible changes in joint morphology, due to a hypothetic weight bearing overload of this limb.

It was hypothesized that there would be marked changes both in the kinetic and the kinematic parameters after the amputation, but that those changes would not impair the ability of the animal to lead a normal life. Based on our clinical experience and some of the aforementioned studies [4–7], it was also hypothesized that there would not be any changes in the contralateral stifle on the MR examination. Thus, after the initial reluctance to the amputation, owners would be satisfied with the procedure.

Methods
This study was carried out in accordance with the German Animal Welfare Guidelines and was approved by the Ethics Committee of the Lower Saxony State Office for Consumer Protection and Food Safety (Approval Number: 10A071). All owners agreed to their dogs participation in the study and signed a consent form.

Patients
All dogs presented to the Small Animal Hospital of the University of Veterinary Medicine Hannover, Foundation (Germany), between March 2010 and October 2011, for a hind limb amputation were included in the study. In total, 12 patients were enrolled. Two additional patients were not included due to aggressiveness in one case, and presence of metallic orthopedic implants in both stifle joints, making it unadvisable to perform the MR examination, in the other case.

Before surgery a thorough physical examination, including an orthopedic and neurologic examination of all remaining limbs and the spine, was performed to rule out any disease which might obscure the results. This examination was repeated 10, 30, 90 and 120 days after the amputation. It was planned that, in case an abnormality was suspected, all necessary diagnostic examination tools would be used to determine the type and location of such an abnormality and its possible relationship with the amputation.

Surgical procedure
On the amputation day, physical status was determined based on the physical examination, blood work and other diagnostic tests as needed. Based on the American Society of Anesthesiologists (ASA) physical status classification system, all patients were classified as ASA 2 (patients with local or mild systemic disease). The animals were premedicated using a combination of levo-methadone (0.6 mg/kg) [1] and diazepam (0.5 mg/kg) [2]; anesthesia was induced with propofol dosed to effect (1–4 mg/kg) [3] After orotracheal intubation, anesthesia was maintained with isoflurane [4] in a 1:1 oxygen: air mixture adjusted according to the physical signs of anesthetic depth (end-tidal isoflurane 0.7-1.5 vol %) and a continuous rate infusion (CRI) of fentanyl (0.16 µg/kg/min),[5] lidocaine (50 µg/kg/min) [6] and ketamine (10 µg/kg/min).[7] Additionally, a preoperative epidural anesthesia with bupivacaine (0.5 mg/kg) [8] and morphine (0.1 mg/kg) [9] and a intraoperative sciatic nerve block with lidocaine (1 mg/kg) [10] were performed. For postoperative analgesia the aforementioned CRI of fentanyl, lidocaine and ketamine was used for 24 h, and carprofen (4 mg/kg)[11] was initiated the day of the surgery and continued for 10 additional days.

The surgical procedure was performed by disarticulation of the hip, as described elsewhere [2]. The dogs remained in the hospital for approximately 5 days.

Kinetic and kinematic gait evaluation
Kinetic (forces) and kinematic (movement) gait analysis was performed one to three days before the amputation, as well as 10, 30, 90 and 120 days after surgery.

Kinetics were measured using a specially designed treadmill[12] consisting of four separate belts, each of them with an integrated force plate underneath. This design allowed the simultaneous measurement of all limb forces.

Kinematic analysis was performed with the aid of retro-reflective markers (Ø 16 mm reflective markers)[13] positioned on 24 anatomic landmarks (8 per remaining limb), using double-sided adhesive tape; the location of these markers has been previously described [10, 11] and is illustrated in Fig. 1. Six high-speed infrared cameras[14] were used to record marker movement in all three remaining limbs simultaneously, as the animals were walking at a controlled speed (measurement frequency: 100 Hz). Before each measurement, static and dynamic camera calibration was performed using an L-shaped calibration device.[15]

On each gait analysis session, patients were gently introduced to the gait on the treadmill; on the first day, a speed at which each individual patient walked comfortably on the treadmill was determined; on each subsequent session the patient was evaluated using the same speed, ranging from 0.5 to 0.8 m/s. During each gait analysis session, two to six trials were recorded, each with a duration of approximately 30 s, until at least one valid trial was obtained. A valid trial was defined as 10 consecutive regular steps, in which the dog walked smoothly, without any external forces from the handler being applied, with all paws landing on the appropriate

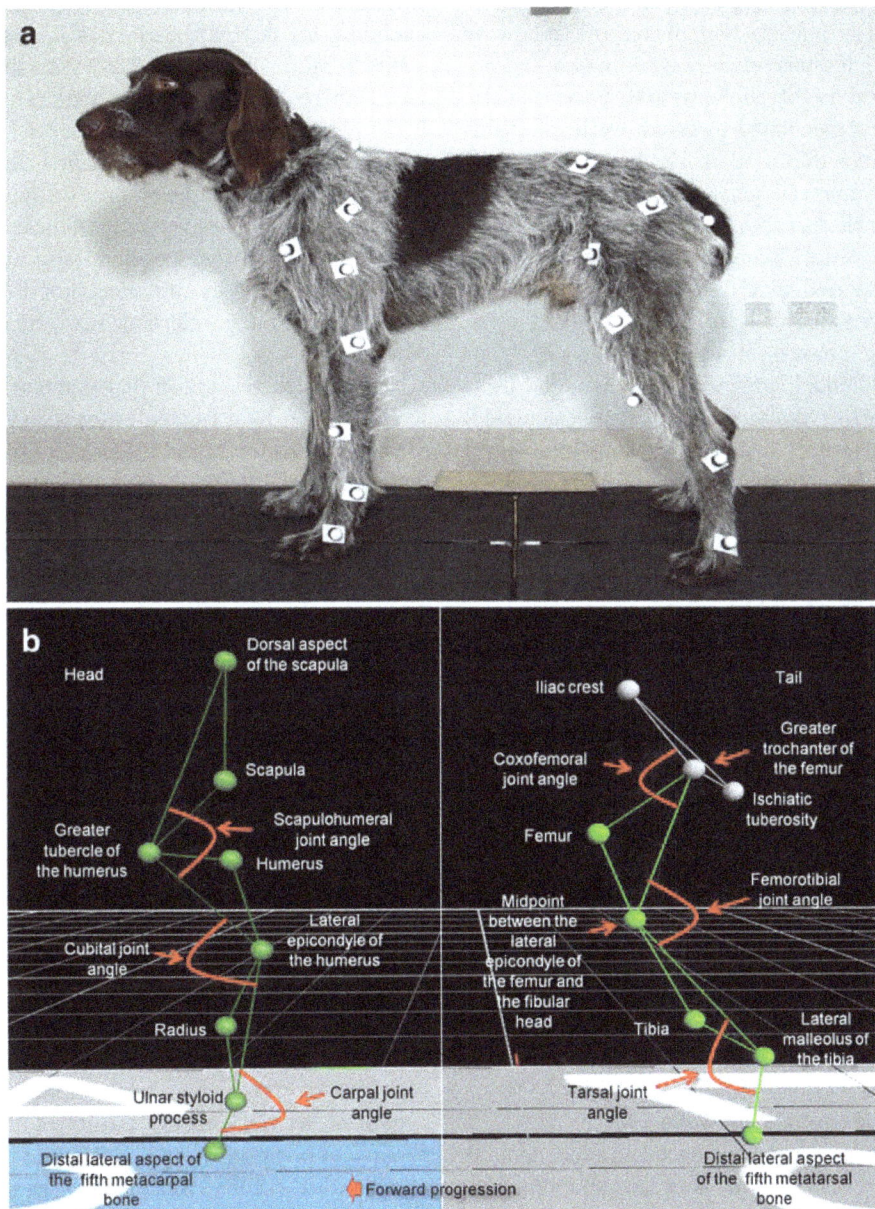

Fig. 1 a Example of the localization of the retro-reflective markers on a healthy patient; **b** Illustration of the localization of the retro-reflective markers on the anatomical reference points and the measured angles

force plate, without overstepping. Video recording was performed, to ensure that the steps were appropriate for analysis.

Both kinetic and kinematic data were simultaneously recorded using commercially available software.[16]

Ten consecutive steps were afterwards analyzed for the following kinetic parameters: peak vertical force (PFz), mean vertical force (MFz), and vertical impulse (integral [IFz]). All forces were normalized to the individual body weight of each dog and data were expressed as percentage of body weight (%BW). Mean ± standard deviation (SD) was calculated from 10 valid consecutive steps. Afterwards, load redistribution (LR) was calculated for each forelimb and remaining hind limb, for each measured parameter (PFz, MFz, IFz), using the following equation (according to Steiss et al. [12]): % load bearing = Fz of the limb/total Fz of all limbs*100. Other kinetic parameters were not calculated to avoid overloading this section with too much information. The kinetic data were processed using commercial software[17] and exported to a commercially available spreadsheet.[18]

In order to process the kinematic data in Vicon Nexus, all markers were labeled in a trial. Then, 10 valid foot strikes were marked manually to define the gait cycle (stance and swing phases) of each limb. Using a 2-dimensional (2-D) model, projected flexion and extension angles of each remaining joint were calculated: contralateral (with respect to the amputated hind limb) scapulohumeral joint, contralateral cubital joint, contralateral carpal joint, ipsilateral (with respect to the amputated hind limb) scapulohumeral joint, ipsilateral cubital joint, ipsilateral carpal joint, contralateral coxofemoral joint, contralateral femorotibial joint and contralateral tarsal joint. Measured angles are illustrated in Fig. 1. In order to compare the movement pattern of each analyzed joint, the gait cycles were normalized to 100 in all dogs and displayed as percentage of one whole stride. The mean joint angle (±SD) and the range of motion (±SD) of the aforementioned joints were calculated from the mean joint angle progression curves (MJAPC) calculated from the 10 strides per dog. Mean joint angles and range of motion were used since the reader can easily understand their comparison between sessions and to avoid overloading the manuscript with too much data. The kinematic data were processed using commercial software[19] and then exported to a commercially available spreadsheet[18].

MR evaluation of the contralateral stifle joint

The MR examination was performed under general anesthesia before and 120 days after amputation. The anesthetic protocol was the same described above, excluding local anesthetics and CRIs. The animals were positioned in lateral recumbency with the limb to be examined in a non-dependent position and the stifle joint at an angle of ~135°. Using a state-of-the-art 3 T MR scan,[20] images were obtained from the contralateral stifle. Small (11 cm Ø) surface ring coils (Achieva 3.0 T Musculoskeletal SENSE Flex S coil 2 elements) were used as image enhancers; these were positioned parallel to each other, lateral and medial to the examined stifle, with the joint centered between the two coils. The MR protocol used included a 3-D (3-dimensional) PDW (proton-density weighted) acquisition sequence, which was afterwards reconstructed in sagittal, dorsal (parallel to patella ligament) and transversal (parallel to tibial plateau) planes (slices every 2 mm), a PDW HR (high-resolution) TSE (turbo spin echo) SENSE (sensitivity encoding for fast MR) sequence in sagittal plane (slices every 2 mm),, a PDW HR SPAIR (spectrally adiabatic inversion recovery) SENSE in sagittal plane (slices every 2 mm), and a T1-weighted TSE clear (constant level appearance) sequence in sagittal plane (slices every 1.8 mm).

This protocol had been previously standardized and regarded as suitable for use in clinical cases, since diagnostic image quality is optimal and acquisition time is only 22 min (total examination time is about 40 min including positioning, reference scan, survey, and sequence planning).

Using a high-resolution diagnostic screen[21] the images were assessed by a trained evaluator (VGZ), who looked for changes in the signal intensity of the cranial cruciate ligament (CrCL), the caudal cruciate ligament (CdCL) and the lateral and medial menisci. Possible changes in the cartilage surfaces, as well as evidence of osteoarthritic changes were also evaluated in the lateral and medial femoral condyles, femoral trochlear groove, patella and tibial plateau.

It was expected that, due to a possible underlying metastatic disease, some patients could die or be euthanized before the end of the study; if that was the case, it was planned to ask the owner to authorize the MR examination postmortem.

Owner evaluation of patient comfort

The owner was requested to fill out an evaluation form (modified from Hielm-Björkman et al. [13]) before the amputation and 10, 30, 90 and 120 days after the procedure, in order to gather his/her (subjective) impressions with regard to patient comfort and recovery. At the end of the study (day 120), owners filled out a questionnaire to assess their final impression regarding the degree of activity and life quality of the dog, and their general impression of and satisfaction with the procedure; besides, owners were encouraged to make further comments. It was planned that if the animal died before the end of the study, an appropriate moment would be looked for to ask the owner to fill out the questionnaire.

The questions of the questionnaire were adapted from Carberry and Harvey [4], Withrow and Hirsch [5], von Werthern et al. [6] and Kirpensteijn et al. [7]. The owners' assessment of patient comfort and the final questionnaire were made in German and translated into English as accurately as possible.

Statistical methods

Due to the small sample size and very heterogeneous patient population included in this study, it was decided to use non-parametric statistics. Thus, data were analyzed using a Kruskal-Wallis one-way ANOVA test to compare between sessions; when statistically significant differences were found, a Wilcoxon signed-rank test for paired observations was performed to determine which session was different. All tests were considered statistically significant if $p < 0.05$ and were performed using standard statistical software.[22] Descriptive statistics were calculated using a commercially available spreadsheet[18], where appropriate.

Results

Clinical data

Breed, sex, age, reason to amputate and performed evaluations of the 12 patients enrolled in this study are illustrated in Table 1. As can be seen in this table, the most common reason for performing the amputation was a tumor, followed by trauma and one surgical complication. Six right and six left hind limbs were amputated. Nine patients survived until the end of the study. Due to the underlying metastatic disease, one animal (patient 5) was euthanized 36 days after the amputation and another one (patient 6) died 120 days after the procedure. One dog (patient 8) died unexpectedly 22 days after the amputation due to abdominal bleeding caused by a previously asymptomatic and undiagnosed hepatic hemangiosarcoma.

Patient 12 presented bilateral hip osteoarthritis; however, it was asymptomatic, and no signs of pain, lameness or difficulty to stand up were detected before or after the amputation. All other patients showed no abnormalities in the physical examination of the remaining limbs. No patient showed abnormalities on the physical examination of the spine throughout the study.

Kinetic and kinematic gait evaluation

The results of the kinetic and kinematic evaluations are presented in Figs. 2, 3, 4 and 5 and Tables 3 and 4. It should be noted that, although nine patients survived until the last examination day, the kinetic and kinematic data were not available from all of them. One animal (Patient 7) refused to walk on the treadmill and others (e.g. Patient 4) walked intermittently in such a way that some trials were not valid for analysis; even though these animals could walk and run perfectly fine on solid ground, they were afraid of walking on the treadmill, apparently due to the movement of the belts. Moreover, although all owners were extremely cooperative, when some of them had the impression that their dog was afraid or tired, they were reluctant to allow their pets to be walked on the treadmill long enough to record valid trials. The number of patients evaluated on each session is also indicated in Tables 3 and 4.

Kinetic data showed that 10 days after amputation there was redistribution of the load to all remaining limbs (Fig. 2 and Table 2). The values and pattern of load shifting are represented in Fig. 2. The recorded PFz, MFz and IFz values showed no remarkable changes during the remaining examination time points, indicating that 10 days after the amputation the patient had already reached its

Table 1 Patients included in this study

Patient	Breed	Sex	Age (Years)	Weight (kg)	Reason to amputate	Gait analyses					PO MR
						Pre	10	30	90	120	
1	Boxer	Male	8	32	Osteosarcoma	+	+	+	+	+	+
2	Labrador	Female	3	31	Rhabdomyosarcoma	+	+	+	+	+	+
3	Mixed-breed dog	Female	4	32	Osteosarcoma	+	+	+	+	+	+
4	Mixed-breed dog	Male	1	20	Severe soft tissue trauma	+	+	+	+	+	+
5	Mixed-breed dog	Male	12	31	Osteosarcoma	+	+	+	E	-	-
6	Swiss Mountain dog	Female	10	39	Osteosarcoma	+	+	+	+	E	-
7	Bernese Mountain dog	Male	2	40	Femoral fracture nonunion	-	-	-	-	-	+
8	German Shepherd mix	Male	7	26	Severe soft tissue trauma	+	+	E	-	-	-
9	Mixed-breed dog	Female	8	13	Osteosarcoma	+	+	+	+	+	+
10	Mixed-breed dog	Female	11	8	Malignant sarcoma	+	+	+	+	+	+
11	Landseer	Female	2	54	Fibrosarcoma	+	+	+	+	+	-
12	Mixed-breed dog	Female	8	49	Osteosarcoma	+	+	+	+	+	+

PO MR: Postoperative magnetic resonance scan; +: Performed; −: Not performed; E: Euthanasia

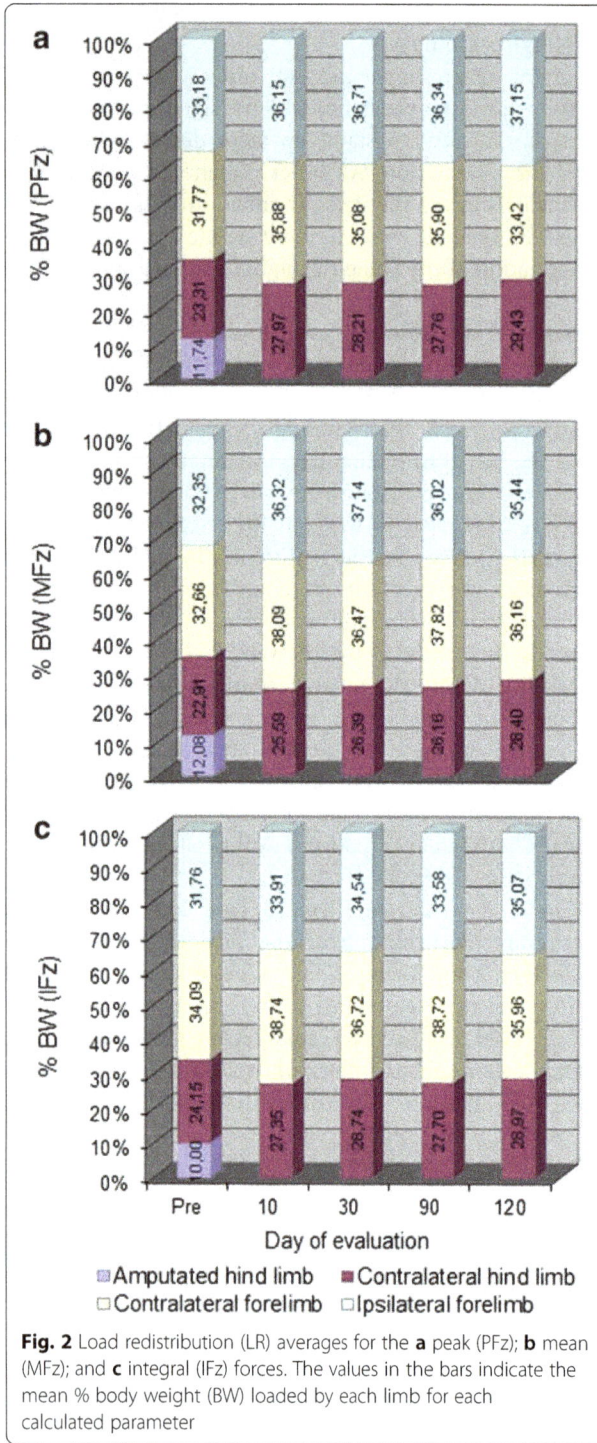

Fig. 2 Load redistribution (LR) averages for the **a** peak (PFz); **b** mean (MFz); and **c** integral (IFz) forces. The values in the bars indicate the mean % body weight (BW) loaded by each limb for each calculated parameter

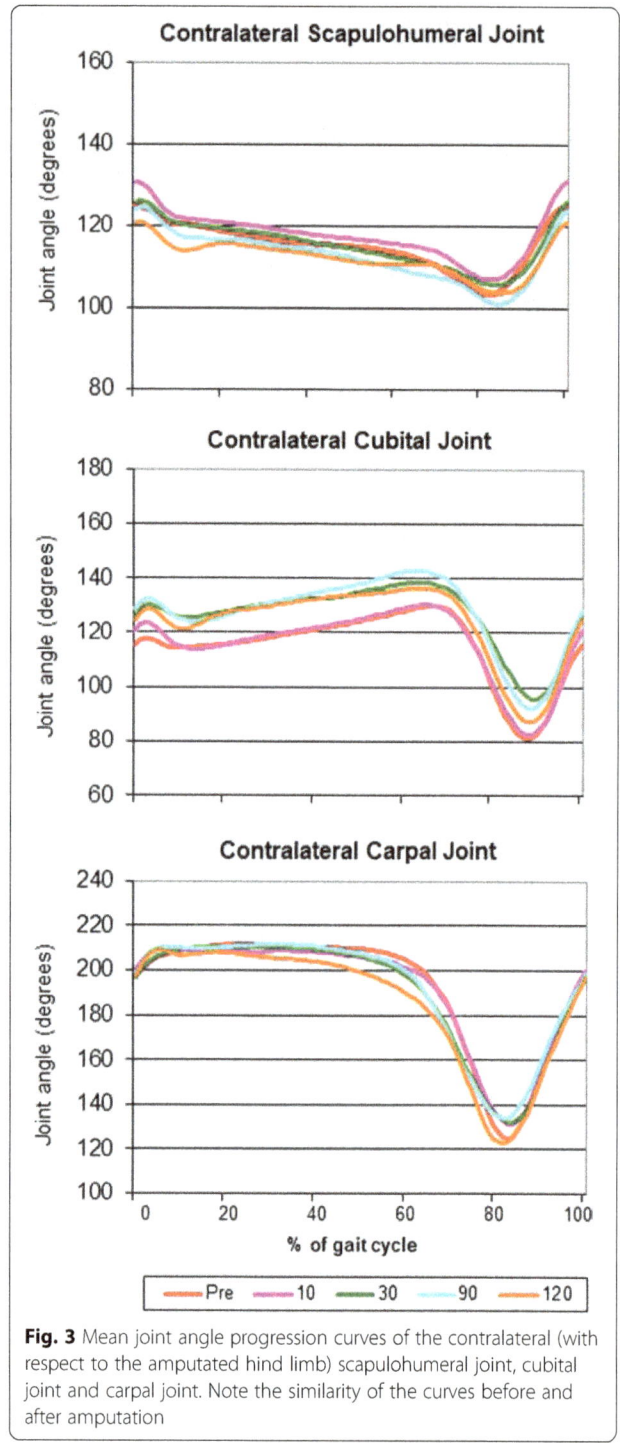

Fig. 3 Mean joint angle progression curves of the contralateral (with respect to the amputated hind limb) scapulohumeral joint, cubital joint and carpal joint. Note the similarity of the curves before and after amputation

new locomotory pattern. This was true for all patients including the lightest (8 kg) and the heaviest (54 kg) ones. There were no statistically-significant differences between sessions (Table 2).

With regard to the kinematic gait analysis, even though the patients walked smoothly on the treadmill (Additional file 1: Video 1), there were significant differences between sessions in the means of almost all joint angles (Table 3). It is important to note that there were also marked variations within a patient in the same session (not shown in Table 3). The MJAPC showed a similar pattern between sessions (Figs. 3, 4 and 5), but these showed marked individual variations (not shown).

Despite all these different kinematic results, ROMs of all analyzed joints were very similar before and after

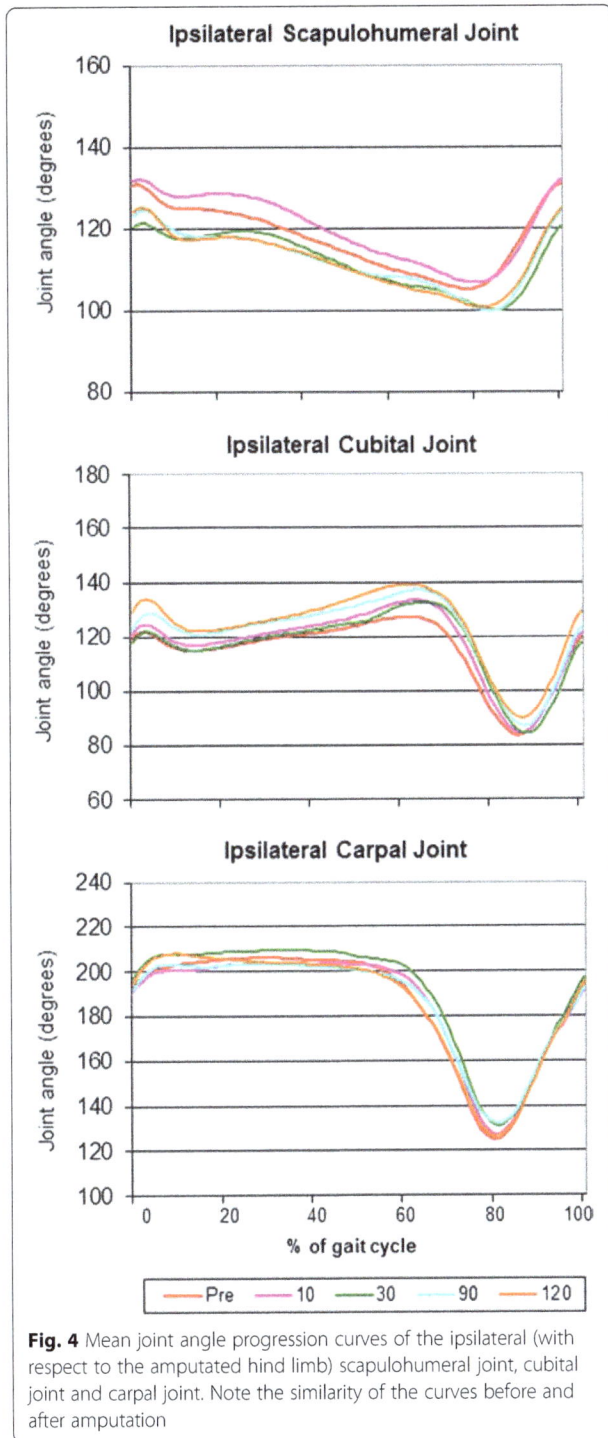

Fig. 4 Mean joint angle progression curves of the ipsilateral (with respect to the amputated hind limb) scapulohumeral joint, cubital joint and carpal joint. Note the similarity of the curves before and after amputation

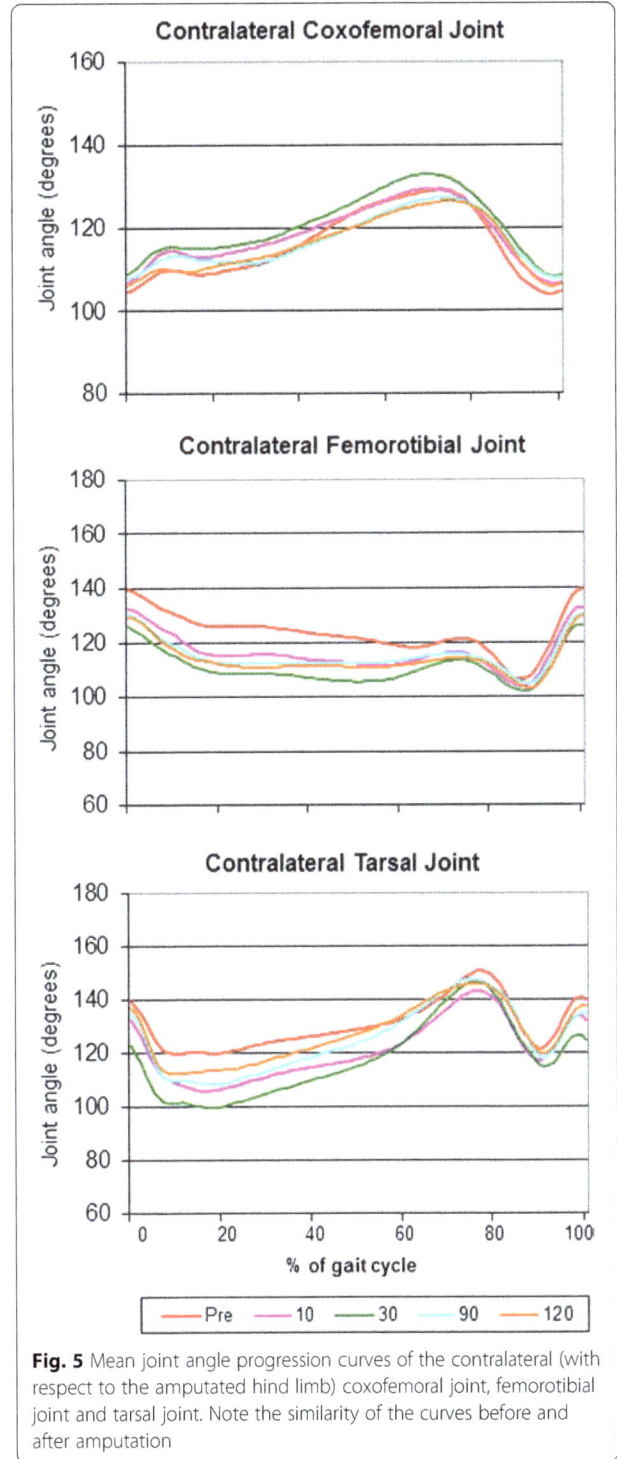

Fig. 5 Mean joint angle progression curves of the contralateral (with respect to the amputated hind limb) coxofemoral joint, femorotibial joint and tarsal joint. Note the similarity of the curves before and after amputation

amputation and remained constant in the subsequent sessions after the amputation, without significant differences between sessions (Table 3).

MR evaluation of the contralateral stifle joint

Postoperative MR examination was possible in eight patients. Although nine patients survived until the end of the study, severe metastatic disease was detected in

patient 11 on day 120, and the MR examination was not performed. Postmortem MR examination was not possible in any case, as the owners were very sensitive about their pet's death, and they elected to dispose the patients' dead bodies themselves. No changes in the signal intensity of the CrCL, CdCL or the lateral and medial menisci were found, in comparison with the preoperative MR

Table 2 Results of the kinetic analysis

		Pre (n = 11)	10 (n = 11)	30 (n = 10)	90 (n = 9)	120 (n = 8)	p
PFz contralateral forelimb							
	Mean	64.88	71.45	67.69	69.78	66.74	0.252
	SD	7.00	4.73	8.71	6.44	8.27	
PFz ipsilateral forelimb							
	Mean	67.78	71.97	70.86	70.64	74.18	0.796
	SD	9.03	5.90	9.29	5.60	11.56	
PFz contralateral hind limb							
	Mean	47.60	55.68	54.44	53.96	58.75	0.454
	SD	11.71	10.07	9.62	13.69	15.36	
MFz contralateral forelimb							
	Mean	47.55	52.71	49.33	50.70	48.49	0.327
	SD	7.13	4.71	6.84	4.37	7.45	
MFz ipsilateral forelimb							
	Mean	47.10	50.27	50.25	48.30	47.53	0.816
	SD	6.93	5.30	7.79	3.43	9.55	
MFz contralateral hind limb							
	Mean	33.37	35.41	35.70	35.08	38.09	0.865
	SD	7.02	6.27	6.42	10.38	10.48	
IFz contralateral forelimb							
	Mean	30.28	32.09	30.41	30.07	28.82	0.945
	SD	7.28	7.46	9.10	8.45	7.54	
IFz ipsilateral forelimb							
	Mean	28.20	28.09	28.61	26.08	28.10	0.967
	SD	5.90	7.12	6.57	6.31	6.81	
IFz contralateral hind limb							
	Mean	21.45	22.65	23.81	21.51	23.21	0.999
	SD	7.28	7.00	8.19	5.23	7.62	

p: p value of the Kruskal-Wallis test; PFz: Peak vertical force; MFz: Mean vertical force; IFz: vertical impulse (integral); SD: Standard deviation

images. No changes in the cartilage surface and no evidence of osteoarthritic changes were found (Fig. 6).

Owner evaluation of patient comfort

The results of the owners' assessment of patient comfort are presented in Table 4 and show a clear tendency of the patients to improve after amputation. Patient movement after amputation is exemplified with Additional file 2: Video 2. Ten owners answered the final questionnaire (Table 5). This questionnaire revealed a high degree of owner satisfaction with the amputation result.

Discussion

The main goal of this study was to provide owners and veterinarians with accurate, objective information, not existing previously, about the outcome of the amputated

patient (i.e. how the dog adapted to the new locomotory status).

Examination times were chosen using the data of a previous study [7] which indicated that most dogs adapted to the amputation within a month, some within a week, and all within 3 months after surgery. With the last follow-up 120 days after the procedure, a final attempt was made to find any evidence of further gait changes. Since there is the belief that orthopedic disease might occur in the remaining limb after amputation, as a result of a theoretical overload, the contralateral stifle was morphologically assessed using MR images, to evaluate this likelihood. The femorotibial (stifle) joint was chosen, instead of the coxofemoral or tarsal joint, as the former has been extensively investigated, and there is a whole body of literature exemplifying normal and pathologic MR images to compare [14–19].

Table 3 Results of the kinematic analysis

		Pre (n = 11)	10 (n = 11)	30 (n = 10)	90 (n = 9)	120 (n = 8)	p
Contralateral scapulohumeral joint	Mean ± SD	115.2 ± 5.67	117.9 ± 5.83	115.4 ± 5.54	112.7 ± 6.09	112.3 ± 4.24	<0.001
	ROM ± SD	27.68 ± 7.48	31.46 ± 8.12	29.51 ± 6.73	31.49 ± 6.26	26.07 ± 6.04	0.478
Contralateral cubital joint	Mean ± SD	114.9 ± 12.93	115.9 ± 12.82	126.5 ± 11.59	127.2 ± 13.67	123.6 ± 13.91	<0.001
	ROM ± SD	57.98 ± 15.56	61.8 ± 11.64	56.51 ± 14.74	60.75 ± 13.06	62.74 ± 9.60	0.898
Contralateral carpal joint	Mean ± SD	192.2 ± 26.85	191.5 ± 24.89	190.1 ± 26.03	191.5 ± 25.66	185.8 ± 26.88	<0.001
	ROM ± SD	99.38 ± 19.62	97.45 ± 11.28	104.7 ± 10.83	94.25 ± 13.65	101.1 ± 8.17	0.666
Ipsilateral scapulohumeral joint	Mean ± SD	117.5 ± 7.92	120.1 ± 8.33	111.9 ± 6.87	112.4 ± 6.94	112.1 ± 7.12	<0.001
	ROM ± SD	34.11 ± 5.69	32.2 ± 4.35	29.77 ± 4.80	32.17 ± 2.71	31.06 ± 5.03	0.654
Ipsilateral cubital joint	Mean ± SD	114.6 ± 12.28	117.6 ± 13.33	116.7 ± 12.94	121.5 ± 13.63	123.8 ± 13.58	<0.001
	ROM ± SD	55 ± 11.81	57.96 ± 11.92	57.23 ± 12.69	59.84 ± 12.73	57.78 ± 11.82	0.916
Ipsilateral carpal joint	Mean ± SD	185.5 ± 26.36	185.6 ± 24.54	190.6 ± 25.54	185.9 ± 23.23	185.5 ± 26.05	<0.001
	ROM ± SD	92.65 ± 19.14	91.83 ± 18.76	91.01 ± 15.71	82.42 ± 12.51	93.36 ± 10.05	0.630
Contralateral coxofemoral joint	Mean ± SD	116.1 ± 8.37	118.4 ± 6.96	120.8 ± 7.516	116.8 ± 6.29	116.1 ± 6.64	<0.001
	ROM ± SD	30.25 ± 6.22	27.47 ± 9.90	30.08 ± 9.71	25.17 ± 9.09	24.89 ± 6.27	0.501
Contralateral femorotibial joint	Mean ± SD	123.2 ± 7.48	115.8 ± 6.62	110.4 ± 5.76	114.7 ± 5.55	113.3 ± 5.68	<0.001
	ROM ± SD	42.4 ± 4.28	37.67 ± 8.44	37.82 ± 7.34	40.8 ± 12.16	34.83 ± 8.31	0.299
Contralateral tarsal joint	Mean ± SD	130.5 ± 8.98	121 ± 10.93	117.8 ± 14.07	124.9 ± 12.21	127.2 ± 10.75	<0.001
	ROM ± SD	47.74 ± 10.2	50.57 ± 10.52	61.27 ± 14.25	57.73 ± 11.24	48.04 ± 14.17	0.143

Mean: mean joint angle calculated from the mean joint angle progression curves; SD: Standard deviation; ROM = Range of Motion; p = p value of the Kruskal-Wallis test

As expected, a very heterogeneous population was found in this study: different breeds, ages and weights. The main reason for amputating a patient was the presence of a tumor, which agrees with previous studies [6, 7]. The mortality seen in this study was not related the amputation itself.

The kinetic and kinematic analyses revealed that the patients had begun adapting to the new locomotory situation even before the amputation was performed, and that 10 days after the procedure, all major changes had already taken place. It was unfortunate that it was not possible to perform all examinations on all patients.

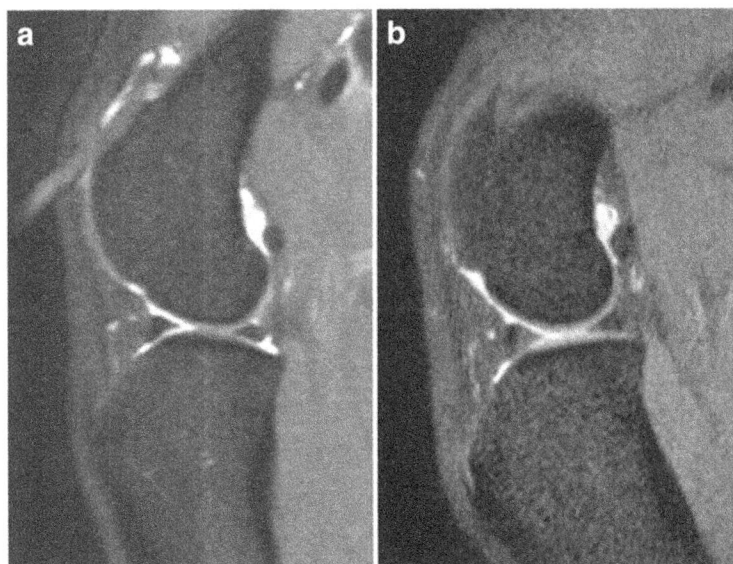

Fig. 6 Example of the magnetic resonance examination of the stifle in one patient before (**a**) and 120 days after the amputation (**b**). No changes could be detected in the joint 120 days after the procedure

Table 4 Owner assessment of patient comfort[a] (first part)

	Pre ($n = 12$)	10 ($n = 12$)	30 ($n = 11$)	90 ($n = 10$)	120 ($n = 10$)
Attitude					
Very bright (score 0)	4	2	6	4	3
Alert (score 1)	5	8	5	6	7
Neither alert nor indifferent (score 2)	3	2	0	0	0
Indifferent (score 3)	0	0	0	0	0
Depressed (score 4)	0	0	0	0	0
Cumulative score for attitude	*11*	*12*	*5*	*6*	*7*
Willingness to move (general)					
Very willing (score 0)	2	3	6	5	5
Willing (score 1)	4	8	5	4	5
Hesitant (score 2)	4	1	0	1	0
Reluctant (score 3)	1	0	0	0	0
Does not move (score 4)	1	0	0	0	0
Cumulative score for willingness to move (general)	*19*	*10*	*5*	*6*	*5*
The dog …					
… lies down …					
Easily (score 0)	3	4	7	9	9
Carefully (score 1)	5	7	4	1	1
Slowly (score 2)	1	1	0	0	0
with difficulty (score 3)	2	0	0	0	0
with a lot of difficulty (score 4)	1	0	0	0	0
Cumulative score for the dog lies down…	*17*	*7*	*4*	*1*	*1*
… stands up …					
Easily (score 0)	4	2	4	5	6
Carefully (score 1)	3	10	6	4	2
Slowly (score 2)	2	0	1	1	2
with difficulty (score 3)	2	0	0	0	0
with a lot of difficulty (score 4)	1	0	0	0	0
Cumulative score for the dog stands up…	*17*	*10*	*8*	*6*	*6*
Willingness to move after resting					
Very willing (score 0)	0	4	4	4	4
Willing (score 1)	5	7	6	5	5
Hesitant (score 2)	6	0	1	1	1
Reluctant (score 3)	1	1	0	0	0
Does not move (score 4)	0	0	0	0	0
Cumulative Score for willingness to move after resting	*20*	*10*	*8*	*7*	*7*
Willingness to move after exercising					
Very willing (score 0)	0	0	1	3	2
Willing (score 1)	3	9	6	4	6
Hesitant (score 2)	4	2	3	3	2
Reluctant (score 3)	3	1	1	0	0
Does not move (score 4)	2	0	0	0	0
Cumulative score for willingness to move after exercising	*28*	*16*	*15*	*10*	*10*
Mean score (sum of cumulative scores / patients evaluated)	*9.3*	*5.4*	*4.1*	*3.6*	*3.6*

[a]Modified from Hielm-Björkman et al. [13]

Table 5 Final owner questionnaire[a] (n = 10)

1. Please indicate how satisfied you are with the results of the amputation			
Very satisfied: 8	Satisfied: 2	Not satisfied: 0	Very dissatisfied: 0

2. Please indicate how well the dog adapted to the amputation			
Very good: 7	Good: 2	Fair: 1	Poor: 0

3. The time the dog took to recover was:		
More than expected: 0	As expected: 3	Less than expected: 7

4. Were behavioral changes observed?	
Yes: 3	No: 7

5. Would you make a similar decision in the future, in case an amputation would be needed in another pet?		
Yes: 10	Not sure: 0	No: 0

6. Before the amputation, were you reluctant to allow this procedure being performed in your dog?	
Yes: 8	No: 2

7. The degree of activity of your dog after the amputation was:		
Increased: 2	The same: 6	Decreased: 2

8. In general, you think that the life quality of the dog after the amputation:		
Increased: 6	Is the same: 4	Decreased: 0

[a]Adapted from Carberry and Harvey [4], Withrow and Hirsch [5], von Werthern et al. [6] and Kirpensteijn et al. [7]

However, exclusively using "good" trials allowed us to obtain reliable results. It should be noted that, even though a valid trial implied that the handler did not exert any external forces, it was not possible to have the animals completely free on the treadmill (see Additional file 1: Video 1). Unfortunately, the willingness to walk or trot or overall activity of the patient were not evaluated in the present study; these factors would have brought additional information about the outcome. It is remarkable that the largest patient (patient 11–54 kg) and the smallest one (patient 10 – 8 kg) adapted equally well. These results agree with the study of Kirpensteijn et al. [7], indicating that, even though subjective, the observations made by the owners of such study were actually very precise. The present study has the advantage of looking at the patients objectively and prospectively, leaving no doubt about the fast adaptation of all animals. The fact that there were no significant changes in the load redistribution after amputation was initially surprising; however, it is easily explainable: all patients were severely lame before the amputation, meaning that the adaptation and compensation to the lack of a hind limb had begun to take place before the amputation was performed. This was even clearer when looking only at those patients which did not load the affected limb at all before surgery. It should also be kept in mind, that the lack of statistically significant changes could have resulted from the low number of dogs included in this study, and therefore in the lack of power of the tests.

The kinematic results (including the statistical analysis) should be interpreted with caution. The fact that significant differences were found in the absolute values of the different joint angles could be explained by the normal variation inherent to motion analysis: marker localization changes lead to changes in joint angles measured. Even though every effort was made to place the markers in the right position, small variations might have occurred, leading to different measurements. However, also huge variations were seen within a session (not shown in Table 3 or Figs. 3, 4 and 5), possibly indicating that the patients adapted to every step they made and in a very irregular manner. Affected balance of the dog during movement and the resulting instability might cause these variations. Another possible explanation is the fact that several gait patterns are possible at a given speed and by a permanent adjustment of the speed of the animal to the treadmill speed [20]. It should also be taken into account that slow speeds were used before the amputation, in order to avoid worsening the pain that patients were already experiencing. After the amputation the animals could have walked on the treadmill more comfortably at faster speeds (personal observations). Even though this might have caused an irregular walking pattern after the procedure, speeds were kept constant to avoid adding a variance factor when measuring the GRF [21]. Finally, the angles measured here can be used to illustrate the movement patterns for the patients in this study, and they cannot be extrapolated to other patient populations. However, our study focuses on determining whether there are variations in the different kinematic parameters before and after amputation in this particular patient population, and that does not seem to be the case.

The similarity in the ROMs before and after surgery is a remarkable finding. The measurement of ROMs seems to be less susceptible to the sources of error commonly found in kinematic studies (misplacement of markers and skin movement), at least in the hind limb [22]. Therefore, the results of the ROMs are more accurate than the absolute measurement of joint angles. That being said, the lack of significant differences between sessions suggests that the patient had also begun to adapt to the new movement situation before amputation, and that this remained stable after the procedure. However, it should also be taken into consideration that joint angular curves in each measurement points are very similar in shape, resulting in stable ROMs; this could also explain why the ROMs showed much less variation than mean joint angles.

The lack of changes in the MR examination of the remaining contralateral stifle after amputation could indicate that an overload in the remaining contralateral hind limb, leading to joint pathology, is not very likely. It was decided to investigate this point, as it is commonly believed by the general public, and even by some veterinarians, that amputating a dog might predispose it to orthopedic abnormalities; the results of our MR (and also our physical examinations) proved otherwise, at least for the stifle. Although 4 months after amputation might possibly be a short time to evaluate joint changes,

a previous study describing the experimentally induced rupture of the CrCL in 5 crossbred dogs showed that it is possible to see changes in the cartilage and subchondral bone as early as 4 weeks after the rupture [17]. It is of course difficult to extrapolate such findings to this study, but it could indicate that, if there were ongoing changes in joint morphology, they would be visible 4 months after amputation. Besides, most of our research subjects were oncologic patients, with a (likely) short life span. Measuring cartilage thickness would have been a more accurate method to evaluate subtle joint changes [17]. Unfortunately, this could not be done due to software limitations. In any case, we did not expect to see any changes, as our clinical experience indicates that no changes are seen in the contralateral limb after a hindlimb amputation; nevertheless, it is not known what kind of changes an amputation would cause in patients suffering from degenerative joint disease in the remaining limbs.

With regard to the owner evaluation assessment of the patient after the procedure, the results were as expected: in Table 4, the positive outcome of most patients can be clearly seen. The improvement is especially remarkable in the ability of the dog to lie down and stand up. The lack of improvement or worsening of some parameters for some patients seemed to be related more to the declining general condition of the patient, than to the effects of the amputation itself. The use of an objective tool to measure patient activity, such as an accelerometer, could have provided more accurate information about the outcome and they have been previously used in animals [23]; however, this tool was not available to us.

The responses to the final questionnaire were also as expected: most owners were initially reluctant to have their dogs amputated, but were satisfied with the overall result and the quality of life was considered good; this is in agreement with other studies [4–7]. In the present study, some owners even considered that their pet's quality of life improved after the amputation, and this might have been related to the removal of the source of pain. The behavioral changes reported by the owners in this study were more small disabilities than behavioral problems. The behavioral problems previously reported [7], such as aggression and anxiety, were not seen in the patients of the present study.

As in previous studies [4, 7], all owners responded that they would have another pet amputated, and none regretted the decision. We believe that an evaluation made by owners whose pets died shortly after the procedure would have been negatively biased and they were not gathered.

The favorable responses of most owners can be explained by the fact that the dogs adapted very soon to their new locomotory situation (kinetic and kinematic analyses) and to the lack of morphologic changes in other joints (as it might be inferred from the lack of morphologic changes in the stifle).

Limitations

Our study provides new information; however, there were important limitations in this study: the lack of a homogeneous population prevented us from comparing the kinetic and kinematic data with other studies looking at normal patient populations or using a control group. However, it is virtually impossible to perform such a clinical study using a homogeneous population. Additionally, kinematic data are breed-specific [24], and not all breeds have been studied yet. In any case, in the present study there were a high number of mixed-breed dogs, which are very difficult to characterize. The small sample size is another important limitation, which also possibly led to lack of statistical power. The effect of missing measurements for some patients might have also obscured the results. Finally, even though the evaluator was experienced in reading MR images of canine stifles, the lack of a board-certified radiologist for interpretation of the images may have also been a limitation of this study.

Conclusions

In spite of the limitations, this study provides objective evidence indicating that dogs have a quick adaptation process after a hind limb amputation. The adaptive processes to the new locomotion begin even before the amputation is performed. Since the veterinarian is responsible for providing accurate information before an amputation [2], we strongly believe that this study provides useful information, that will allow veterinarians the possibility to give dog owners more realistic expectations of a hind limb amputation.

Endnotes

[1]L-Polamivet®: Intervet Deutschland GmbH, Unterschleißheim, Germany

[2]Diazepam-ratiopharm®: Ratiopharm GmbH, Ulm, Germany

[3]Narcofol® 10 mg/mL: CP-Pharma Handelsgesellschaft GmbH, Burgdorf, Germany

[4]Isofluran CP®: CP-Pharma Handelsgesellschaft GmbH, Burgdorf, Germany

[5]Fentanyl-Janssen® 0.05 mg/mL: Janssen-Cilag GmbH, Neuss, Germany

[6]Xylocain® 2 %: AstraZeneca GmbH, Wedel, Germany

[7]Ketamin 10 %: Selectavet Dr. Otto Fischer GmbH, Weyarn-Holzolling, Germany

[8]Bupivacain-RPR-actavis® 0.5 %: Actavis Deutschland GmbH & Co. KG, Langenfeld, Germany

[9]Morphin Hexal® 10 mg/mL: Hexal AG, Holzkirchen, Germany

[10]Xylocain® 2 %, AstraZeneca GmbH, Wedel, Germany

[11]Rimadyl® Injektionslösung: Pfizer GmbH, Berlin, Germany

[12]Treadmill model 4060–80: Bertec Corporation, Columbus, OH, USA

[13]Vicon Motion Systems Ltd., Oxford, UK

[14]MX3+ camera system: Vicon Motion Systems Ltd., Oxford, UK

[15]Vicon Calibration Device: Vicon Motion Systems Ltd., Oxford, UK

[16]Vicon Nexus: Vicon Motion Systems Ltd., Oxford, UK

[17]MyoResearch XP Master Edition, Noraxon U.S.A. Inc., Scottsdale, AZ, USA

[18]Microsoft® Excel 2007

[19]Vicon Nexus and Bodybuilder: Vicon Motion Systems Ltd., Oxford, UK

[20]Philips Achieva 3.0 T X-series MRI: Philips Healthcare, Hamburg, Germany

[21]EIZO RadiForce™ RX211 Medical color LCD monitor: Enzo Nanao Corporation, Hakusan, Ishikawa, Japan

[22]GraphPad Prism® Version 4: GraphPad Software, Inc. La Jolla, California, USA

Additional files

Additional file 1: Video 1. Thirty-two kilogram patient walking on the treadmill at 0.8 m/s. Although the walking pattern is very similar between sessions, evident differences can be observed.

Additional file 2: Video 2. Forty-kilogram dog (patient 7) walking and running 4 months after the amputation. Note that the dog has no difficulty in its movements whatsoever, neither when walking nor when running.

Competing interests
The authors declare that no competing interests exist.

Authors' contributions
Conceived the study: IN. Designed the study: VGZ, VvB, NE, DB, IN, PW. Performed data collection: VGZ, VvB, NE. Analyzed the data: VGZ, PW. Wrote the paper: VGZ. Critical revision of the manuscript: VGZ, VvB, NE, DB, IN, PW. Final approval of the version to be published: VGZ, VvB, NE, DB, IN, PW.

Acknowledgements
The authors wish to thank Peter Dziallas, Beate Länger and Davina Wolf for performing the MRs, Martin Beyerbach for his statistical assistance and the patients' owners for their cooperation.
Partially funded by the National University of Colombia and the Colombian government in cooperation with the German Academic Exchange Service (DAAD) by a research scholarship awarded to VGZ.

Author details
[1]Small Animal Hospital, University of Veterinary Medicine Hannover, Foundation, Bünteweg 9, D-30559 Hannover, Germany. [2]Small Animal Clinic, Faculty of Veterinary Medicine, National University of Colombia, Carrera 30 # 45-03 (Ciudad Universitaria), Bogotá, Colombia.

References

1. Stone EA. Amputation. In: Newton CD, Nunamaker DM, editors. Textbook of small animal orthopaedics. New York: IVIS Ithaca; 1985. p. 577–88.
2. Weigel JP. Amputations. In: Slatter DH, editor. Textbook of small animal surgery Saunders. Philadelphia: Saunders; 2003. p. 2180–90.
3. Lipowitz AJ. Complications in small animal surgery: diagnosis, management, prevention. Media: Williams & Wilkins; 1996. p. 606–609.
4. Carberry CA, Harvey HJ. Owner Satisfaction with Limb Amputation in Dogs and Cats. J Am Anim Hosp Assoc. 1987;23:227–32.
5. Withrow SJ, Hirsch VM. Owner response to amputation of a pet's leg. Vet Med Small Anim Clin. 1979;74:332. 334.
6. von Werthern J, Horst C, Schwartz G. Zur Gliedmaßenamputaiton bei Hund und Katze: Eine Besitzerbefragung. Kleintierpraxis. 1999;44:169–76.
7. Kirpensteijn J, van den Bos R, Endenburg N. Adaptation of dogs to the amputation of a limb and their owners' satisfaction with the procedure. Vet Rec. 1999;144:115–8.
8. Schulz M. Coping psychologically with amputation. Vasa. 2009;38 Suppl 74:72–4.
9. Kirpensteijn J, van den Bos R, van den Brom WE, Hazewinkel HAW. Ground reaction force analysis of large breed dogs when walking after the amputation of a limb. Vet Rec. 2000;146:155–59.
10. Böddeker J, Drüen S, Meyer-Lindenberg A, Fehr M, Nolte I, Wefstaedt P. Computer-assisted gait analysis of the dog: Comparison of two surgical techniques for the ruptured cranial cruciate ligament. Vet Comp Orthop Traumatol. 2012;25:11–21.
11. Hottinger HA, DeCamp CE, Olivier NB, Hauptman JG, Soutas-Little RW. Noninvasive kinematic analysis of the walk in healthy large-breed dogs. Am J Vet Res. 1996;57:381–8.
12. Steiss JE, Yuill GT, White NA, Bowen JM. Modifications of a force plate system for equine gait analysis. Am J Vet Res. 1982;43:538–40.
13. Hielm-Bjorkman AK, Kuusela E, Liman A, Markkola A, Saarto E, Huttunen P, et al. Evaluation of methods for assessment of pain associated with chronic osteoarthritis in dogs. J Am Vet Med Assoc. 2003;222:1552–8.
14. Baird DK, Hathcock JT, Rumph PF, Kincaid SA, Visco DM. Low-field magnetic resonance imaging of the canine stifle joint: normal anatomy. Vet Radiol Ultrasound. 1998;39:87–97.
15. D'Anjou MA, Moreau M, Troncy E, Martel-Pelletier J, Abram F, Raynauld JP, et al. Osteophytosis, subchondral bone sclerosis, joint effusion and soft tissue thickening in canine experimental stifle osteoarthritis: Comparison between 1.5T magnetic resonance imaging and computed radiography. Vet Surg. 2008;37:166–77.
16. Blond L, Thrall DE, Roe SC, Chailleux N, Robertson ID. Diagnostic accuracy of magnetic resonance imaging for meniscal tears in dogs affected with naturally occuring cranial cruciate ligament rupture. Vet Radiol Ultrasound. 2008;49:425–31.
17. Boileau C, Martel-Pelletier J, Abram F, Raynould J-P, Troncy E, D'Anjou M-AD, et al. Magnetic resonance imaging can accurately assess the long-term progression of knee structural changes in experimental dog osteoarthritis. Ann Rheum Dis. 2008;67:926–32.
18. Gavin PR, Holmes SP. Orthopedic. In: Practical small animal MRI. Gavin PR, Bagley RS, editors. Ames: John Wiley & Sons; 2009. p. 233–272.
19. Winegardner KR, Scrivani PV, Krotscheck U, Todhunter RJ. Magnetic resonance imaging of subarticular bone marrow lesions in dogs with stifle lameness. Vet Radiol Ultrasound. 2007;48:312–17.
20. Maes LD, Herbin M, Hackert R, Bels VL, Abourachid A. Steady locomotion in dogs: temporal and associated spatial coordination patterns and the effect of speed. J Exp Biol. 2008;211(Pt 1):138–49.
21. Riggs CM, DeCamp CE, Soutas-Little RW, Braden TD, Richter MA. Effects of subject velocity on force plate-measured ground reaction forces in healthy greyhounds at the trot. Am J Vet Res. 1993;54:1523–6.
22. Kim SY, Kim JY, Hayashi K, Kapatkin AS. Skin movement during the kinematic analysis of the canine pelvic limb. Vet Comp Orthop Traumatol. 2011;24:326–32.
23. Yam PS, Penpraze V, Young D, Todd MS, Cloney AD, Houston-Callaghan KA, et al. Validity, practical utility and reliability of Actigraph accelerometry for the measurement of habitual physical activity in dogs. J Small Anim Pract. 2011;52:86–91.
24. Bockstahler B, Muller M, Henninger W, Mayrhofer E, Peham C, Podbregar I. Kinetic and kinematic motion analysis of the forelimbs in sound Malinois dogs - sampling of basic values. Wien Tierarztl Monatsschr. 2008;95:127–38.

2

Regeneration of dermal patterns from the remaining pigments after surgery in *Eublepharis macularius*

Noriyuki Nakashima[1,2] (iD)

Abstract

Background: Dermal injury of the *Eublepharis macularius* (leopard gecko) often results in a loss of the spotted patterns. The scar is usually well recovered, but the spots and the tubercles may be lost depending on the size and part of the lesion. This report presents a surgical attempting, in which the pigments in the edge of the remaining skin flap are partially preserved to maximally restore the natural pigmentation patterns during the course of dermal regeneration.

Case presentation: A four-year-old female lizard *E. macularius* was evaluated due to a subcutaneous tumor in the occipito-pterional portion behind its right eye. A solid tumor beneath the skin was surgically enucleated under general anesthesia. Then, the ulcerated skin was dissected away together with the tumor. The necrotic edge of the remaining skin flap was carefully trimmed to leave as much of the pigmented portions as possible on the outskirt of the skin flap. The scar was covered with the remaining skin flap, and the uncovered lesion was protected with Vaseline containing gentamicin. The lesion was rapidly covered with regenerated dermis within a week, and the epidermis with round and well-oriented pigmented spots were almost completely restored in four months.

Conclusion: The surgical suture of the skin flap after removal of the ulcerated margins resulted in the scar-free regeneration of the scales and the pigmented spots. And the pigmented spots of the remaining skin close to the lesion site might be a source of the regenerated spots.

Keywords: *Eublepharis macularius*, Dermal scar, Pigment regeneration, Pigment preservation

Background

Eublepharis macularius (*E. macularius*, also known as a leopard gecko) becomes popular since this exotic reptile is docile in nature and is easy to handle; moreover, it is very unique and diverse in its coloration and dermal patterns [1]. Scientifically, *E. macularius* is considered a good model for the study of regeneration, because of its tremendous potential for epimorphic scar-free regeneration at the wound site in the body skin and the tail [2–5]. And pigment pattern regeneration is of interest to both practitioners and researchers [6].

When the loss of the skin tissue of *E. macularius* was large, the lost scales were usually replaced by the deformed and small scales, meanwhile the large cone-like scales (tubercles: defined in Fig. 3 in this report) were not regenerated on the tail or trunk [3–5]. Another study on the tail regeneration after autotomy reported the incomplete recovery of the *de-novo* pigmentation in the newly regenerated tail [3, 4], but the coloration was somewhat blurred and different from the original patterns [3, 4]. The skin regeneration was also studied by experimental excision [5], it was reported that the skin also underwent the scar-free regeneration and restored rather complex patterns of coloration. And interestingly, the regenerated skin close to the pre-existent pigments was also slightly pigmented (see Fig. 2 in [5]), implying that the pigment cells would migrate to the lesion site from the nearby pigmented spots.

Correspondence: nakashima@nbiol.med.kyoto-u.ac.jp;
nakashima_noriyuki@med.kurume-u.ac.jp
[1]Department of Physiology, Graduate School of Medicine, Kyoto University, Yoshida-Konoe, Sakyo-ku, Kyoto 606-8501, Japan
[2]Department of Physiology, School of Medicine, Kurume University, 67, Asahi-machi, Kurume-shi, Fukuoka 830-0011, Japan

In clinical situations, for a variety of diseases are known for *E. macularius*, and surgerical resection is often an inevitable medical option [6]. In the course of surgery, the spotted portion of the skin is sometimes removed due to severe dermal damage or subcutaneous adhesion as will be shown in the present report. Inspired by a series of the previous reports [3–5], the author proposed to preserve a portion of the pigmented skin edge to regenerate as much the same pigment patterns as possible in a case in which the tumor should be excised together with the ulcerated.

Case presentation

A four-year-old female leopard gecko *E. macularius* suffered from a subcutaneous tumor in the occipito-pterional portion behind its right eye. The subject weighed 35 g at the date of surgery and was fed daily with commercial mealworms supplemented with calcium and vitamin D powder and housed in a 60 (width) x 30 (depth) x 35 (height) cm³ acryl cage, equipped with a floor panel heater, calcium-containing sand bedding, and a 75 W night-light lamp throughout the observation. Room temperature was maintained at 27–30 °C, with the humidity at 60–80 %.

Surgical operation

Upon first inspection, the tumor mass (T in Fig. 1a and b) was palpable, motile, and smooth but had already developed to an ulcerated lesion. The appetite, activity and consciousness level were normal. The wound was bleeding, and the rear edge of the tumor was cracked and fused to the molting skin (Fig. 1a). Thus, an immediate surgical resection was performed under general anesthesia. A mixture of the following anesthetics was used: 8.0 mL midazolam (Dormicam, Astellas Pharma Inc., Tokyo, Japan), 1.5 mL medetomidine hydrochloride and 0.4 mL butorphanol tartrate (Domitol and Vetorphale, Meiji Seika Pharma Co., Ltd., Japan) was adjusted to 30 mL with normal saline. Prior to the operation, the patient was calmed in a dark box, and 100 μL of the anesthetic mixture was slowly injected subcutaneously twice within ten minutes (200 μL total) into the lateral part of the right femur using a 30-G needle (Terumo, Japan).

The incision was made from the crack at the outer perimeter of the ulcerated skin at the occipito-pterional area (Fig. 1b). The skin flap was partially trimmed with scissors to preserve five pigmented regions in the margin (red arrows; Fig. 1c). The isolated mass was easily enucleated. Note that no communicating fistula was found towards the ocular region (Fig. 1c). The wound was rinsed twice with saline and sutured using a 14 mm curved needle with a 7–0 nylon string (Nazme Seisakusho Co., Ltd., Japan).

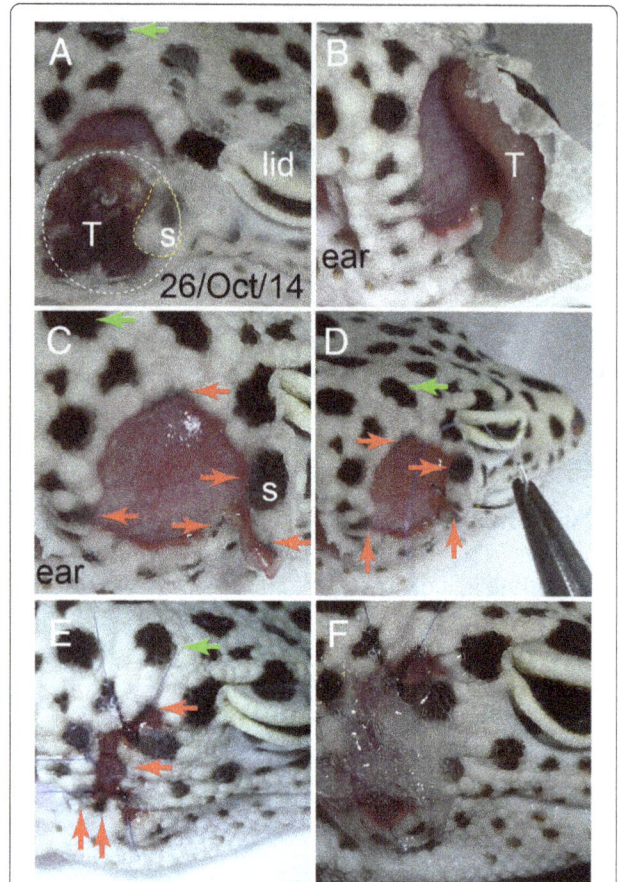

Fig. 1 Photographic review of the pigment regeneration. **a** The cracked and ulcerated skin due to the tumor observed from the occipital direction. The white dotted circle indicates the rim of the tumor (T). The *yellow dotted line* indicates the skin flap. A *green arrow* pointing an ecliptic spot is used as a landmark to identify the orientation of the other spots in all the panels hereafter. **b** Appearance of the tumor attached to the flapped skin together with the necrotic tissue. **c** The subcutaneous appearance after the tumor excision. Red arrows, in all the figures hereafter, indicate the preserved dermal spots in the skin margin. **d**, **e** The remaining skin flap was stretched and sutured to the remaining caudal skin rim with strong tension. **f** The scar was covered with ointment containing gentamicin

The exposed sub-dermal area (E in Fig. 1c) was about 46 mm² large, and the remaining skin flap (s in Fig. 1a) was about 6 mm² large without tension. Consequently, the skin flap was sutured with a sufficient margin from the edge of the incision (Fig. 1d) because the shortened skin needed extensive stretching to cover as much lesion area as possible (Fig. 1e). The uncovered wound (about 2 mm²) was plastered with artificial ointment containing Vaseline, saline, and gentamicin (50 μg/mL) to avoid infection and dehydration (Fig. 1f).

A total of 100 μL gentamicin solution (100 μg/mL) was also orally administered twice a day for one post-operative week. The post-operative course was stable and uneventful. The dermal wound epithelium was rapidly regenerated by post-operative day 5 as previously reported [5], but the pigmented spots had not changed much (Fig. 2a). One month following the surgery, the subject underwent the first post-operative molting (Fig. 2b), and the pigmented spots had grown from the remaining pigments with a little bit blurred perimeter (Fig. 2c and d). In the four months since the surgery, the regenerated spots looked almost undistinguishable from the pre-existent spots with a rather vivid border, and the epidermal scales with yellow coloration were restored (Fig. 2e and f). The delayed yellowish coloration should be a general recovery course of the epidermis in *E. macularius* [4].

Followed up for three more months, there were no more changes in the wound healing process in the operated area (Fig. 3a). The newly pigmented spots were

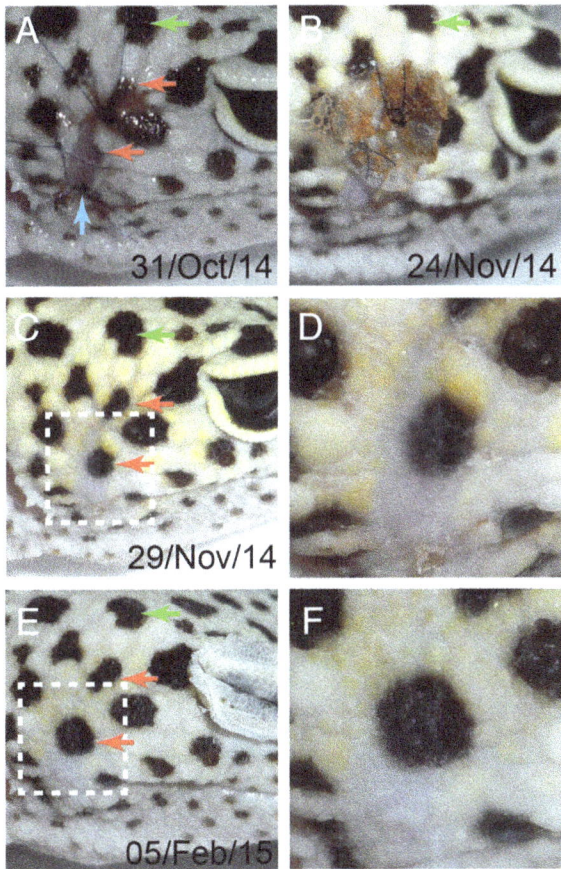

Fig. 3 The close observation of the regenerated skin. **a** The regenerated skin at post-operative month 7. **b** The un-operated side on the same date. **c** and **d** Close-up views of the regenerated scales in the dotted squares in (**a**). **e** and **f** Magnified photos of representative scales in occipito-pterional (**e**) and trunk (**f**) regions. **g** and **h** The distribution patterns of the tubercles in the operated side (**g**) and the intact side (**h**). The pigmented spots became larger and more vivid in four post-operative months. *Green asterisks* in (**d**) and (**g**) indicate the regenerated tubercles. *Pink asterisks* in (**e**)-(**h**) are the intact tubercles. The colored letters indicates as follows: R, right; L, left. The green arrow is the same landmark scale shown in Fig. 1a

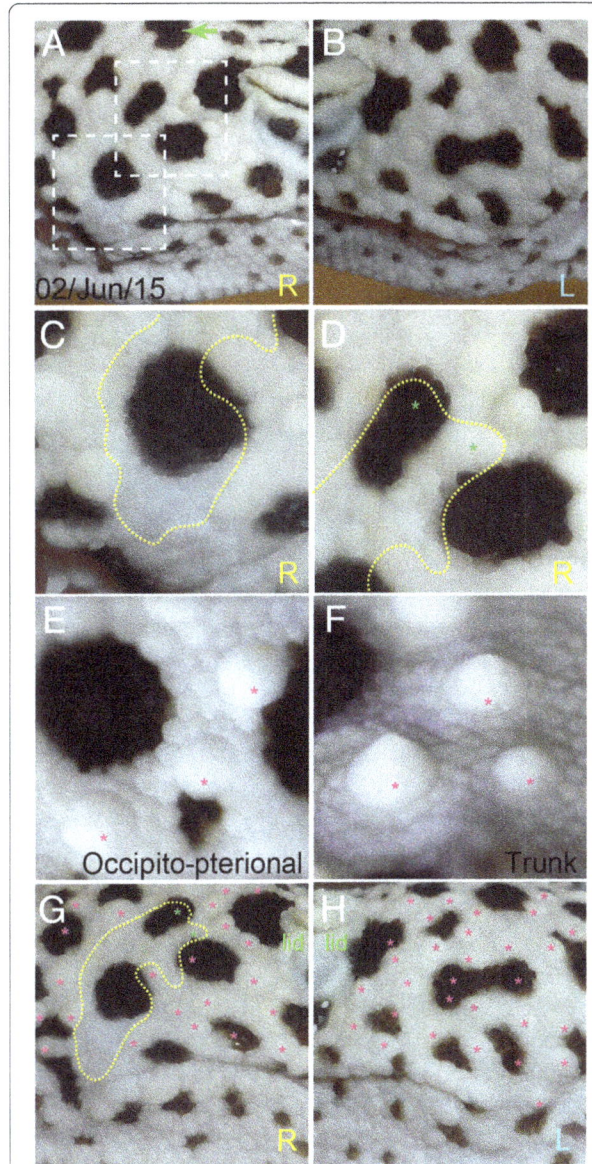

Fig. 2 The time-course of the regeneration of the skin. **a** The scar at post-operative day 5. Newly regenerated dermis was observed in the open wound cleft (*blue arrow*). Two out of the four remaining pigmented scales were visible in this panel (*red arrows*). The glistening appearance was due to the remaining ointment. **b** The first molting a month after the surgery. **c** The large and clear spots reappeared in a post-operative month (red arrows). **d** Close-up view of the dotted square area in (**c**). **e** The spots became larger and more vivid at 4 post-operative months. **f** Close-up view of the dotted square area in (**e**). Green arrow is the same landmark scale shown in Fig. 1a

distributed evenly and the appearance looked rather natural compared to the un-operated side (Fig. 3b). The regenerated area surrounded by the imaginary borders of the surgical margin (yellow dotted line: Fig. 3c, d and g) was about 20 mm^2. On higher magnification, the skin in *E. macularius* is tessellated with two different types of scales (Fig. 3e and f): small polygonal scales and cone-like large interspersing scales with round perimeters (defined as tubercles). The tubercles are rather flattened at the occipito-pterional region (pink asterisks in Fig.ure 3e) compared to those on the trunk (pink asterisks in Fig. 3f). The regenerated skin comprised of the small mosaic scales with no obvious scar as reported previously [3–5]. However, much of the large cone-like tubercles were not regenerated but only sparsely located in the operated side (pink asterisks in Fig. 3g), whereas such tubercles were evenly distributed in the intact side (pink asterisks in Fig. 3h). But, it is noteworthy that two tubercles were newly formed in the dorsal area of the operated region (green asterisks in Fig. 3d and g: compare with Fig. 1c).

Discussion

Although a large portion of the dermal tissues was completely lost and disconnected because of the surgical operation, the regenerated spots grew rapidly and re-localized again evenly and clearly (Fig. 3a). These new spots were also equally away from the pre-existing adjacent spots, so the potential of the color restoration might be influenced by the remaining chromatophores in the vicinity. In addition, a few tubercles were restored in the dorsal part of the occipito-pterional portion, but not near the corner of the mouth (Fig. 3d and g). Considering that the tubercles on the tail or trunk of *E. macularius* do not regenerate [3–5], the skin regeneration at the occipito-pterional portion behind the eye is rather unique. The mechanism how the tubercles could regenerate at the occipito-pterional portion is unclear, but the regeneration potential might differ between the rostral and caudal parts of the body of *E. macularius*. Importantly, not all the reptilian species have the remarkable potentials of scar-free regeneration like *E. macularius* [7]. So, the pattern restoration after the skin damage needs further investigation across the species.

Conclusion

The surgical suture of the skin flap after removal of the ulcerated margins resulted in the scar-free regeneration of the scales and the pigmented spots. And the pigmented spots of the remaining skin close to the lesion site might be a source of the regenerated spots.

Abbreviation
E. macularius, *Eublepharis macularius*

Acknowledgement
The author thanks Yumiko Nishinaka for her technical assistance in the surgery and nursing of the subject animal.

Funding
This report was supported by Grants-in-Aid for Young Investigator at Kyoto University (to NN).

Authors' contribution
NN designed and performed all of the procedures, analyzed the data, and wrote the manuscript.

Competing interests
Noriyuki Nakashima declares no conflicts of interests with respect to the present article.

Ethics approval and consent to participate
Written informed consent was obtained from the animal owner for the benefits, outcomes and side-effects of the surgical procedures and the publication of this case report and any accompanying images. The animal owner was also continuously informed of the condition of the animal throughout the treatments. The experimental and surgical procedures were performed according to the Regulation on Animal Experimentation at Kyoto University established by Animal Research Committee, Kyoto University and under the permission of the Animal Experimentation Committee at Kyoto University. The author also conformed to the CARE guideline and the Animal Research: Reporting In Vivo Experiments (ARRIVE) guideline.

References
1. De Vosjoli P., Ron Tremper R., Klingenberg R. The Herpetoculture of Leopard Geckos. California: Advanced Visions Inc.; 2005.
2. Carlson BM. Principles of regenerative biology. Massachusetts: Academic Press-Elsevier Ltd; 2007.
3. McLean KE, Vickaryous MK. A novel amniote model of epimorphic regeneration: the leopard gecko, Eublepharis macularius. BMC Dev Biol. 2011;11:50.
4. Delorme SL, Lungu IM, Vickaryous MK. Scar-free wound healing and regeneration following tail loss in the leopard gecko, Eublepharis macularius. Anat Rec (Hoboken). 2012;295:1575–95.
5. Peacock HM, Gilbert EA, Vickaryous MK. Scar-free cutaneous wound healing in the leopard gecko, Eublepharis macularius. J Anat. 2015;227(5):596–610.
6. Alworth LC, Hernandez SM, Divers SJ. Laboratory reptile surgery: principles and techniques. J Am Assoc Lab Anim Sci. 2011;50:11–26.
7. Wu P, Alibardi L, Chuong CM. Regeneration of reptilian scales after wounding: neogenesis, regional difference, and molecular modules. Regeneration (Oxf). 2014;1(1):15–26.

3

Prognostic indicators for perioperative survival after diaphragmatic herniorrhaphy in cats and dogs: 96 cases (2001-2013)

Claire Legallet[1], Kelley Thieman Mankin[1*] and Laura E. Selmic[2]

Abstract

Background: To determine associations between perioperative mortality after surgery for traumatic diaphragmatic hernia, medical records of 17 cats and 79 dogs that underwent diaphragmatic herniorrhaphy were reviewed.

Results: The combined perioperative survival rate was 81.3% (88.2% in cats and 79.8% in dogs). Data from acute and chronic cases was assessed separately. Of the acute cases (12 cats and 48 dogs), 10 cats (83.3%) and 38 dogs (79.2%) survived to discharge. Of the chronic cases (5 cats and 31 dogs), 5 cats (100%) and 25 dogs (80.6%) survived to discharge. The time between trauma and surgery, trauma and admission, and admission and surgery were not associated with survival. For cats and dogs, increased duration of anesthesia and surgical procedure were associated with increased mortality ($P = 0.0013$ and 0.004, respectively). Animals with concurrent soft tissue injuries had a 4.3 times greater odds of mortality than those without soft tissue injury ($P = 0.01$). Animals with concurrent soft tissue and orthopedic injuries had a 7.3 times greater odds of mortality than those without soft tissue and orthopedic injuries ($P = 0.004$). Animals that were oxygen dependent had a 5.0 times greater odds of mortality than those that were not ($P = 0.02$). No other variables were significantly associated with survival.

Conclusions: For cats and dogs that underwent surgery for traumatic diaphragmatic hernia, increased anesthetic duration, increased duration of surgical procedure, concurrent soft tissue injuries, concurrent soft tissue and orthopedic injuries, and perioperative oxygen dependence were associated with increased mortality.

Keywords: Cat, Diaphragmatic herniorrhaphy, Dog, Surgery, Trauma

Background

Diaphragmatic hernia is a common injury occurring in cats and dogs. Trauma caused by motor vehicle injury is the most common cause of diaphragmatic hernia and leads to a variety of clinical signs, with the most common being respiratory difficulty [1–12]. Following surgical treatment, the reported survival rate is 54–90% [1, 3, 5, 7–11, 13].

Multiple factors have been reported to influence the rate of survival, including the timing of surgical intervention [1, 2, 6–8, 10, 11]. In one study, surgical intervention within 24 h of trauma, or more than 1 year after trauma resulted in significantly higher mortality rates in dogs [1].

However, the aforementioned study was flawed in design and power [1]. Dogs with acute and chronic herniation, and congenital and traumatic herniation were analysed together [1]. Additionally, the authors of this study report that the 62.5% chronic herniation mortality rate was falsely increased by including dogs that died of unrelated medical problems [1]. Further, only 8 dogs underwent surgery over a year following trauma for chronic hernia repair. Therefore, conclusions drawn from this data should be viewed with suspicion. 40 dogs underwent surgery within 24 h of trauma. Although stabilization procedures were not discussed, the primary cause of death was listed as "shock". As a result of this previously published study, some investigators recommend delaying surgical intervention for a minimum of 24 h to permit stabilization of the patient prior to surgery [1, 7]. Stabilizing animals prior to anesthesia and surgery may reduce the mortality rates due to complications from dehydration, hypovolemic

* Correspondence: kthieman@cvm.tamu.edu
[1]Department of Small Animal Clinical Sciences (Thieman Mankin, Legallet), College of Veterinary Medicine, Texas A&M University, College Station, TX 77843-4474, USA
Full list of author information is available at the end of the article

and distributive shock, and hypoxemia [11]. However, a more recent study has shown no significant impact of early surgical intervention on perioperative mortality rate [8]. This study evaluated 92 dogs and cats undergoing diaphragmatic herniorrhaphy for traumatic herniation [8]. Animals with acute and chronic herniation were evaluated separately [8]. In animals with acute herniation, this study found no associations between perioperative survival and time from trauma to admission, time between admission and surgery, or time from trauma to surgery [8]. Contrary to the previous study, this study suggests early intervention is not associated with poor survival outcomes [8].

The purpose of this retrospective study was to examine factors influencing survival in dogs and cats undergoing diaphragmatic herniorrhaphy.

Methods
Criteria for selection of cases
An electronic medical record search was performed to identify cats and dogs undergoing diaphragmatic herniorrhaphy as treatment for traumatic diaphragmatic hernia at Texas A&M Veterinary Teaching Hospital between 1st October 2001 and 31st April 2014. Criterion for inclusion was surgical treatment of a traumatic diaphragmatic hernia. Diagnosis of diaphragmatic hernia was made by use of radiography and/or ultrasonography, and confirmed by surgical exploration. In order to determine if the diaphragmatic hernia was traumatic or congenital, the medical record was reviewed and a combination of history, location of hernia, concurrent injuries detected, and surgical findings (presence of adhesions) were used.

Procedures
The following information was obtained from medical records: age, sex and neuter status, and body weight; respiratory rate, pulse oximetry (SpO$_2$), and blood lactate at presentation; cause of diaphragmatic hernia (if known); concurrent soft tissue and/or orthopedic injuries; times from trauma to admission (TA), trauma to surgery (TS), and admission to surgery (AS); duration of anaesthesia and surgery; organs herniated; additional surgical procedures performed during herniorrhaphy; intraoperative and postoperative complications; times from admission to discharge, and surgery to discharge. TA time was based on information provided by the owner or referring veterinarian. For animals without known trauma, TA was calculated from the onset of symptoms. Acute and chronic diaphragmatic hernias were defined as TA periods ≤ 14 days and > 14 days, respectively [8, 10]. Respiratory distress was considered to be present if "dyspnea" or "respiratory distress" were recorded in the medical record [8]. Animals were also evaluated for respiratory distress based on respiratory rate and SpO$_2$ at admission: Animals with respiratory rates > 40 breaths per minute and/or SpO$_2 < 95\%$ [14] were defined as being in respiratory distress. Animals were classified into survival groups as alive to discharge from hospital or death prior to discharge from hospital, including animals euthanized during or after surgery.

Treatment
All animals underwent general anesthesia, manual ventilation and diaphragmatic herniorrhaphy by standard ventral midline abdominal approach.

Pre- and postoperative care
After surgery, all of the animals were recovered in the intensive care unit (ICU). All of the animals were closely monitored while in the ICU. All animals had their respiratory rate monitored at least every 2 h. All animals were treated with an opiate. The opiate was administered on presentation, as a premedication and/or induction agent, and intra- or postoperatively. Different types of opiates and a range of doses were used based on clinician preference. Many animals also received a non-steroidal anti-inflammatory drug (NSAID), while some received steroids. Many animals underwent electrolyte monitoring and received fluids and additional supportive care as clinically indicated.

Statistical analyses
Continuous variables were tested for normality using histograms, skewness, kurtosis, and Shapiro-Wilk tests. If the variables were normally distributed, the mean and standard deviations were presented. For non-normally distributed variables, the median and range were presented. Categorical variables were presented by frequency and percentages.

Kaplan-Meier methodology was used to calculate the median and 95% confidence interval for time from TA, TS, AS, anesthetic duration, surgery duration, and admission to discharge or death for all cases and stratified by species, duration of hernia (acute vs. chronic and for whether animals survived or died in the perioperative period. Log-rank tests were used to assess for differences in these time-to-event variables for species, duration of hernia and for animals that survived to discharge and those that did not survive.

Univariable logistic regression analysis was used to test for associations between mortality and patient demographics (sex and neuter status, age, weight, and species), characteristics at presentation (duration of diaphragmatic hernia, presence of dyspnea, tachypnea >40bpm, pulse oximetry <95%, necessity of thoracocentesis, elevation of serum lactate, number of injuries, presence of concurrent orthopedic injuries, and orthopedic and soft tissue injuries). In addition, associations between different operative factors (time < 24 h following admission, number of anesthetic procedures or number of surgical procedures, number of organs herniated, and which organs were herniated) were tested. A logistic regression model was used with variables of duration or hernia and whether surgery was performed within 24 h of trauma to evaluate effect of these variables on mortality given the findings of previous studies. Multivariable logistic regression analysis was not performed given the low number of animals that died (18). Odds ratios (OR) were calculated with 95% Wald confidence intervals (CI) for each variable.

Statistical significance was set at $p < 0.05$. Statistical analyses were performed using commercially available software[1].

Results

Ninety-six animals, 17 cats and 79 dogs, were included in the study. The most common cause of diaphragmatic hernia was motor vehicle accident (Table 1).

Seventeen cats were included in the study. Breeds included domestic mix breed cat ($n = 16$, 94.1%) and Rag Doll ($n = 1$, 5.9%). Sex, neuter status, age, and weight were not associated with mortality (Table 2).

Two cats with acute herniation died. Both of the cats that died had concurrent injuries, which were treated surgically. One cat underwent nephrectomy due to an avulsed renal vein, artery and ureter. This cat underwent cardiopulmonary arrest once prior to celiotomy and was successfully resuscitated, but arrested again intraoperatively and died. The other cat that died suffered a penetrating thoracic wound and multiple abdominal punctures after being attacked by a dog. The cat underwent celiotomy and thoracotomy, diaphragmatic herniorrhaphy, two partial lung lobectomies, and repair of the thoracic and abdominal wounds, but became septic and was euthanized 4 days postoperatively.

Seventy-nine dogs were included in the study. The commonly represented breeds were mixed breed (10, 12.7%), Labrador retriever (9, 11.4%), and Chihuahua (5, 6.3%). Other breeds included Alaskan Malamute, Australian Shepherd, Basset Hound, Beagle, Black Mouth Cur, Bloodhound, Border Collie, Boston Terrier, Boxer, Cairn Terrier, Cardigan Welsh Corgi, Catahoula Hog Dog, Cocker Spaniel, Coton de Tulear, English Bulldog, Fox Terrier,

German Shepherd, Golden Retriever, Great Pyrenees, Italian Greyhound, Jack Russell Terrier, Maltese, Miniature Dachshund, Miniature Pinscher, Miniature Poodle, Pembroke Welsh Corgi, Pomeranian, Rat Terrier, Shetland Sheepdog, Shih Tzu, Standard Dachshund, Standard Poodle, Treeing Walker Coon Hound, Weimaraner and West Highland Terrier. Sex, neuter status, age, and weight were not associated with mortality (Table 2).

For all animals, oxygen dependence at any time during hospitalization was associated with increased mortality (Table 3). Oxygen dependence preoperatively and postoperatively were associated with increased mortality (Table 3). However, respiratory rate, presence of dyspnoea, pulse oximetry, thoracocentesis, serum lactate levels at presentation, and hernia duration were not associated with mortality (Table 3).

For all animals, presence of concurrent soft tissue injuries were associated with increased mortality (Table 4). Additionally, presence of concurrent orthopedic and soft tissue injuries were associated with increased mortality (Table 4). However, concurrent orthopedic injuries, number of injuries, number of surgeries, number of anesthetic episodes, number of organs herniated and organs herniated had no association with mortality (Table 4). The most common concurrent surgery performed with diaphragmatic herniorrhaphy was amputation in cats and ovariohysterectomy or orchiectomy in dogs (Table 5).

For all animals, increased duration of surgical procedure was associated with increased mortality (Table 6). Additionally, increased anesthetic duration was associated with increased mortality (Table 6). TA, TS, AS, and duration of surgical procedure were not associated with mortality (Table 6). Following adjustment for duration of hernia (acute vs. chronic), there was no association with mortality for patients with TA >24 h vs. ≤ 24 h.

Discussion

The perioperative survival rate in the study reported herein was 81.3% overall, with 88.2% of cats and 79.8% of dogs surviving to discharge. The perioperative survival rates following surgical treatment of acute and chronic diaphragmatic herniae was 83.3% and 100% in cats, respectively, and 79.2% and 80.6% in dogs, respectively. These survival rates are consistent with recent reports [1, 3, 5, 7–10, 13]. Chronic diaphragmatic herniae have been associated with a significantly worse prognosis in older reports. The difference in survival rates for chronic diaphragmatic hernia between more recent and older reports may be due to the definition of a chronic diaphragmatic hernia with Gibson et al [8] and Minihan et al [10] defining any hernia treated > 2 weeks after trauma as chronic, while Boudrieau and Muir [1] defined this as > 1 year [1].

Table 1 Cause of diaphragmatic hernia in cats and dogs that underwent diaphragmatic herniorrhaphy

Cause	Cats $n = 17$	Dogs $n = 79$	All animals ($n = 96$)
Motor vehicle accident	5 (29.4%)	39 (49.4%)	44 (45.8%)
Unknown/suspected trauma	9 (52.9%)	33 (41.8%)	42 (43.8%)
Other trauma	3 (17.6%)	7 (8.9%)	10 (10.4%)

Table 2 Patient characteristics of cats and dogs that underwent diaphragmatic herniorrhaphy and associations with mortality

Characteristic	Category	Dogs (n = 79)	Cats (n = 17)	All cases (n = 96)	OR (95% CI)	P-value
Species	Cat	–	–	–	Ref	0.42
	Dog				1.9 (0.4–9.2)	
Sex and neuter status	Female spayed	31 (39.2%)	4 (23.5%)	35 (36.5%)	0.8 (0–6.6)	0.84
	Female intact	9 (11.4%)	1 (5.9%)	10 (10.4%)	2.9 (0.5–30.7)	0.33
	Male castrated	20 (25.3%)	12 (70.6%)	32 (33.3%)	2.3 (0.4–25.8)	0.53
	Male intact	19 (24.1%)	0 (0.0%)	19 (19.8%)	Ref	–
Sex	Female	40 (50.6%)	5 (29.4%)	45 (46.9%)	–	–
	Male	39 (49.4%)	12 (70.6%)	51 (53.1%)		
Age at diagnosis (yr)	Median, range	3.0 (0.2–12.9)	4.7, 1.5–8.5	3.1, 0.2–12.9	1.1 (1.0–1.3)	0.10
Weight (kg)	Median, range	10.6, 2.2–52.0	4.6, 2.3–8.0	8.0, 2.2–52.0	1.0 (1.0–1.1)	0.33

Results are for univariable logistic regression analysis. Values were considered significant at $p < 0.05$. OR Odds ratio, CI Confidence interval, Ref Reference category, yr years, kg kilograms

In the present study, the mortality rate for cats and dogs was significantly associated with increased duration of surgical procedure, increased anesthetic duration, concurrent soft tissue injuries, concurrent soft tissue and orthopedic injuries, and perioperative oxygen dependence. Animals with increased duration of surgical procedure or anesthetic duration had an increase in mortality. It is possible that increased duration of surgical procedure and anesthetic duration themselves actually lead to an increase in mortality. However, we suspect that animals with more severe injuries and additional intrathoracic trauma may have been slower to recover from anesthesia, and therefore had longer anesthetic times and

increased mortality. It is also possible that more severe trauma lead to more significant diaphragmatic disruption and resultant difficulty performing the herniorrhaphy, and therefore longer surgery and anesthetic times. Alternatively, extended anesthetic duration may have been due to comorbidities, unforeseen surgical complications, and/or concurrent surgical procedures. As concurrent surgical procedures increase surgical time and anaesthetic time, this variable was evaluated separately but was not correlated with mortality ($P = 0.09$). However, this may be due to a type II statistical error.

Animals with concurrent orthopedic and soft tissue injuries had a 7.3 times greater odds of mortality than those

Table 3 Presenting characteristics of cats and dogs that underwent diaphragmatic herniorrhaphy and associations with mortality

Characteristic	Category	Dogs (n = 79)	Cats (n = 17)	All cases (n = 96)	OR (95% CI)	P-value
Hernia duration	Acute	48 (60.8%)	12 (70.6%)	60 (62.5%)	1.3 (0.4–3.7)	0.69
	Chronic	31 (39.2%)	5 (29.4%)	36 (37.5%)	Ref	-
Survival	Acute	38/48(79.2%)	10/12 (83.3%)	48/60 (80.0%)	-	–
	Chronic	25/31(80.6%)	5/5 (100.0%)	30/36 (83.3%)		
	All	63/79(79.8%)	15/17(88.2%)	78/96 (81.3%)		
Respiratory rate at presentation	Mean (SD)	54 (19.0)	52 (17.0)	53 (18.0)	0.3 (0.1–1.0)	0.05
	>40bpm	55 (73.3%)	4 (23.5%)	68 (73.9%)	Ref	–
	≤40bpm	20 (26.7%)	13 (76.5%)	24 (26.1%)		
Dyspnoea at presentation	Dyspnoeic	13 (16.5%)	4 (23.5%)	17 (17.7%)	0.9 (0.2–3.6)	0.90
	Non–dyspnoeic	66 (83.5%)	13 (76.5%)	79 (82.3%)	Ref	
Pulse oximetry at presentation	<95%	25 (31.7%)	5 (29.4%)	30 (31.3%)	0.6 (0.2–1.9)	0.36
	≥95%	54 (68.4%)	12 (70.6%)	66 (68.8%)	Ref	–
Thoracocentesis at presentation	Performed	10 (13.2%)	4 (23.5%)	14 (15.0%)	0.8 (0.2–3.9)	0.75
	Not performed	66 (86.8%)	13 (76.5%)	79 (85.0%)	Ref	
Oxygen dependent	Yes	46 (58.3%)	9 (53.0%)	55 (57.3%)	5.0 (1.3–18.7)	0.02*
	No	33 (41.8%)	8 (47.0%)	41 (42.7%)	Ref	
Oxygen dependent	Preoperative	28 (35.4%)	8 (47.1%)	36 (37.5%)	4.2 (1.0–17.1)	0.04*
	Postoperative	18 (22.8%)	1 (5.9%)	19 (19.8%)	5.8 (1.3–26.8)	0.02*
	None	33 (41.8%)	8 (47.1%)	41 (42.7%)	Ref	–
Serum lactate	Elevated	14 (17.7%)	7 (41.1%)	21 (21.9%)	0.9 (0.2–3.5)	0.89
	Normal	36 (45.6%)	3 (17.6%)	39 (40.6%)	Ref	
	Unknown	29 (36.7%)	7 (41.1%)	36 (37.5%)	–	

Results are for univariable logistic regression analysis
OR Odds ratio, CI Confidence interval, Ref Reference category, SD Standard deviation
*Indicates statistically significant difference

Table 4 Anesthesia and operative details of diaphragmatic herniorrhaphy in cats and dogs and associations with mortality

Characteristic	Category	Dogs ($n = 79$)	Cats ($n = 17$)	All cases ($n = 96$)	OR (95% CI)	P value
Anesthetic episodes during hospitalization	Median (range)	1 (0–2)	1 (1)	1.0 (0–2)	0.2 (0.0–1.8)	0.15
Concurrent surgeries	Median (range)	1 (1–4)	1 (1–3)	1 (1–4)	1.8 (0.9–3.7)	0.09
Number of injuries	Median (range)	1 (1–5)	2 (1–4)	1 (1–5)	1.5 (1.0–2.4)	0.05
Concurrent orthopedic injuries	Yes	30 (38.0%)	7 (41.2%)	37 (38.5%)	1.8 (0.6–5.0)	0.27
	No	49 (62.0%)	10 (58.8%)	59 (61.5%)	Ref	
Concurrent soft tissue injuries	Yes	11 (13.9%)	6 (35.3%)	17 (17.7%)	4.3 (1.4–13.8)	0.01*
	No	68 (86.1%)	11 (64.7%)	79 (82.3%)	Ref	
Concurrent orthopedic and soft tissue injuries	Yes	7 (8.9%)	4 (23.5%)	11 (11.5%)	7.3 (1.9–27.7)	0.004*
	No	72 (91.1%)	13 (76.5%)	85 (88.5%)	Ref	
Number of organs herniated	Median (range)	3 (0–6)	3 (0–5)	3 (0–6)	0.8 (0.6–1.1)	0.22
Organs herniated	Liver	51 (64.6%)	9 (52.9%)	60 (62.5%)	0.5 (0.2–1.5)	0.23
	Small intestine	43 (54.4%)	8 (47.1%)	51 (53.1%)	0.9 (0.3–2.4)	0.77
	Gallbladder	40 (50.6%)	6 (37.5%)	46 (48.4%)	0.5 (0.2–1.4)	0.16
	Stomach	34 (43.0%)	9 (52.9%)	43 (44.8%)	0.6 (0.2–1.6)	0.28
	Spleen	31 (39.2%)	7 (41.2%)	38 (39.6%)	0.5 (0.2–1.6)	0.26
	Omentum	17 (21.5%)	1 (5.9%)	18 (19.0%)	0.8 (0.2–3.2)	0.78
	Colon	8 (10.1%)	1 (5.9%)	9 (9.4%)	1.3 (0.2–6.7)	0.78
	Pancreas	3 (3.8%)	1 (5.9%)	4 (4.2%)	4.7 (0.6–35.8)	0.14
	Kidney	4 (5.1%)	2 (12.5%)	6 (6.3%)	4.9 (0.9–26.8)	0.06
	Cecum	3 (3.8%)	0 (0.0%)	3 (3.2%)	–	–

Results are for univariable logistic regression analysis
OR Odds ratio, CI Confidence interval, Ref Reference category
*Indicates statistically significant difference

Table 5 Concurrent surgical procedures in cats and dogs that underwent surgery for traumatic diaphragmatic herniorrhaphy

Concurrent surgical procedure	Cats 6/17	Dogs 28/79
Neuter (OHE/castration)	1 (1/0)	9 (5/4)
Resection and anastomosis	0	5
Splenectomy (Partial or complete)	1	4
Wound closure/debridement	1	3
Gastropexy	0	3
Body wall herniorrhaphy	1	2
Intrathoracic surgery (Median sternotomy/Thoracotomy)	0	2 (1/1)
Amputation	2	0
Bladder repair	1	0
Bronchoscopy	0	1
Oesophageal feeding tube placement	1	0
Gastrotomy	0	1
Jejunal feeding tube placement	0	1
Liver lobectomy	0	1
Lung lobectomy	1	0
Nephrectomy	1	1
Prepubic tendon avulsion repair	0	1
PSS ameroid constrictor placement	0	1

OHE Ovariohysterectomy, PSS Portosystemic shunt. Some animals underwent more than one concurrent surgical procedure

without orthopedic and soft tissue injuries (Table 4). Additionally, animals with concurrent soft tissue injuries had a 4.3 times greater odds of mortality than those without soft tissue injuries (Table 4). The severity of polytrauma may be associated with the number and severity of injuries and increased mortality rate. However, there was no association with mortality for animals with only diaphragmatic hernia and orthopedic injures.

Animals that were oxygen dependent during hospitalization had a 5.0 times greater odds of mortality than those that were not oxygen dependent (Table 3). Animals that were oxygen dependent were likely to have more severe clinical signs. We suspect that oxygen dependent animals had more significant pulmonary and/or intrathoracic disease than animals that were not oxygen dependent, making it understandable that they were more likely to die during the perioperative period. Animals that were oxygen dependent preoperatively had a 4.2 times greater odds of mortality than those that were not oxygen dependent preoperatively whereas animals that were oxygen dependent postoperatively had a 5.8 times greater odds of mortality than those who were not oxygen dependent postoperatively (Table 3). We do not recommend that oxygen therapy be withheld from animals that require it, but instead the requirement for oxygen supplementation should be recognized as a risk factor for mortality.

Our study did not find an association in perioperative survival rates with timing of surgery. In older reports

Table 6 Diaphragmatic herniorrhaphy surgery and anesthesia timing in cats and dogs and associations with mortality

Characteristic	Category	Animals alive ($n = 78$)	Animals that died ($n = 18$)	All cases ($n = 96$)	P-value
Time from trauma to admission (hrs)	Median, 95% CI	102.8, 22.1–178.8	38.6, 2.4–421.9	87.1, 22.1–177.6	0.64
Time from trauma to surgery (hrs)	Median, 95% CI	132.0, 58.6–207.5	47.9, 16.2–429.0	113.8, 48.2–201.0	0.63
Time from admission to surgery (hrs)	Median, 95% CI	16.3, 9.9–21.2	15.2, 7.0–20.1	16.3, 10.3–20.1	0.57
Anaesthesia duration (hrs)	Median, 95% CI	3.0, 2.7–3.2	4.3, 3.2–4.7	3.1, 2.8–3.3	0.0013*
Duration of surgical procedure (hrs)	Median, 95% CI	1.4, 1.3–1.6	1.9, 1.5–2.3	1.53, 1.40–1.67	0.004*

P–values reports are the results of the log–rank univariable analysis assessing association with mortality
Hrs hours, CI Confidence interval
*Indicates statistically significant difference

[1, 7], dogs treated < 24 h after trauma had a significantly increased risk of mortality. However, in the present study and the study by and Gibson et al [8], the timing of surgery did not have a significant impact on survival rates. We expect this finding is due to improvements in critical care pre- and postoperatively, and improvements in anaesthetic management intraoperatively. The original report finding that animals with diaphragmatic hernia have an increased mortality rate when undergoing surgery within 24 h of trauma concluded that herniorrhaphy should be delayed until the animal is stabilized [1]. We refute that the mortality rate is correlated with the timing of surgery.

Many limitations are present in this study due to the retrospective nature. Some medical records were incomplete. Although dyspnea and respiratory distress were qualified with respiratory rate and oxygen saturation, these are subjective assessments. The exact time of trauma was often unclear, and occasionally, no history of a traumatic event was reported by the owner. Therefore, it is possible that a congenital diaphragmatic hernia was mistaken for a traumatic diaphragmatic hernia. While possible, we consider this unlikely. Diaphragmatic hernia was discovered in two dogs after surgical fracture repair, thus prolonging time from admission to surgery and increasing median and maximum time from admission to surgery. There were a low number of cats that underwent diaphragmatic herniorrhaphy, and no associations were made with perioperative survival. Advancements in anesthetic protocol occurred over the 12 years of the study and may have increased perioperative survival. Due to variability of anesthetic protocol and low numbers of cases per year, statistics were not performed to assess the impact of anesthetic protocols. If this study was prospective, a trauma score may have been assessed which may have been correlated with perioperative survival.

Conclusion

Cats and dogs that underwent longer surgical procedures, underwent longer anesthesia, those with concurrent soft issue injuries, those with concurrent soft tissue and orthopedic injuries, and those that were oxygen dependent during hospitalization had a higher mortality rate. Based on our findings, we do not recommend that every animal with a diaphragmatic hernia be stabilized for 24 h or more prior to surgery. Instead, we recommend that preoperative stabilization be performed, with surgery to follow as indicated clinically.

Endnotes

[1] SAS software, Version 9.3 of the SAS System for PC. SAS and all other SAS Institute Inc. product or service names are registered trademarks or trademarks of SAS Institute Inc., Cary, NC, USA.

[2] Nova Critical Care Xpress, Nova Biomedical, Waltham, MA.

[3] VITROS 250, Ortho-Clinical Diagnostics, Rochester, NY.

Abbreviations
AS: Time from admission to surgery; CI: Confidence intervals; Hr: Hours; Kg: Kilograms; NSAID: Non-steroidal anti-inflammatory drug; OHE: Ovariohysterectomy; OR: Odds ratio; PSS: Portosystemic shunt; Ref: Reference category; SD: Standard deviation; SpO_2: pulse oximetry; TA: Time from trauma to admission; TS: Time from trauma to surgery; Yr: Years

Acknowledgements
The authors wish to thank Dr. Julius Liptak and Dr. Charles Bruce for scientific advice and technical editing.

Funding
This research received no specific grant from any funding agency in the public, commercial or not-for-profit sectors. The open access publishing fees for this article have been covered by the Texas A&M University Open Access to Knowledge Fund (OAKFund), supported by the University Libraries and the Office of the Vice President for Research.

Authors' contributions
CL performed the data collection by record acquisition and review. CL performed manuscript preparation. KTM performed the study design and concept as well as assisted in data collection, manuscript preparation and review. LS completed the statistical analysis and assisted in manuscript preparation and review. All authors read and approved the final manuscript.

Competing interests
The authors declare that they have no competing interests.

Consent for publication
Not applicable.

Author details
[1]Department of Small Animal Clinical Sciences (Thieman Mankin, Legallet), College of Veterinary Medicine, Texas A&M University, College Station, TX 77843-4474, USA. [2]The Department of Veterinary Clinical Medicine (Selmic), College of Veterinary Medicine, University of Illinois at Urbana-Champaign, Urbana, IL 61802, USA.

References

1. Boudrieau RJ, Muir WM. Pathophysiology of traumatic diaphragmatic hernia in dogs. Compend Contin Educ Pract Vet. 1987;9:379–85.
2. Hunt GB, Johnson KA. Diaphragmatic Hernias. In: Tobias KM, Johnston SA, editors. Veterinary Surgery: Small Animal. St. Louis: Elsevier Saunders; 2012. p. 1380–90.
3. Wilson GP, Newton CD, Burt JK, et al. A review of 116 diaphragmatic hernias in the dog and cat. J Am Vet Med Assoc. 1971;159:1142–5.
4. Wilson GP, Hayes Jr HM. Diaphragmatic hernia in the dog and cat: a 25-year overview. Semin Vet Med Surg (Small Anim). 1986;1:318–26.
5. Walker RG, Hall LW. Rupture of the diaphragm: Report of 32 cases in dogs and cats. Vet Rec. 1965;77:830–7.
6. Fossum TW. Surgery of the lower respiratory system: pleural cavity and diaphragm. In: Fossum TW, Hedlund TS, Hulse DA, et al., editors. Small Animal Surgery. 3rd ed. St Louis: Mosby Elsevier; 2007. p. 896–929.
7. Sullivan M, Reid J. Management of 60 cases of diaphragmatic rupture. J Small Anim Pract. 1990;31:425–30.
8. Gibson TWG, Brisson BA, Sears W. Perioperative survival rates after surgery for diaphragmatic hernia in dogs and cats: 92 cases (1990-2002). J Am Vet Med Assoc. 2005;227:105–9.
9. Garson HL, Dodman N, Baker GJ. Diaphragmatic hernia. Analysis of fifty-six cases in dogs and cats. J Small Anim Pract. 1980;21:469–81.
10. Minihan AC, Berg J, Evans KL. Chronic diaphragmatic hernia in 34 dogs and 16 cats. J Am Anim Hosp Assoc. 2004;40:51–63.
11. Schmiedt CW, Tobias KM, McCrackin Stevenson MA. Traumatic diaphragmatic hernia in cats: 34 cases (1991-2001). J Am Vet Med Assoc. 2003;222:1237–40.
12. Crowe DT. The acute and delayed diaphragmatic hernia. In Mazzaffero E, editor. Proceedings of the 10th International Veterinary Emergency Critical Care Symposium; 2004 Sep 8-12; San Diego, California. San Antonio, Texas: American College of Veterinary Emergency and Critical Care: Veterinary Emergency and Critical Care Society; 2004. p. 795–9.
13. Brody RS, Sauer RM. Clinico-pathologic conference. J Am Vet Med Assoc. 1964;145:1213–22.
14. Hendricks JC. Pulse Oximetry. In: King LG, editor. Textbook of Respiratory Diseases in Dogs and Cats. St. Louis: Elsevier; 2004. p. 193–7.

4

Course of serum amyloid A (SAA) plasma concentrations in horses undergoing surgery for injuries penetrating synovial structures

Eva Haltmayer[1][*] [iD], Ilse Schwendenwein[2] and Theresia F. Licka[1,3]

Abstract

Background: Injuries penetrating synovial structures are common in equine practice and often result in septic synovitis. Significantly increased plasma levels of serum amyloid A (SAA) have been found in various infectious conditions in horses including wounds and septic arthritis. Plasma SAA levels were found to decrease rapidly once the infectious stimulus was eliminated. The purpose of the current study was to investigate the usefulness of serial measurements of plasma SAA as a monitoring tool for the response to treatment of horses presented with injuries penetrating synovial structures. In the current study plasma SAA concentrations were measured every 48 hours (h) during the course of treatment.

Results: A total of 19 horses with a wound penetrating a synovial structure were included in the current study. Horses in Group 1 ($n = 12$) (injuries older than 24 h) only needed one surgical intervention. Patients in this group had significantly lower median plasma SAA levels ($P = 0.001$) between 48 h (median 776 mg/L) and 96 h (median 202 mg/L) after surgery. A significant decrease ($P = 0.004$) in plasma SAA levels was also observed between 96 h after surgery (median 270 mg/L) and 6 days (d) after surgery (median 3 mg/L). Four horses (Group 2) required more than one surgical intervention. In contrast to Group 1 patients in Group 2 had either very high initial plasma concentrations (3378 mg/L), an increase or persistently high concentrations of plasma SAA after the first surgery (median 2525 mg/L). A small group of patients ($n = 3$) (Group 3) were admitted less than 24 h after sustaining a wound. In this group low SAA values at admission (median 23 mg/L) and peak concentrations at 48 h after surgery (median 1016 mg/L) were observed followed by a decrease in plasma SAA concentration over time.

Conclusions: A decrease in plasma SAA concentrations between two consecutive time points could be associated with positive response to treatment in the current study. Therefore, serial measurements of plasma SAA could potentially be used as an additional inexpensive, quick and easy tool for monitoring the treatment response in otherwise healthy horses presented with injuries penetrating synovial structures. However further studies will be necessary to ascertain its clinical utility.

Keywords: Equids, Serum amyloid A (SAA), Injury synovial structure, Septic synovitis, Wound infection

* Correspondence: Eva.Haltmayer@vetmeduni.ac.at
[1]Department of Small Animals and Horses, Clinic for Horses, Equine Surgery, University of Veterinary Medicine Vienna, Veterinärplatz 1, A-1210 Vienna, Austria
Full list of author information is available at the end of the article

Background

Injuries penetrating synovial structures are common in equine practice [1, 2, 3]. These injuries cause contamination of the affected synovial structure and can subsequently lead to septic synovitis. Septic synovitis is a serious and potentially lethal condition in horses that requires immediate diagnosis and subsequent treatment [4–6]. Arthroscopic lavage is the recommended treatment of choice [2, 7–9]. However, more invasive approaches have been described in severely affected cases [10–12]. With adequate treatment, survival rates in adult horses range from 84% [6] to 90% [2] with 54% [6] to 81% [2] of horses returning to previous levels of performance [2, 4–6], except horses where solar foot penetration caused septic synovitis. In one larger scale study by Findley et al. [3] survival to discharge was only 56 and 36% returned to their previous athletic function. Introduction of pathogens into a synovial cavity causes a strong inflammatory response resulting in local swelling, heat and pain and eventually leading to enzymatic breakdown of hyaluronic acid and cartilage [7]. The inflammatory response is mainly driven by the release of cytokines from macrophages and monocytes at the site of injury. These pro-inflammatory mediators especially interleukin-1 (IL-1), tumor necrosis factor alpha (TNF-α) and interleukin-6 (IL-6) stimulate the hepatic acute phase protein synthesis [13] once released into circulation. In horses, serum amyloid A (SAA) was shown to be a reliable marker of various septic and non-septic inflammatory conditions [13–18]. SAA is a major acute phase protein in equids and characterized by a rapid and remarkable increase (up to several 1000-fold) from low to undetectable baseline values in plasma concentration and a rapid decrease, once inflammatory or infectious stimuli are eliminated [13, 18]. SAA reaches peak concentrations in plasma about 48 h after the onset of inflammation [18]. Jacobsen et al. [17] were the first to document that septic arthritis elicits a prominent acute phase response with significantly higher SAA concentrations in serum compared to healthy horses and horses with non-septic arthritis. Diagnosis and monitoring of successful treatment in patients with injuries penetrating synovial structures commonly relies on repeated synoviocentesis of the affected structure and subsequent synovial fluid analysis [19] as well as clinical signs such as lameness, heat and swelling. Synovial fluid analysis can be inconclusive under certain circumstances especially after repeated synoviocenteses [17, 20, 21] or drug application [20, 21]. Moreover, repeated synoviocentesis and subsequent collection of synovial samples can be difficult, especially under field conditions. Fibrin formation, synovial hypertrophy, and loss of synovial fluid via drainage through an open wound can also interfere with successful collection of a synovial fluid sample. To our knowledge, there are only limited reports about serial SAA measurements [17] over the course of treatment for assessment of treatment success.

The aim of the present study was to evaluate the course of plasma SAA over time in patients undergoing treatment for injuries penetrating synovial structures and to evaluate plasma SAA as a potential marker for treatment response. Hypothesis tested is that plasma SAA concentrations decrease significantly in response to successful treatment.

Methods

Animals

Horses over 1 year of age admitted to the Equine Hospital, University of Veterinary Medicine Vienna, Austria for investigation and treatment of injuries penetrating synovial structures between May 2012 and January 2013 were included in the study. Inclusion criteria were injuries (lacerations, open fractures, puncture wounds and street nail injury) penetrating synovial structures and requiring surgical intervention. Pregnant mares and horses younger than 1 year, as well as horses with clinically relevant medical conditions prior to the development of the presenting complaint such as horses with additional, not wound associated infections or inflammatory conditions were excluded from the study.

Remnants of plasma samples obtained for routine blood work were used for SAA measurements, or blood was withdrawn from a previously placed intravenous (IV) catheter. No invasive procedure was performed for study purposes only. Owner's written consent was obtained at admission.

For description of results and statistical analysis horses were divided into three Groups. Group 1 ($n = 12$) consisted of horses with injuries older than 24 h, Group 2 ($n = 4$) were horses that required more than one surgical intervention/one lavage and Group 3 ($n = 3$) consisted of horses with fresh (< 24 h) injuries. Decision for further lavages was taken by the clinician in charge of the case based on clinical findings and results of synovial fluid analysis.

Initial assessment

A thorough clinical examination and routine blood work (complete blood count, creatinine, total protein, glutamate dehydrogenase, gamma-glutamyl transferase, creatinine kinase, potassium and fibrinogen) was performed on each patient. Samples for routine blood work were obtained by venipuncture of the jugular vein using a vacutainer system (Vacuette, Greiner Bio-One GmbH, Frickenhausen, Germany) or from a venous catheter. On admission, horses underwent a limited orthopaedic examination, as was decided relevant by the clinician in charge of the case. No evaluation at trot, no flexion tests and no diagnostic anaesthesia was performed, as the horses were lame at the walk and/or had obvious wounds and swellings. Additionally, radiographic and/or ultrasonographic examinations were performed.

Centesis of at least 1 synovial structure adjacent to the injury was carried out, and when possible synovial fluid was collected. If no synovial fluid sample could be obtained, the involved synovial structure was distended with sterile saline solution to identify communication with a wound. In cases where no synovial fluid sample could be aspirated sterile saline solution was injected and immediately re-aspirated to obtain a synovial lavage sample. Synovial samples were analysed at the Clinical Pathology Unit, University of Veterinary Medicine Vienna, Austria by one of the authors (IS). A smear and a cytospin were prepared from native and lavage samples and stained with a Romanowsky-type stain (Haemafix™ Biomed Labordiagnostik GmbH, Oberschleißheim, Germany) for verification of automated cell counts, cell differentiation and evaluation of mucin precipitate. The concentration of nucleated cells (TNCC) was determined in undiluted samples with a laser based hematology system (Advia 2120™, Siemens Diagnostics, Erlangen, Germany). To samples with high viscosity, which were inappropriate for automated counting a grain of hyaluronidase powder was added, so that they could be analysed. In diluted samples only the ratio of neutrophils and monocytes was analysed. Total protein concentration was evaluated by refractometry from undiluted samples. An injury penetrating synovial structures was confirmed when communication of the injury with a synovial cavity was found (positive pressure test) and/or synovial fluid analysis results showed TNCC $>20 \times 10^3/\mu L$ and/or neutrophils >80% and total protein >4 g/dL [19, 22]. Pathological findings on physical examination (lameness, swelling, heat, fever) were also taken into account.

Preoperative treatment and surgery

All treatment decisions were carried out by the clinician in charge of the case. Preoperatively, an intravenous catheter was placed in a jugular vein, and all patients received systemic broad spectrum antimicrobials: penicillin (30.000 IU/kg, IV, every 6 h) and gentamicin (6.6 mg/kg, IV, once daily). When indicated by results of antimicrobial susceptibility tests, marbofloxacin (2 mg/kg, IV, once daily) or cefquinome (2.2 mg/kg, IV, once daily) were used. All patients received non-steroidal anti-inflammatory drugs (NSAIDs): flunixin meglumine (1.1 mg/kg, IV, twice daily) or phenylbutazone (2 mg/kg, PO, twice daily). Patients were treated surgically by standard wound debridement and lavage of the affected synovial structure under general anaesthesia or standing under sedation and regional anaesthesia. Lavage was performed either through 16G and 18G needles or arthroscopically. All affected synovial structures were closed after lavaging. Details about patients and treatment procedures are displayed in Table 1.

Postoperative management

After surgery horses were kept on systemic antimicrobials and NSAIDs. Antimicrobials, a combination of 250 IU bacitracin and 5000 IU neomycin or 500 mg amikacin were instilled into the synovial structure after lavage and after each synovial centesis. In some cases distal regional limb perfusions (DRLP) with 500 mg amikacin were performed in addition. During hospitalization, horses were examined clinically at least once a day (lameness assessment at the walk and physical examination). Horses received bandage changes every 2–3 days or as needed.

SAA samples and assay

Blood samples for plasma SAA measurements were taken at admission (before initial surgical treatment) and subsequently every 48 h until infection was considered to be resolved (improved clinical presentation, synovial fluid analysis within normal limits)-this was taken as a favourable response to treatment. Samples were collected from a previously placed intravenous catheter or where routine blood work was taken at time point representing the 48 h interval remnants of plasma samples from this routine blood work were used. Venous blood samples were collected into blood tubes containing heparin and centrifuged. The supernatant was either analysed immediately, if the clinician in charge of the case decided to include SAA analysis in the routine blood work, or frozen at $-20\,°$C and stored for a maximum of 60 days until analysis. Analyses were performed at the Clinical Pathology Unit, University of Veterinary Medicine Vienna, Austria, using a commercially available immunoturbidimetric assay (LZ test SAA, Eiken Chemical Co, Tokyo, Japan) validated for use in horses in a prior study [23] and re-evaluated and adapted on a fully selective autoanalyser for clinical chemistry (Cobas ™501c, Roche Diagnostics, Vienna, Austria) by the Department for Clinical Pathology [24]. Cut-off value of <10 mg/L was established for the local population of healthy horses prior to the present study [24].

Statistical methods

Patients of Group 2 and Group 3 were excluded from statistical analysis due to the low number of patients.

Statistical analyses were performed using MedCalc 11.3.1.0 package (MedCalc Software bvba, Ostend, Belgium). All probabilities were two-tailed and P values <0.05 were regarded significant. To test for normality a Kolmogorov-Smirnov test was performed. Univariate comparisons of two consecutive plasma SAA measurements were performed with the non-parametric Wilcoxon test for paired samples (respective P-values were not adjusted for multiple comparisons).

Course of serum amyloid A (SAA) plasma concentrations in horses undergoing surgery for injuries...

29

Table 1 Detailed patient information reporting age (in years), breed, sex, diagnosis, treatment, complications and synovial fluid parameters

Group	Patient	Signalement	Diagnosis	Surgical treatment	Repeated AL/ standing lavage	Complications	Duration of injury	Synovial parameters at admission[a]	Duration of treatment
1	2	Trotter, 6y, S	Pastern laceration right hind, septic digital flexor tendon sheath	Wound debridement; standing needle lavage digital flexor tendon sheath		None	>24 h	Positive pressure test; >80% neutrophils; 3200 TNC/ μL; TP 4 g/dL	4 days treatment was continued by referring veterinarian
1	5	Gidran, 13y, G	Laceration left tarsus, septic tarsal sheath	Wound debridement; AL tarsal sheath; GA		None	2 days	>85% neutrophils; and positive pressure test	9 days
1	6	Cob, 13y, M	Street nail injury right front, septic distal interphalangeal joint	AL distal interphalangeal joint; GA		Euthanasia d 30 of hospitalization after developing septic navicular bursitis right front	2 days	>95% neutrophils; 200 TNC /400xHPF; TP 7,2 g/dL	15 days for septic interphalangeal joint
1	8	Nonius, 9y, G	Street nail injury left hind, septic navicular bursa	BL navicluar bursa:; GA		none	5 days	>95% neutrophils; positive pressure test	14 days
1	11	WB, 18y, G	Puncture wound left hind fetlock, cellulitis	Debridement and standing needle lavage metatarsophalangeal joint		Euthanasia after discharge due to laminitis right hind	>2 days	80% neutrophils; 3200 TNC/ μL; TP 3 g/dL	16 days
1	12	Cob, 16y, M	Laceration left tarsus septic tarsometatarsal joint	needle lavage tarsometatarsal joint: GA		Euthanasia on d 27 of hospitalisation due to osteomyelitis left Mt. IV	4 days	>95% neutrophils; positive pressure test	19 days for septic tarsometatarsal joint
1	13	Pony, 20y, G	Laceration, bone sequester left humerus, septic bicipital bursa	Needle lavage, sequestrectomy, standing		None	>24 h	Positive pressure test	28 days
1	14	Icelandic horse, 15y, M	Laceration left elbow; septic elbow joint, open intraarticular olecranon fracture Type II	AL elbow joint, fracture repair; GA		None	>24 h	Positive pressure test	26 days
1	15	WB, 24y, G	Laceration SDFT and DDFT right hind, septic digital flexor tendon sheath	TVL digital flexor tendon sheath; GA		Scar tissue formation SDFT	2 days	Positive pressure test; >75% neutrophils; 21,910 TNC/ μL; TP 4 g/dL	10 days
1	16	Icelandic horse, 2y, M	Laceration right carpus septic carpal joints	AL carpal joints; GA		None	>36 h	Positive pressure test; >80%	12 days

Table 1 Detailed patient information reporting age (in years), breed, sex, diagnosis, treatment, complications and synovial fluid parameters *(Continued)*

								neutrophils; 26,670 TNC/µL; TP 3,4 g/dL	
1	18	Arab, 17y, M	Laceration left tarsus, septic tarsocrural joint/open comminuted calcaneus fracture	standing needle lavage tarsocrural joint;		Euthanasia on d 7 of hospitalisation due to pleural effusion, heart failure	>36 h	Positive pressure test; >96% neutrophils; 10,270 TNC/µL; TP 5 g/dL	6 days
1	20	WB, 12y, G	Laceration right front fetlock septic digital flexor tendon sheath	TVL digital flexor tendon sheath; GA		Adhesions formation SDFT and digital tendon sheath;	7 days	Positive pressure test; >88% neutrophils; 310 TNC/400× HPF; TP 3,5 g/dL	18 days
2	4	WB, 8y, G	Laceration right stifle; septic femoropatellar joint	Wound debridement; AL femoropatellar joint: GA	Yes; AL; GA; 48 h after first surgery	None	36 h	Positive pressure test; >80% neutrophils; 8700 TNC/µL; TP 4,6 g/dL	9 days
2	7	QH, 4y, G	Laceration right carpus septic middle carpal joint; osteomyelitis carpal accessory bone	AL middle carpal joint: GA	8 days after first surgery; curettage of carpal accessory bone, GA; no AL indicated	Osteomyelitis accessory carpal bone	>2 days	positive pressure test; >80% neutrophils; 120 TNC/400× HPF; TP 6,4 g/dL	28 days
2	17	Polo Pony, 16y, G	Puncture wound left tarsus; septic tarsal sheath	AL tarsal sheath; GA	Yes; AL; GA 96 h after initial surgery		4 days	>95% neutrophils; >100 TNC/400× HPF; TP 7,2 g/dL	23 days
2	19	Trotter, 8y, M	Laceration right carpus septic carpal joints	AL carpal joints; GA	Yes; 3 ALs GA 48 h, 96 h and 6 days after initial surgery		5 days	>90% neutrophils; 36,600 TNC/µL; TP 6 g/dL	36 days
3	1	WB, 3y, M	Laceration left tarsus, contaminated tarsocrural joint	wound debridement; AL tarsocrural joint: GA		None	5 h	>90% neutrophils; 35,880 TNC/µL; TP 5 g/dL	12 days
3	3	Criollo, 20y, M	Street nail injury right hind; contaminated navicular bursa	BL navicular bursa; GA		None	6 h	Positive pressure test	20 days
3	9	WB, 9y, M	Pastern laceration left hind, contaminated digital flexor tendon sheath	TVL digital flexor tendon sheath; GA		None	4 h	Positive pressure test; >95% neutrophils; 14,220 TNC/µL; TP 2,4 g/dL	10 days

M mare, *S* stallion, *G* gelding, *WB* warmblood, *QH* quarter horse, *Mt. IV* fourth metatarsal bone, *DDFT* deep digital flexor tendon, *SDFT* superficial digital flexor tendon, *GA* general anaesthesia, *DRLP* distal regional limb perfusion, *AL* arthroscopic lavage, *TVL* tendovaginoscopic lavage, *BL* bursoscopic lavage, *HPF* high power field, *TP* total protein
[a]not all parameters were available for each patient, dependent on the amount of synovial fluid/if synovial fluid was obtained

Results

Study population and samples

Nineteen horses admitted to the University Clinic for Horses, University of Veterinary Medicine Vienna, Austria, between May 2012 and January 2013 matched the inclusion criteria. Horses were of mixed breed and age. Females and males were evenly distributed.

Patient details including clinical data and surgical procedures are displayed in Table 1.

In 15 patients an arthroscopy/bursoscopy/tendovaginoscopy and lavage of the affected synovial structure was performed under general anaesthesia.

In 5 patients wound revision and lavage of the affected synovial structure was performed standing under sedation and regional anaesthesia through 16G or 18G needles. Decision on needle lavage was based on the presence of a calcaneal fracture in case 18, on the risk of a humeral fracture during recovery in case 13, on the anatomy of the joint involved in case 12 and on financial considerations in the remaining cases.

Post operatively horses were kept on systemic broad-spectrum antimicrobials and NSAIDs for a median of 10.5 days (range 7–25 days). Four patients received a median of 3 (range 2–4) DRLPs with antimicrobials. In 9 patients repeated synoviocentesis was performed to monitor treatment success and intrasynovial antimicrobials were administered after each procedure.

Plasma SAA concentrations

Statistical analysis was not performed in Group 2 and 3 due to the limited number of patients.

Median plasma SAA values of all Groups are displayed in Table 2.

Patients in Group 1 showed a significant decrease in plasma SAA concentrations over the course of treatment: Patients in that group had two different rise and fall pattern. Four individuals showed the peak concentration at time of admission and the remaining patients had peak concentrations at 48 h after surgery. Time of injury to admission was not connected to one of the rise and fall pattern in Group 1 (Fig. 1a).

The median percentage decrease of plasma SAA in this group was 70% (range 18–100%) between 48 and 96 h and 99% (range 17–100%) between 96 h and 6 days after initial surgical intervention. Results of pairwise comparison of two time points of measurement are displayed in Fig. 1b.

Patients in Group 2 showed variable patterns of plasma SAA concentration over time. Two horses (4, 19) showed persistently high or even increased levels of SAA after the first surgery, patient 17 showed a very high increase between the first and the second surgery and patient 7 showed very high initial SAA values and only a minor decrease before the second surgery (Fig. 2). This represents a median increase in plasma SAA concentrations of 24% (range – 40 – +100%) between 48 and 96 h and a median decrease of only 60% (range 15–85%) between 96 h and 6 days after the first surgery. Especially in Patient 19 the increase before surgery can be well observed (Fig. 2).

Patients in Group 3 showed typical rise and fall pattern with a peak at 48 h after initial surgical treatment. In that Group injuries happened <24 h before admission (Fig. 3). The median decrease of plasma SAA levels was 60% (range 9–84%) between 48 and 9 h post initial treatment and 98% (range 61–100%) between 96 h and 6 days after surgery.

Discussion

In the current study we monitored the course of plasma SAA concentrations in response to treatment in 19 otherwise healthy horses with injuries penetrating synovial structures. Plasma SAA concentrations in cases with injuries penetrating synovial structures decreased rapidly in response to treatment and returned to levels below the reference value (10 mg/L) during the course of successful treatment (Figs.1a, 3). Therefore SAA analysis offers a timely and useful tool for monitoring the effect of treatment of injuries penetrating synovial structures. Jacobsen et al. [17] mentioned in their study that plasma SAA concentration in one horse with septic arthritis decreased during the course of treatment. This could also be observed in the present study in horses treated for injuries penetrating synovial structures. To the authors' knowledge, this is the first study investigating the utility of serial plasma SAA measurements for

Table 2 Median (range) of plasma SAA values (mg/L) of horses over their course of treatment for injuries penetrating synovial structures. Group 1: horses with injuries older than 24 h requiring only a single surgical intervention, Group 2: horses that required more than one surgical intervention, Group 3: horses with wounds of less than 24 h

	pre OP	48 h	96 h	6 days*
Group 1 (n = 12)	454 (275–6378) a	776 (422–2100) a	201 (19–864) b	5 (0–17) c
Group 2 (n = 4)	940 (16–3378)	2525 (495–4000)	2593 (811–3370)	1000 (122–2618)
Group 3 (n = 3)	23 (7–77)	1016 (273–1666)	297 (159–500)	5 (0–17)

pre OP preoperative
Different letters indicate significant difference (P < 0.05) between time-points of SAA measurements during treatment
*At time point 6 days data was available from 9 horses in Group 1, 4 horses in Group 2 and 2 horses in Group 3.

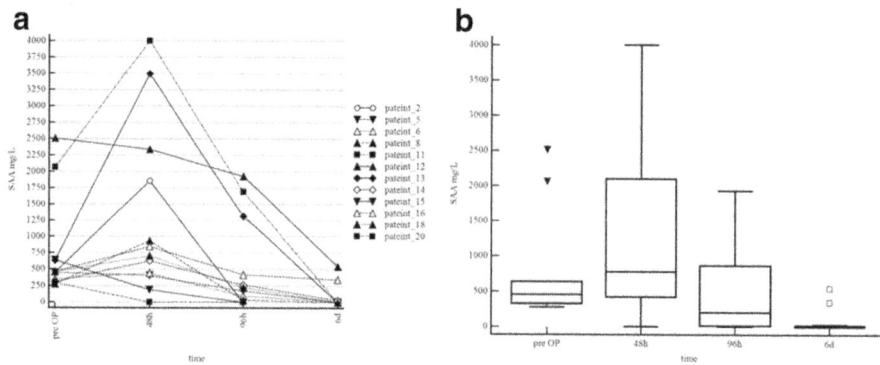

Fig. 1 a Course of plasma SAA of all patients in Group 2. Peak values could be observed between pre OP (n = 4) and 48 h after surgery (n = 7). Notice the continuous decrease of plasma SAA concentrations after surgery. **b** Box and *whisker plots* of course of plasma SAA concentration during treatment of patients of Group 1 Explanations: In *box-and-whisker plots*, *central box* represents values from lower to upper quartile, *middle line* represents the median; *whiskers* extend from minimum to maximum value, excluding outside and far out values which are displayed as separate points

monitoring treatment response in patients with injuries penetrating synovial structures in a clinical set up. Data indicates that the course of plasma SAA concentration reflects the response to treatment well. Patients of Group 1 and 3 with a highly favourable response to initial surgical treatment showed a continuous decrease of SAA concentrations between 48 and 96 h after surgery as well 6 days after surgery. In contrast in cases with ongoing infection (Group 2) different patterns of SAA could be observed. Two horses (4, 19) showed persistently high or even increased levels of SAA after the first surgery, one horse (17) showed a very high increase between the first and the second surgery and the other horse (7) showed very high initial SAA values and only a

minor decrease before the second surgery. However this has to be interpreted with care due to the low number of patients and no conclusion can be drawn from the data at this point.

Persistently high concentrations of SAA have been previously reported in horses with complications after elective and emergency surgery [14, 25, 26]. In the present study this was considered to be an indication for lack of treatment response. However, further surgical treatment was instigated only with corresponding clinical signs and synovial fluid analysis and was not based on SAA values. This does not preclude that animals could have potentially improved without additional intervention. However, such an experimental set up cannot be used in client owned

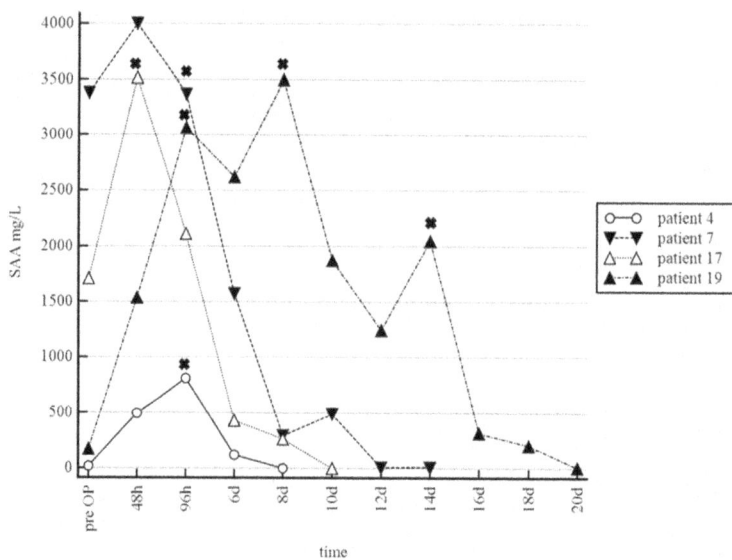

Fig. 2 Course of plasma SAA in horses of Group 2 Timepoints of surgery are marked (+). In patients 4 and 19 an increase of plasma SAA was observed before the following surgical treatment. Patient 7 showed very high initial SAA values with only a minor decrease before the second surgical intervention. Patient 17 showed an unusual high increase after the first surgery

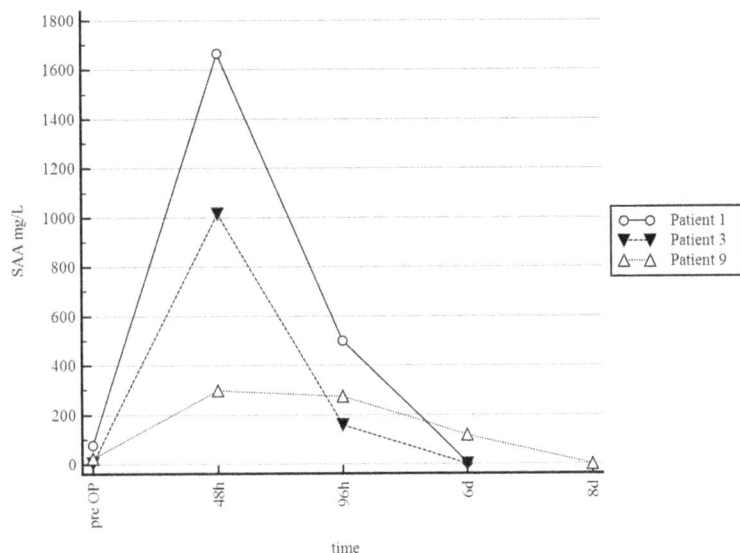

Fig. 3 Illustration of the typical rise and fall pattern of plasma SAA concentrations of patients with injuries <24 h. Peak concentrations are observed 48 h after surgery. Notice the relative low pre OP plasma SAA values

horses. The time interval of 48 h for SAA sample collection in the present study was chosen because SAA shows peak concentration 48 h after onset of infection [13, 18]. Concentrations of SAA correspond to the severity of tissue damage as well as to the volume of damaged tissue [18] and drop rapidly as soon as synthesis stops [18]. Due to these unique features of SAA sequential measurements of plasma SAA concentrations were suggested as a useful aid in patient management, planning of treatment strategies and in decision-making whether to perform surgery or not [13, 18].

Duration of the disease process prior to admission as well as the stage of the disease process at admission have to be carefully considered when interpreting SAA concentrations in a patient [17, 18]. In the current study patients in Group 3 had normal or very low SAA concentrations (range from 6.7 mg/L to 23.1 mg/L) at the time of admission, despite a positive pressure test and/or neutrophil counts >90% in synovial fluid. In these patients the reported duration between detection of injury by the owner and hospital admission was <24 h thus below the reported lag time for SAA increase. Jacobsen et al. [17] also described one case where the authors assumed that the time from injury to sample collection was too short for the local inflammatory response to induce hepatic SAA synthesis. In this particular case the delay between injury and sample collection was only 2 h. The three patients in Group 3 support this suggestion [17]. Therefore care has to be taken when interpreting single SAA values, especially in early stages of disease and results of the current study strongly suggest that SAA values obtained at a single time point should not be used for diagnostic purposes. Also low-grade infections [14] and well sequestrated

infections [14] were previously reported to cause a retarded response in plasma SAA in relation to clinical signs. This can be explained by a local inflammatory response that is not "strong" enough to trigger SAA synthesis in the liver and incite a systemic inflammatory response. In contrast Belgrave et al. [14] reported that SAA values were increased 24 h prior to onset of clinical signs in horses with colic and metritis [13] and therefore SAA could potentially aid in early detection of inflammation. However due to the limited number of patients in Group 3 no conclusions can be drawn at this point.

In the present study most patients showed peak concentration of plasma SAA 48 h after surgery. In all cases surgery was performed on the day of hospital admission. Therefore, peak values might have been influenced by the degree of infection of the injury site and/or the synovial structure, as well as by surgical trauma [25–27], general anaesthesia [28, 29] or antimicrobial treatment [30]. Jacobsen et al. [27] reported slightly increased plasma SAA values up to 5 days after arthroscopy (up to 100 mg/L), however these levels remain much lower than in the cases of the present study [26]. Sanchez-Teran et al. [31, 32] recently suggested in their study that in healthy adult horses neither arthroscopic lavage nor through-and-through joint lavage with needles influenced plasma SAA concentrations 48–120 h after surgery. Moreover, Pollock et al. [26] described that healthy horses undergoing an elective surgery responded similar to surgical trauma than horses with elevated plasma SAA concentrations undergoing emergency surgery. In four patients in Group 1 a decrease in plasma SAA could be observed between admission and 48 h after surgery (Fig. 1a). These results do not support the suggestion that surgical trauma alone led to the typical rise and fall pattern post-surgery, however due to the low number of cases no conclusion can be drawn.

Currently little and controversial information is available regarding the effects of general anaesthesia on plasma SAA concentrations. One study reported no increase in plasma SAA concentrations after general anaesthesia [28], another study reported values of up to 520.7 mg/l in horses 24 h after general anaesthesia of a maximum of 2 h duration without surgery [29]. However, the latter study also reported high inter-individual differences so that high and low responders among horses could be discussed.

All patients enrolled in the current study received NSAIDs during the course of treatment. The effect of non-steroidal anti-inflammatory drugs on the acute phase response has been investigated studies in various species (dogs, ruminants, humans) other than horses [33–35]. These studies showed that administration of non-steroidal anti-inflammatory drugs did not affect the acute phase response in comparison to a non-treated control group. On the other hand some studies exist that state the opposite [36, 37]. Based on these contradictory information it remains unclear whether the course of SAA was affected by administration of NSAIDs in horses in the current study. This leaves room for further studies investigating the effect of NSAIDs on SAA response in horses with injuries penetrating synovial structures. Increased plasma SAA concentrations were observed in pregnant mares starting 1 week before parturition until 1 month post partum [16]. Therefore pregnant mares were excluded from the present study. Horses younger than 1 year were also excluded from the present study because differentiation between traumatic septic arthritis and septic arthritis/physitis in foals was deemed to be potentially imprecise.

Nunokawa et al. [38] described in their study that various inflammatory and infectious diseases lead to increased plasma SAA concentrations in horses. Therefore in patients with multiple inflammatory processes plasma SAA concentrations are only of limited use for monitoring response to treatment for injuries penetrating synovial structures. In horses with postoperative complications unrelated to the site of injury that reportedly lead to an increase in plasma SAA concentration such as gastrointestinal pathologies [39, 40] (eg. colitis) interpretation of SAA concentrations regarding the state of infection of the primary injury by a single measurement might be challenging or even impossible.

One limitation of the present study is that patients presented with a variety of wounds and different types of tissues involved. This, however, reflects a typical hospital population and therefore allows testing the hypothesis in a routine clinical setting.

These wounds led to various amounts of tissue damage and infection of tissue surrounding the synovial structure. Therefore it stands to reason that the pattern of SAA during the course of treatment was likewise influenced by resolution of infection from the wound and/or synovial structure.

In the present study two patients had fractures in addition to the injuries penetrating synovial structures. Plasma SAA concentrations therefore may have been influenced by the surgical trauma due to fracture repair in patient 14 and trauma to the bone itself in both patients. In patient 14 serial SAA measurements showed a decrease over the course of treatment which was considered a reflection of favourable response to treatment. Patient 18 was euthanized due to heart failure. However synovial analysis prior to euthanasia revealed no synovial sepsis. In Patient 12 osteomyeltis of the fourth metatarsal bone was diagnosed after synovial sepsis of the tarsometatarsal joint was considered to be improved (clinical improvement, low SAA). Consent for further treatment was not given by the owner and the patient was euthanised. In this case plasma SAA was within normal limits despite the presence of osteomyelitis. The reason for the lack of increased plasma SAA could not be determined in this case. Another limitation of the present study is, that due to the clinical design, the number of plasma samples obtained per horse could not be standardised more stringently. Number of samples obtained depended on the time required for resolution of infection.

Conclusions

In summary the results of the present study suggest that sequential measurement of SAA exhibiting continuously declining concentrations seems to indicate a favourable response to treatment. Serial plasma SAA concentrations potentially offer a relatively inexpensive, non-invasive and rapid method to monitor response to treatment in injuries penetrating synovial structures. However due to the small number of patients and the variation in the data of the current study further investigations will be necessary to ascertain the clinical value of plasma SAA as a complementary monitoring tool in horses with injuries penetrating synovial structures.

Abbreviations

AL: Arthroscopic lavage; BL: Bursoscopic lavage; d: Day (s); DDFT: Deep digital flexor tendon; DRLP: Distal regional limb perfusion; G: Gelding; GA: General anaesthesia; h: Hour (s); HPF: High power field; IL-1: Interleukin-1; IL-6: Interleukin-6; IQR: Interquartile range; IV: Intravenous; M: Mare; Mt. IV: Fourth metatarsal bone; NSIAD: Non steroidal anti-inflammatory drug; preOP: Preoperative; QH: Quarter horse; S: Stallion; SAA: Serum amyloid A; SDFT: Superficial digital flexor tendon; TMT: Tarsometatarsal joint; TNC: Total nucleated cells; TNCC: Total nucleated cell count; TNF-α: Tumor necrosis factor alpha; TP: Total protein; TVL: Tendovaginoscopic lavage; WB: Warmblood

Funding

This study was funded from T. Licka's research allowance of the Veterinary University Vienna Austria. No external funding (neither private nor corporate) was used for this study.

Authors' contributions
The study was designed by EH, TFL and IS. Data collection and study execution were done by EH and TFL. Laboratory analysis was performed by IS. All Authors contributed to the data analysis and interpretation, to preparation and final approval of the manuscript.

Competing interests
The authors declare that they have no competing interests.

Consent for publication
Not applicable.

Author details
[1]Department of Small Animals and Horses, Clinic for Horses, Equine Surgery, University of Veterinary Medicine Vienna, Veterinärplatz 1, A-1210 Vienna, Austria. [2]Department of Pathobiology, Clinical Pathology, University of Veterinary Medicine Vienna, Veterinärplatz 1, A-1210 Vienna, Austria. [3]Department of Veterinary Clinical Studies, Royal (Dick) School of Veterinary Studies, University of Edinburgh, Easter Bush Campus, Midlothian EH25 9RG, Scotland.

References
1. Gibson KT, McIlwraith CW, Turner AS, Stashak TS, Aanes WA, Trotter GW. Open joint injuries in horses: 58 cases (1980-1986). J Am Vet Med Assoc. 1989;194:398–404.
2. Wright IM, Smith MRW, Humphrey DJ, Eaton-Evans TC, Hillyer MH. Endoscopic surgery in the treatment of contaminated and infected synovial cavities. Equine Vet J. 2003;35:613–9.
3. Findley JA, Pinchbeck GL, Milner PI, Bladon BM, Boswell J, Mair TS, Suthers JM, Singer ER. Outcome of horses with synovial structure involvement following solar foot penetrations in four UK veterinary hospitals: 95 cases. Equine Vet J. 2014;46:352–7.
4. Milner PI, Bardell DA, Warner L, Packer LMJ, Senior JM, Singer ER, Archer DC. Factors associated with survival to hospital discharge following endoscopic treatment for synovial sepsis in 214 horses. Equine Vet J. 2014;46:701–5.
5. Schneider RK, Bramlage LR, Moore RM, Mecklenburg LM, Kohn CW, Gabel AA. A retrospective study of 192 horses affected with septic arthritis/tenosynovitis. Equine Vet J. 1992;24:436–42.
6. Walmsley EA, Anderson GA, Muurlink MA, Whitton RC. Retrospective investigation of prognostic indicators for adult horses with infection of a synovial structure. Aust Vet J. 2011;89:226–31.
7. Bertone A. Infectious arthritis. In: McIlwraith C, Trotter G, editors. Joint disease in the horse. Philadelphia: WB, Saunders; 1996. p. 397–409.
8. LaPointe J, Laverty S, La Voie J. Septic arthritis in 15 Standardbred race horses after intraarticular injection. Equine Vet J. 1992;24:430–4.
9. Meijer M, van Weeren P, Rijkenhuizen A. Clinical experiences of treating septic arthritis in the equine by repeated joint lavage: a series of 39 cases. J Am Vet Med Assoc. 2000;47:351–65.
10. Booth TM, Abbot J, Clements A, Singer ER, Clegg PD. Treatment of septic common digital extensor tenosynovitis by complete resection in seven horses. Vet Surg. 2004;33:107–11.
11. Marsh CA, Watkins JP, Schneider RK. Intrathecal deep digital flexor tenectomy for treatment of septic tendonitis/tenosynovitis in four horses. Vet Surg. 2011;40:284–90.
12. Mc Nally TP, Slone DE, Hughes FE, Lynch TM. Tenosynoviotomy for sepsis of the digital flexor tendon sheath in 9 horses. Vet Surg. 2013;42:114–8.
13. Petersen HH, Nielsen JP, Heegaard PMH. Application of acute phase protein measurements in veterinary clinical chemistry. Vet Res. 2004;35:163–87.
14. Belgrave RL, Dickey MM, Arheart KL, Cray C. Assessment of serum amyloid A testing of horses and its clinical application in a specialized equine practice. J Am Vet Med Assoc. 2013;243:113–9.
15. Cohen ND, Chaffin MK, Vandenplas ML, Edwards RF, Nevill M, Moore JN, Martens RJ. Study of serum amyloid A concentrations as a means of achieving early diagnosis of Rhodococcus equi pneumonia. Equine Vet J. 2005;37:212–6.
16. Coutinho da Silva MA, Canisso IF, MacPherson ML, Johnson AE, Divers TJ. Serum amyloid A concentration in healthy periparturient mares and mares with ascending placentitis. Equine Vet J. 2013;45:619–24.
17. Jacobsen S, Thomsen MH, Nanni S. Concentrations of serum amyloid A in serum and synovial fluid from healthy horses and horses with joint disease. Am J Vet Res. 2006;67:1738–42.
18. Jacobsen S, Andersen PH. The acute phase protein serum amyloid A (SAA) as a marker of inflammation in horses. Equine Vet Educ. 2007;19:38–46.
19. Steel CM. Equine synovial fluid analysis. Vet Clin North Am Equine Pract. 2008;24:437–54.
20. Dykgraaf S, Dechant JE, Johns JL, Christopher MM, Bolt DM, Snyder JR. Effect of intrathecal amikacin administration and repeated centesis on digital flexor tendon sheath synovial fluid in horses. Vet Surg. 2007;36:57–63.
21. Sanchez Teran AF, Rubio Martinez LM, Villarino N, Sanz MG. Effects of repeated intra-articular administration of amikacin on serum amyloid A, total protein and nucleated cell count in synovial fluid from healthy horses. Equine Vet J. 2012;44:12–6.
22. Frisbee DD. Synovial joint biology and Pathobiology. In: Auer JA, Stick JA, editors. Equine Surgery. Philadelphia: WB, Saunders; 2012. p. 1096–114.
23. Jacobsen S, Kjelgaard-Hansen M, Hagbard Petersen H, Jensen AL. Evaluation of a commercially available human serum amyloid A (SAA) turbidimetric immunoassay for determination of equine SAA concentrations. Vet J. 2006; 172:315–9.
24. Swancar-Haid P. Implementierung eines serum Amyloid a (SAA) Asseys als früher marker entzündlicher Erkrankungen beim Pferd. MS thesis in biomedical science: FH Fachhochschule campus Wien, 2011.
25. Jacobsen S, Jensen JC, Frei S, Jensen AL, Thoefner MB. Use of serum amyloid A and other acute phase reactants to monitor the inflammatory response after castration in horses: a field study. Equine Vet J. 2005;37:552–6.
26. Pollock PJ, Prendergast M, Schumacher J, Bellenger CR. Effects of surgery on the acute phase response in clinically normal and diseased horses. Vet Rec. 2005;156:538–42.
27. Jacobsen S, Nielsen JV, Kjelgaard-Hansen M, Toelboell T, Fjeldborg J, Halling-Thomsen M, Martinussen T, Thoefner MB. Acute phase response to surgery of varying intensity in horses: a preliminary study. Vet Surg. 2009;38:762–9.
28. Pepys MB, Baltz ML, Tennent GA, Kent J, Ousey J, Rossdale PD. Serum amyloid A protein (SAA) in horses: objective measurement of the acute phase response. Equine Vet J. 1989;21:106–9.
29. Stowasser-Raschbauer B, Kabes R, Moens Y. Serum Amyloid A-Konzentrationen beim Pferd nach einer Allgemeinanästhesie mit und ohne chirurgischen Eingriff. Wien Tierärztl Mschr. 2013;100:127–32.
30. Busk P, Jacobsen S. Martinussen: administration of perioperative penicillin reduces postoperative serum Amyloid A response in horses being castrated standing. Vet Surg. 2010;39:638–43.
31. Sanchez-Teran AF, Bracamonte JL, Hendrick S, Burguess HJ, Duke-Novakovski T, Schott M, Hoff B, Rubio-Martínez LM. Effect of arthroscopic Lavage on systemic and synovial fluid serum Amyloid A in healthy horses. Vet Surg. 2016;45:223–30.
32. Sanchez-Teran AF, Bracamonte JL, Hendrick S, Riddell L, Musil K, Hoff B, Rubio-Martínez LM. Effect of repeated through-and-through joint lavage on serum amyloid a in synovial fluid from healthy horses. Vet J. 2016;210:30–3.
33. Karademir, U, Akin I, Erdogan H, Ural K, Asici GSE: Effect of Ketoprofen on acute phase protein concentrations in goats undergoing castration. BMC Vet Res. 2016. doi: 10.1186/s12917-016-0748-y.
34. Kum C, Voyvoda H, Sekkin S, Karademir U, Tarimcilar T. Effects of carprofen and meloxicam on C-reactive protein, ceruloplasmin, and fibrinogen concentrations in dogs undergoing ovariohysterectomy. Am J Vet Res. 2013; 74:1267–73.
35. Ebersole JL, Machen RL, Steffen MJ, Willmann DE. Systemic acute-phase reactants, C-reactive protein and haptoglobin, in adult periodontitis. Clin Exp Immunol. 1997;107:347–52.
36. Plessersa E, Wynsa H, Watteyna A, Pardonb B, De Baerea S, Sysb SU, De Backera P, Croubels S. Immunomodulatory properties of gamithromycin and ketoprofen inlipopolysaccharide-challenged calves with emphasis on theacute-phase response. Vet Immunol Immunopathol. 2016;171:28–37.
37. Menkes CJ. Effects of disease-modifying anti-rheumatic drugs, steroids and non-steroidal anti-inflammatory drugs on acute-phase proteins in rheumatoid arthritis. Br J Rheumatol. 1993;32:14–8.
38. Nunokawa Y, Fujinaga T, Taira T, Okumura M, Yamashita K, Tsunoda N, Hagio M. Evaluation of serum amyloid A protein as an acute-phase reactive protein in horses. J Vet Med Sci. 1993;55:1011–6.

39. Vandenplas ML, Moore JN, Barton MH, Roussel AJ, Cohen ND. Concentrations of serum amyloid A and lipopolysaccharide-binding protein in horses with colic. Am J Vet Res. 2005;66:1509–16.

40. Pihl TH, Scheepers E, Sanz M, Goddard A, Page P, Toft N, Andersen PH, Jacobsen S. Influence of disease process and duration on acute phase proteins in serum and peritoneal fluid of horses with colic. J Vet Intern Med. 2015;29:651–8.

Biomechanical evaluation of monosegmental pedicle instrumentation in a calf spine model and the role of fractured vertebrae in screw stability

Fuxin Wei[1†], Zhiyu Zhou[1,2†], Le Wang[1†], Shaoyu Liu[1*], Rui Zhong[1], Xizhe Liu[1], Shangbin Cui[1], Ximin Pan[3], Manman Gao[1] and Yajing Zhao[4]

Abstract

Background: Monsegmental pedicle instrumentation (MSPI) has been used to treat thoracolumbar fractures. However, there are few reports about the biomechanical characteristics of MSPI compared with traditional short-segment pedicle instrumentation (SSPI) in management of unstable thoracolumbar fractures, and the influence of vertebral fracture on screw stability is still unclear.

Methods: This study was to compare the immediate stability between MSPI and SSPI in management of unstable L1 fracture, and to evaluate the role of fractured vertebrae in screw stability. Two studies were performed: in the first study, sixteen fresh calf spines (T11-L3) were divided into two groups, in which unstable fractures at L1 were produced and then instrumented with MSPI or SSPI respectively. The range of motion (ROM) and lax zone (LZ) of specimens were evaluated with pure moment of 6 Nm loaded. The second study measured and compared the pullout strength of screws inserted in to 16 intact and fractured vertebrae of calf spines (L1-3) respectively. The correlation of pullout strength with load sharing classification (LSC) of fractured vertebrae was analyzed.

Results: No significant difference in the ROM and LZ of the destabilized segments after fixation between MSPI and SSPI, except in axial rotation of ROM ($P < 0.05$). After fatigue cyclic loading, the MSPI showed a significant increase of ROM during lateral bending and axial rotation ($P < 0.05$); however, there were no significant differences in the LZ during all loading models between groups ($P > 0.05$). The mean pullout strength of pedicle screws in fractured vertebrae decreased by 13.7 %, compared with that of intact vertebrae ($P > 0.05$), and had a low correlation with LSC of the fractured vertebrae ($r = 0.293$, $P > 0.05$).

Conclusions: MSPI can provide effective immediate stability for management of unstable thoracolumbar fractures; however, it has less fatigue resistance during lateral bending and axial rotation compared with SSPI. LSC score of fractured vertebrae is not a major influence on the pullout strength of screws.

* Correspondence: gzsyliu@qq.com
†Equal contributors
[1]Department of Spine Surgery, the First Affiliated Hospital and Orthopedic Research, Institute of Sun Yat-sen University, Guangzhou, China
Full list of author information is available at the end of the article

Background

Most thoracolumbar fractures are stable injuries that can be treated nonoperatively [1]. However, unstable fractures with retropulsed bone fragments and canal compromise usually warrant surgical intervention. The introduction of transpedicular screws by Roy-Camille and Demeulenaer, followed by the development of the internal fixator by Dick et al. [2], has made the short-segment pedicle screw instrumentation (SSPI) a popular method [3, 4]. After the development of the load-sharing classification (LSC) [5], more and more authors believe that on the condition of no severe anterior column defect, treatment of thoracolumbar burst fractures with SSPI can achieve clinical success [6, 7].

Saving motion segments by limiting the number of the fusion segments has been as a fundamental principle of spinal surgery [8]. Some authors have tried using monosegmental pedicle instrumentation (MSPI) with placement of pedicle screws directly into the fractured and normal vertebral body adjacent to the fractured endplate to treat thoracolumbar fractures, especially in cases of flexion distraction injuries [3, 9], and yielded good clinical results [10, 11]. Although the biomechanical properties of various similar approaches have been reported in the literature, there are few reports about the biomechanical characteristics of MSPI and whether the monosegmental pedicle instrumentation can provide immediate stability equivalent to that provided by SSPI is uncertain. In addition, complications of screw loosening and correction loss were not uncommon when performing MSPI in management of thoracolumbar fractures [11], especially for those combined with a load-sharing score of more than 6 points, which was reported in our previous clinical study [12]. To our knowledge, the contribution of the fractured vertebrae to screw stability and the relationship between the screw stability and the load sharing classification of fractured vertebrae has also not been well documented.

To quantify the biomechanical characteristics of MSPI in management of unstable thoracolumbar fractures, we performed two studies: the first study compared the immediate stability of the two pedicle instrumentation methods (MSPI and SSPI) in management of unstable thoracolumbar fractures; the second study investigated the role of fractured vertebrae on the screw stability and analyzed the correlation of the screw stability with load sharing classification of the fractured vertebrae.

Methods

The study protocol was reviewed and approved by the institutional review board and ethics committee of the First Affiliated Hospital of our university (No. 2013–204).

Study 1

Specimen preparation

Sixteen fresh frozen calf spines (T11-L3) were harvested with the age at time of death ranged from 6 to 8 weeks, which has been found to be the age at which calf spines best mimic the adult human spine [13]. In preparation, standard anteroposterior and lateral plain films were obtained and inspected to rule out pathologic abnormalities, and then surrounding soft tissue and muscle were dissected with care to preserve bone, discs and spinal ligaments. Both ends of the specimens were embedded with polymethylmethacrylate(PMMA) in a square aluminum mounting cast. The specimens were wrapped in saline-soaked gauze, kept in double plastic bags, and stored frozen at –30 °C. Before testing, each specimen was thawed at room temperature in a humidity-controlled environment for 12–18 h. To avoid influence on the biomechanical behavior by autolysis and air exposure, all specimens were kept moist during the tests by spraying saline onto them. Handling and storage of cadaver material in this manner, routinely used in vitro biomechanical investigation, does not alter the material characteristics of the bone and soft tissues [14]. All specimens were randomly allocated into two groups: the MSPI and SSPI groups.

Testing protocol

Flexibility of specimens was tested in 4 conditions (Table 1). Unstable 3-column fractures at the L-1 level were created by using a servohydraulic mechanical testing machine (MTS858 Bionix machine, MTS system Inc., Minneapolis, MN). To create a consistent injury pattern, a preinjury was created in each specimen, with reference to the methods reported previously [15, 16]. Minimal osteotomies were made with an osteotome at the upper endplate, and a 2-mm drill bit was used to create eight holes parallel and oblique to the intervertebral discs in the anterior cortex of the L1 vertebral body, extending to the posterior edge of the vertebral body. Then, the specimens were mounted in the MTS spinal fixture and subjected to flexion–compression at a rate of 5 mm/s until the vertebral body was compressed more than 50 %, and lastly were followed by disruption of the posterior longitudinal ligament, ligamentum flavum, and supraspinous and interspinous ligaments with our intension to cause a 3-column injury to

Table 1 Sequence of conditions tested

Step	Condition
1	normal
2	after creating L1 burst fractures
3	after performing T12–L2 pedicle-screw fixation (SSPI) or T12–L1 pedicle-screw fixation (MSPI)
4	after fatigue cyclic loading

SSPI indicates short-segment pedicle instrumentation; MSPI indicates monosegmental pedicle instrumentation

replicate a clinically relevant, challenging condition for fixation hardware to stabilize. Lateral radiographs and CT scans were routinely taken to demonstrate the extent of destabilization (Fig. 1a, b). The anterior body height [17] compression and load sharing classification score (LSC) [5] were used in describing the instability model, and the recovery rate of the anterior body height was calculated as follows: (preoperative compression rate-postoperative compression rate)/preoperative compression rate × 100 %, which were showed in Table 2.

Pedicle screws were inserted using standard techniques by a fellowship-trained, spine surgeon, who was familiar with pedicle screw placement. All the pedicle screws were inserted using a digital torque driver (accuracy ± 0.5 %, Cedar Digital Driver: DSD-4 M; Sugisaki Meter Company, Ltd, Ibaraki, Japan). The insertional torque was monitored continuously during insertion, and the highest torque during insertion was defined as the "maximal insertional torque". The highest torque acquired during the final 360° revolution of the screw was defined as the "seating torque" [18]. Fluoroscopy was used during pedicle screw insertion to ensure adequate placement. We placed the same size screws (5 × 35 mm, general spine system, GSS) at the vertebral bodies followed by interconnection using appropriate-sized connectors between T12-L1 in the MSPI group and T12-L2 in the SSPI group (Fig. 1c, d).

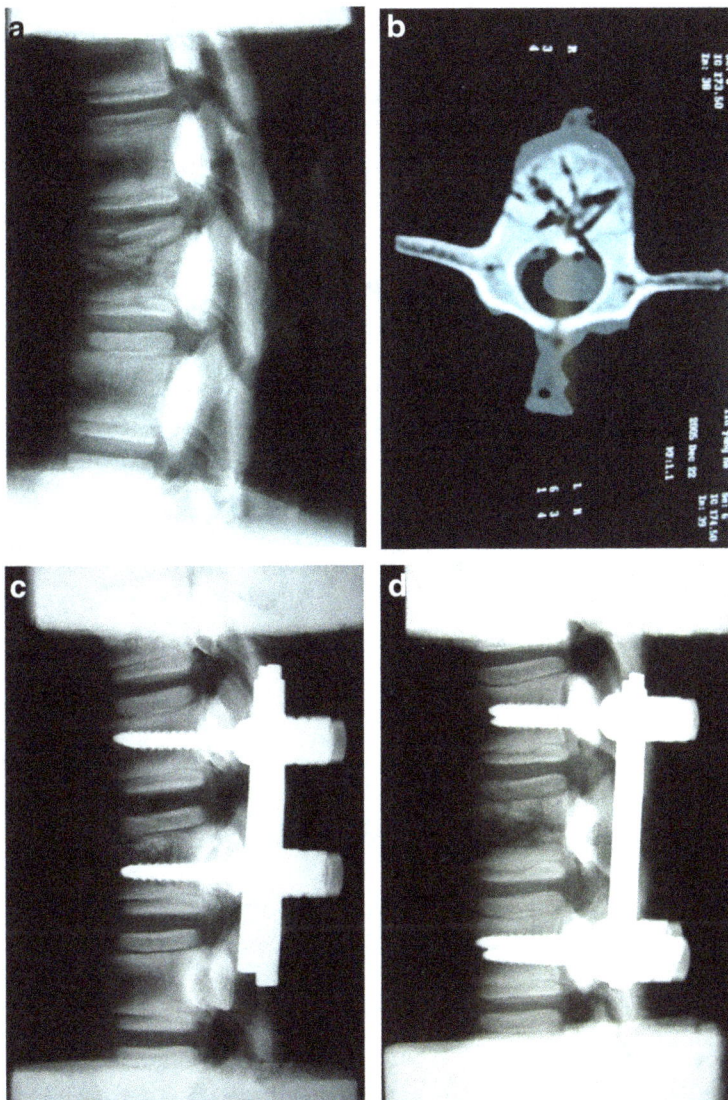

Fig. 1 Radiographs showing post-injury specimens and that after pedicle instrumentation. a Lateral radiographs showing vertebral fractures at L1 level. b Axial computed tomography (CT) scan showing vertebral fractures and disruption of posterior edge of the vertebral body. c Monosegmental pedicle instrumentation (MSPI) with placement of pedicle screws directly into the fractured and normal vertebral body adjacent to the fractured endplate. d Traditional short-segment pedicle instrumentation (SSPI) with placement of pedicle screws into the upper and lower vertebral bodies adjacent to the fractured vertebral body

Table 2 Roentgenographic data of the instability model between the two groups mean (standard deviation)

Parameter	Before fixation	After fixation	Recovering rate (%)
Load sharing Score			
SSPI	6.3 (1.8)	n/a	n/a
MSPI	6.6 (2.1)	n/a	n/a
FG in study 2	6.2 (2.3)	n/a	n/a
Anterior body height compression (%)			
SSPI	40 (11)	4.0 (1.0)	90.0 (11.1)
MSPI	41 (14)	3.0 (1.4)	92.7 (8.0)

SSPI indicates short-segment pedicle instrumentation; MSPI indicates monosegmental pedicle instrumentation; FG indicates fractured group
n/a indicates not available

In each of the 4 conditions listed in Table 1, the specimen was mounted on a spine tester for three-dimensional spinal motion at room temperature (Fig. 2), as described previously [19]. The inferior cast was fixed to the machine, while the loading jig was attached to the superior cast (Fig. 3a). The machine applied six pure moments to the specimen in flexion, extension, bilateral bending, and bilateral axial rotation [19]. Each moment was applied in three load-unload cycles to a maximum 6 Nm and was allowed to creep for 30s at each load-step to account for viscoelastic effects [20, 21]. On the third load cycle, stereo images of the markers inserted into the transverse process and anterior vertebral body of the specimen were recorded by a 3-dimensional laser scanister (3D Digital Corp. United States, Fig. 3b) and stored on a computer. The marker coordinates were digitized using a previously developed computer program, and the motion capabilities of the whole specimen were determined in three-dimension. The accuracy of the measurement system has been determined [19]. The maximum error in marker position was 1.0 mm (1° in segmental angle) for a 60 mm × 60 mm × 150 mm measuring space. Throughout the tests, the specimens were kept wet using 0.9 % physiological saline.

Between the test sequence of step 3 and step 4, the specimens with pedicle instrumentation were fixed on the MTS material testing machine for the fatigue cyclic

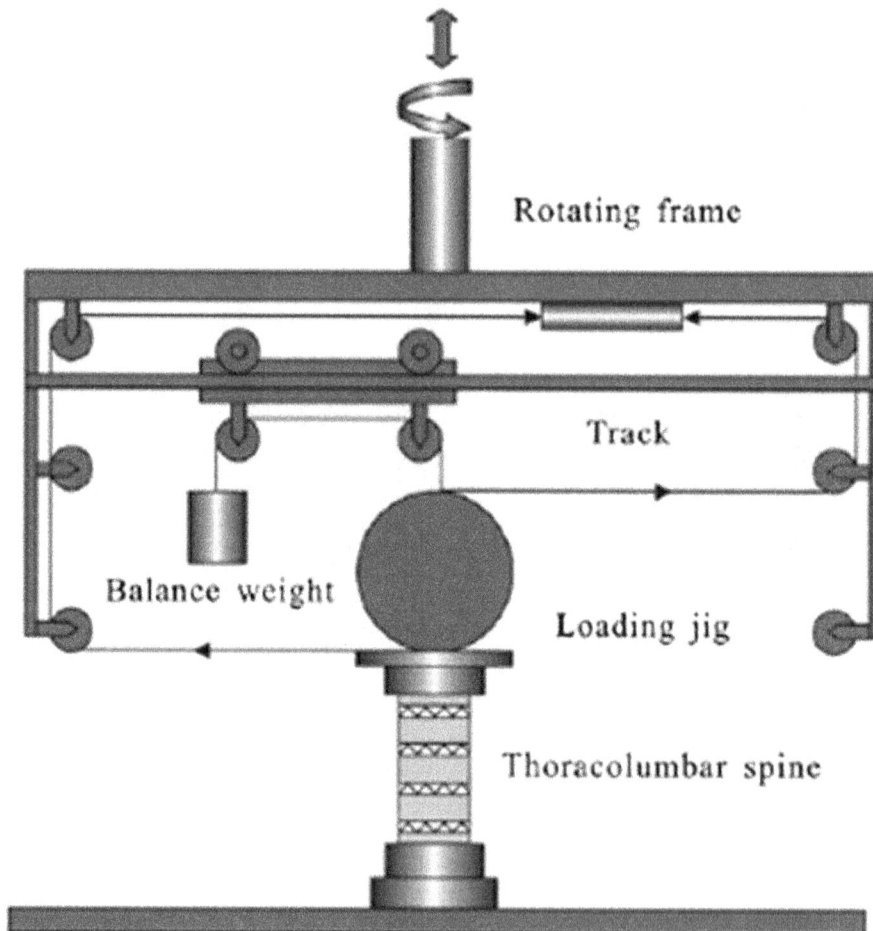

Fig. 2 The diagram of the spine tester for three-dimensional spinal motion

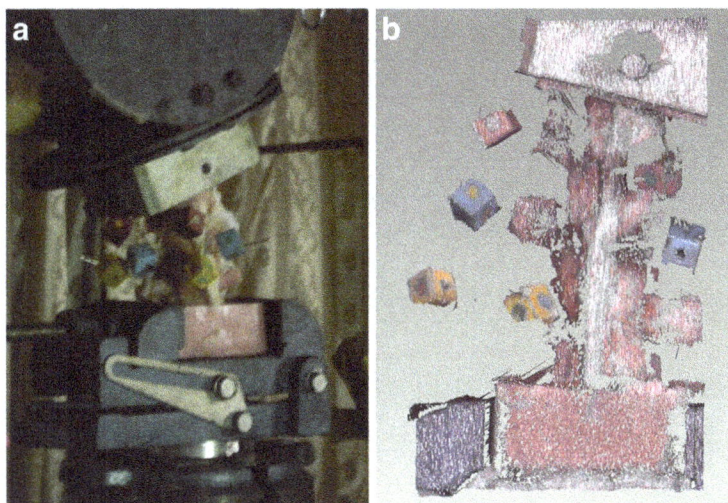

Fig. 3 Calf specimen and stereo image. **a** Calf T12 to L2 specimen with three non-colinear circular marks in the spine tester. **b** Stereo image of the markers on the specimen were recorded by a 3-dimensional laser scanister

loading test. The fatigue parameter applied under torque control was a moment of ± 6 Nm conducted at a rate of 0.5Hz up to 2000 cycles of flexion-extension, lateral bending, and axial rotation respectively. To restore the physiologic hydration of the specimens, the specimens were wrapped in a saline-soaked gauze throughout the test.

From the raw data, the angular ROM across T12–L1 was calculated during motion in all planes. As an additional measure of stability, the angular lax zone (LZ, the portion of the ROM in which ligaments and hardware are not yet substantially loaded) was determined [22].

Study 2
Specimen preparation
Thirty-two fresh frozen vertebrae from 6 to 8 weeks old calf spines with all soft tissue removed (T11-L3) were randomized into two groups: intact group (IG) and fractured group (FG). The vertebral fracture models of the FG were created as described previously, and the load sharing classification scores (LSC) were recorded. The same size pedicle screws were inserted into the vertebral bodies of both groups by the same surgeon, and the "maximal insertional torque", "seating torque" were again measured. Each specimen was then individually potted in a casting mold of PMMA, which encased the vertebral body, leaving the posterior elements and pedicle screws exposed (Fig. 4a).

Axial pullout test
Axial pullout tests were conducted in the specimens using the MTS machine. In brief, the PMMA mold was rigidly secured to the base of the testing apparatus using an angle vise. The long axis of the screw was aligned to the axis of the machine to create a pure axial pullout force on each screw (Fig. 4b). Pull-to-failure tests were

performed with a starting preload of 1 N and crosshead speed of 1 mm/s. Failure load was recorded for each pullout test (Fig. 5). The maximum force to pull the screw out from the pedicle was recorded as the axial pullout strength. The pullout strength of each vertebra was the mean of the sum of pullout strength calculated from both left and right side of pedicle screws.

Data analysis
The SPSS (version16.0, Chicago, IL, USA) package was used for the statistical analysis. The ROM and LZ of the same condition between groups were analyzed using Student's t-test. The ROM and LZ at different conditions in each group were analyzed using one-way ANOVA and the least significant difference test (LSD-t). The "maximal insertional torque", "seating torque" and the axial pullout strength between the normal and fractured vertebrae were compared using Student's t-test, respectively. Pearson correlation coefficient was used to correlate the biomechanical data with LSC score of the specimens. Statistical significance was indicated at $P < 0.05$.

Results
Study 1
There were no significant differences of LSC and anterior body height compression rate between the instability models of the two groups ($P > 0.05$, see Table 2). There was also no significant difference in the recovery rate of the anterior body height compression between groups ($P > 0.05$).

Data for ROM from both right and left lateral bending and axial rotation showed no difference ($P > 0.05$) and were combined when used for comparison. For all three motion planes (lateral bending, flexion/extension, and

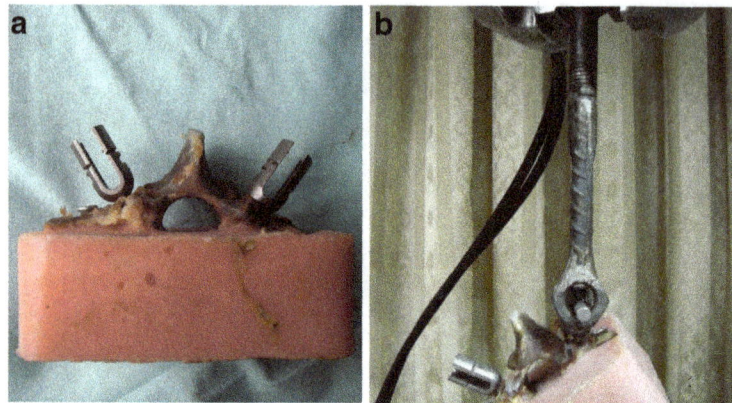

Fig. 4 Pedicle screw pullout. **a** Samples embedded in PMMA. **b** The long axis of the screw was aligned to the axis of the machine to create a pure axial pullout force

axial rotation), the instability model showed an increased ROM and LZ when compared with the intact status in each group respectively (Fig. 6, Fig. 7, P < 0.01). Both of the SSPI and MSPI significantly reduced the ROM and LZ across T12–L1 to within the mean values observed in the intact condition (Fig. 6, Fig. 7, P < 0.05).

After stabilization, the SSPI allowed less ROM than MSPI during any loading model, however, except in the axial rotation, there were no significant differences in the other directions (Fig. 6, P > 0.05). Similarly, the SSPI allowed less LZ than MSPI during any loading model; however, there were no significant differences in all the directions (Fig. 7, P > 0.05).

After fatigue cyclic loading, although both groups allowed greater ROM and LZ than constructs during any loading model, there were no significant differences (P > 0.05), except in the LZ during axial rotation of the MSPI (P < 0.05). Although there were no significant differences in the LZ during all loading models between groups (P > 0.05), the MSPI group showed a significant

increase in ROM than the SSPI group during the lateral bending and axial rotation after fatigue cyclic loading (Fig. 6, Fig. 7, P < 0.05).

Study 2
Insertional torque
Both of the mean maximal insertional torque and seating torque in the fractured vertebrae decreased significantly compared to that in the intact vertebrae (P > 0.01, see Table 3). Although the mean axial pullout strength in the fractured vertebrae decreased compared to that in the intact vertebrae, the difference was not significant (P > 0.05, see Table 3).

Biomechanical data correlation with LSC
The mean load sharing classification score (LSC) of the specimens was 6.2 ± 2.3 points (see Table 2). The maximal insertional torque ($r = 0.713$) and seating torque ($r = 0.735$) for the screws had a high correlation with LSC of the specimens (P > 0.01, Fig. 8). However, the axial pullout strength ($r = 0.293$) had a low correlation with LSC of the specimens (P > 0.05, Fig. 8).

Discussion
Although the surgical method to be selected in the treatment of thoracolumbar fractures remains a matter of discussion [1, 23], instrumented posterior fusion is the most frequently used surgical treatment because of the low morbidity and comorbidity, and surgeons' familiarity with posterior approach compared with anterior approach. Short-segment pedicle instrumentation (SSPI), which typically span the levels immediately adjacent to the fracture, is almost the most widely used [24–26].

With the advent of minimal invasive surgery, an important consideration is achieving stability with fusion of the fewest number of motion segments. Some authors have been using monosegmental pedicle instrumentation

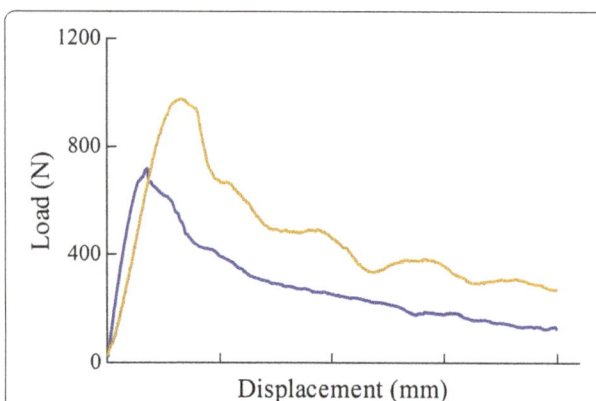

Fig. 5 Two example load–displacement curves acquired from pullout testing. The pullout strength is determined at the maximum value of the curve

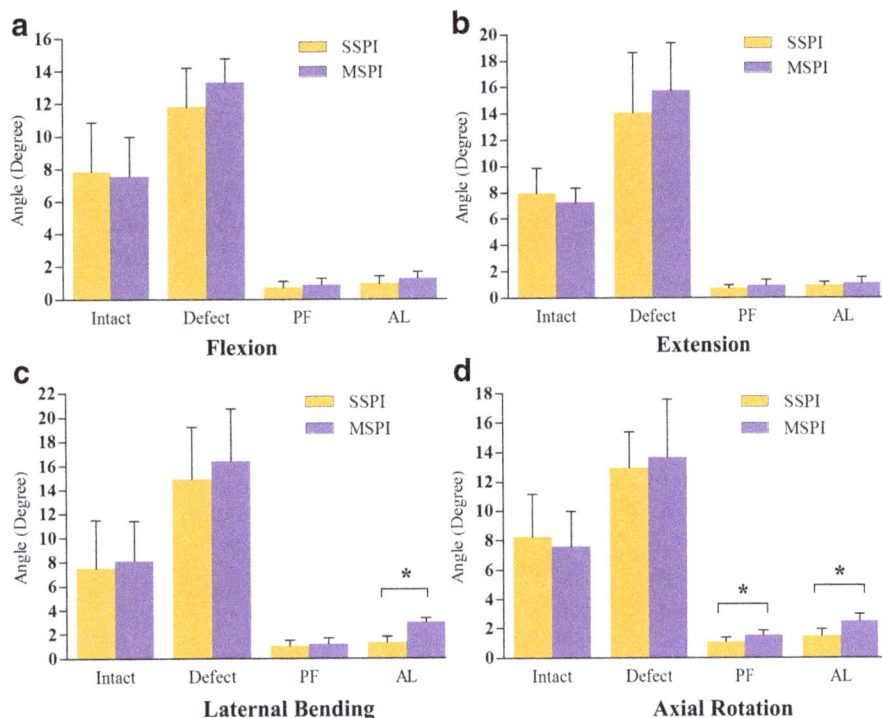

Fig. 6 The mean angular ROM of T12–L1 for all loading directions. **a**. The mean angular ROM of T12–L1 in flexion. **b**. The mean angular ROM of T12–L1 in extension. **c**. The mean angular ROM of T12–L1 in lateral bending. **d**. The mean angular ROM of T12–L1 in axial rotation. Error bars show standard deviation. *: P < 0.05; ROM: range of motion; PF: pedicle fixation; AL: after cyclic loading

(MSPI) to treat thoracolumbar fractures [3, 11, 27]. We also used this method in management of 47 patients with thoracolumbar fractures and compared the clinical and radiologic late results with that of short-segment pedicle instrumentation (SSPI). The results showed no significant differences in the correction rate of local kyphosis and anterior body height compression, and there were also no significant difference in the average correction loss of all radiographic parameters between the two methods [12]. However, the biomechanical characteristics of MSPI in management of unstable thoracolumbar

fractures and whether the MSPI can provide effective immediate stability equivalent to that provided by traditional SSPI is still uncertain.

In this study, we found that both of the SSPI and MSPI significantly reduced the ROM and LZ across T12–L1 to within the mean values observed in the intact condition, which predicted that the MSPI could provide equal immediate stability to that of SSPI with respect to the reconstruction of unstable 3-column fractured models. However, in clinical applications, one of the most commonly observed internal failure is loosing of the pedicle screws due

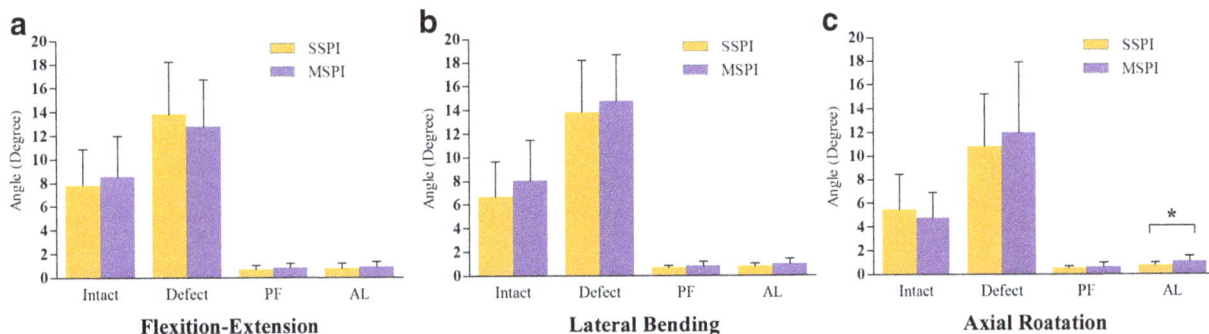

Fig. 7 The mean angular LZ of T12–L1 for all loading directions. **a**. The mean angular LZ of T12–L1 in the direction of flexion-extension. **b**. The mean angular LZ of T12–L1 in the direction of lateral bending. **c**. The mean angular LZ of T12–L1 in the direction of axial rotation. Error bars show standard deviation. *: P < 0.05; LZ: lax zone; PF: pedicle fixation; AL: after cyclic loading.

Table 3 Performance of the screws in intact and fractured vertebrae: Mean (standard deviation)

Parameter	Fractured vertebrae	Intact vertebrae	% Decrease	P value
Maximal insertional torque (Nm)	0.29(0.13)	0.40(0.15)	27.5	0.001
Seating torque in (Nm)	0.23(0.11)	0.28(0.13)	17.9	0.04
Axial pullout strength (N)	558(305)	646(266)	13.7	0.06

to fatigue cyclic loading. Therefore, this study also designed to measure the stability of the pedicle instrumentation after 2000 cyclic loading to represent the early situation of postoperation, as described in previous studies [28–30]. After cyclic loading, the ROM for the lateral bending and axial rotation in the MSPI increased significantly in comparison with the SSPI. The possible reason for this was shear forces of pedicle screw induced in the process of cyclic loading, which could affect the screw stability in the fractured vertebrae. Whatever the reason for the observed outcome, this predicted that the effectiveness of immediate fatigue resistance of MSPI is inferior to SSPI, especially in the lateral bending and axial rotation, which should be paid more attention to in the clinical application.

Previous studies have revealed that high incidence of instrumentation failure and loss of kyphotic correction after SSPI was caused mainly by the structural and mechanical deficiency of the anterior column after indirect reduction of the fracture [4, 31]. A general assessment system of fractured vertebral body, the load sharing score (LSC), is a successful way to predict clinically successful SSPI. Dai et al. [32] proved that the LSC can be applied with excellent reliability for assessing thoracolumbar fractures. Gaines et al. [33] made a conclusion from their clinical experiences that a LSC ≤ 6 indicated adequate sharing of load through the injured vertebral body along with SSPI, whereas a LSC ≥ 6 predicted highly possible failure of SSPI, and should be avoided. In this study, although the average LSC of the instability models in each group was more than 6, no significant increase of ROM after cyclic loading was found in both groups, except in the LZ during axial rotation of the MSPI. This suggested that thoracolumbar fractures with LSC ≥6 could be not a strict contraindication for MPSI. However, this need to be verified by further clinical study.

There are understandable concerns that the pullout strength of the pedicle screw inserted into the fractured vertebral body may not be sufficient for the stability reconstruction. It was illustrated that the pedicle, rather than the vertebral body, contributed ~60 % of the pullout strength at the screw-bone interface [34]. Zindrick et al. [35] reported no difference in pullout strength between similar-size screws inserted to a 50 % depth versus to anterior cortex. So long as there is integrity of both pedicles, the screws inserted into the fractured level are supposed to have fairly tolerable stiffness and pullout strength. To further analyze the contribution of the fractured vertebrae to screw stability, axial pullout was carried out and compared for the screws inserted into the fractured vertebrae and normal vertebrae in this study. The maximal insertional torque and seating torque of screws inserted into the fractured vertebrae decreased significantly compared with that of intact vertebrae ($P > 0.05$), but not resulting in greater drop of axial pullout strength for the screws. The insertion torque is believed to result from resistance of the screw with bone and also from radial compression of the trabecular against cortical bone in the vertebral body [36]; however, the pedicle is denser in the subcortical bone, in which the threads of the screw engage tightly, than in trabecular bone. This may explain

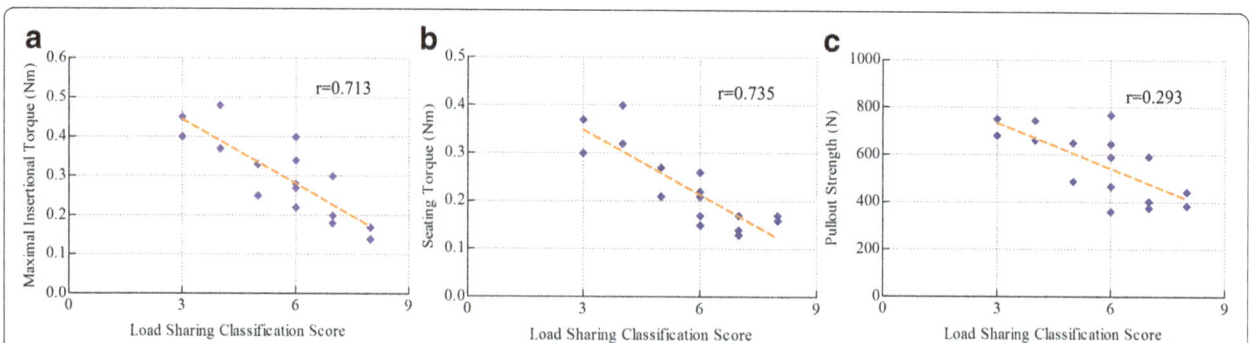

Fig. 8 The correlation between maximum insertional torque, seating torque, pullout strength and the Load Sharing Classification (LSC) score of the fractured vertebrae. **a**. The correlation between the maximum insertional torque and the Load Sharing Classification (LSC) score of the fractured vertebrae. **b**. The correlation between the seating torque and the Load Sharing Classification (LSC) score of the fractured vertebrae. **c**. The correlation between the pullout strength and the Load Sharing Classification (LSC) score of the fractured vertebrae. The axial pullout strength had a low correlation with LSC of the specimens ($r = 0.293$, $P > 0.05$)

why the pullout strength of the pedicle screw is less affected by the vertebral fracture. This finding is also in agreement with data analyzed the correlation of the screw stability with LSC in the current study, where the strength of the correlation with LSC dropped in pullout strength of the screws ($r = 0.293$), compared with maximal insertional torque ($r = 0.713$) and seating torque ($r = 0.735$). Importantly, the axial pullout strength of screws inserted into the fractured vertebrae just dropped by 13.7 % of screws inserted into the normal vertebrae, which showed no significant difference. This result confirmed the previously reported conclusion that the pedicle was the major structure that contributed most of the pull-out strength at the screw-bone interface [34].

This experiment utilized calf spines. Despite the differences between calf and human anatomy [37], the elasticity and anatomical structure of calf spines are similar to human spines. As well, the difference in size is small, and there are no pathological changes, such as joint degeneration and osteoporosis in the calf spines. These characteristics are all useful when doing this experiment, and calf spine was regarded as the most suitable substitute material for the human spine [38]. However, although the unstable fracture model has been widely used in biomechanical experiments, the model does not take into account the stability effect of the neuromuscular structure on the spine. As well, in vitro experiments can only evaluate biomechanical changes during the early post-operative period, unlike clinical observations of the dynamic process of spinal fusion, during which intervertebral stability strengthens as the bone gradually heals. Therefore, designing a suitable model that can simulate the entire spine, as well as the mechanical and loading conditions, remains a challenge. In addition, due to laboratory facility limitations, this experiment did not investigate the rod strain of the instruments and the post-fixation stress of adjacent joints. Given our results, further clinical observation and biomechanical study is warranted.

Conclusion

This current study demonstrated that MSPI can provide effective immediate stability for management of unstable thoracolumbar fractures, however, it has less fatigue resistance during lateral bending and axial rotation compared with SSPI. The axial pullout strength of screws inserted into the fractured vertebrae dropped by 13.7 % of screws inserted into the normal vertebrae. LSC score of fractured vertebrae is not a major influence of the pullout strength of screws.

Competing interests
The authors declare that they have no competing interests.

Authors' contributions
FW, ZZ, and LW performed biomechanical test for the specimens. FW and RZ performed the specimen preparation. XP performed radiological evaluation. MG performed the statistical analysis. SL conceived of the study and participated in its design. FW drafted the manuscript. YZ perfromed the data collection. All authors read and approved the final manuscript.

Acknowledgements
This study was founded by National Natural Science Foundation of China (No.U1032001), Science & Technology Planning Project of Guangdong Province (No. 2010B010800019) and Natural Science Foundation of Guangdong (No. S2013010015775). We thank Weidong Zhao for technical assistance of biomechanical testing.

Author details
[1]Department of Spine Surgery, the First Affiliated Hospital and Orthopedic Research, Institute of Sun Yat-sen University, Guangzhou, China. [2]The medical school of Shenzhen University, Shenzhen, China. [3]Department of Radiology, the First Affiliated Hospital of Sun Yat-sen University, Guangzhou, China. [4]The medical school of Sun Yat-sen University, Guangzhou, China.

References
1. Wood K, Buttermann G, Mehbod A, Garvey T, Jhanjee R, Sechriest V. Operative compared with nonoperative treatment of a thoracolumbar burst fracture without neurological deficit. A prospective, randomized study. J Bone Joint Surg Am. 2003;85-A(5):773–81.
2. Dick W, Kluger P, Magerl F, Woersdörfer O, Zäch G. A new device for internal fixation of thoracolumbar and lumbar spine fractures: the 'fixateur interne'. Paraplegia. 1985;23(4):225–32.
3. Finkelstein JA, Wai EK, Jackson SS, Ahn H, Brighton-Knight M. Single-level fixation of flexion distraction injuries. J Spinal Disord Tech. 2003;16(3):236–42.
4. Gelb D, Ludwig S, Karp JE, Chung EH, Werner C, Kim T, Poelstra K. Successful treatment of thoracolumbar fractures with short-segment pedicle instrumentation. J Spinal Disord Tech. 2010;23(5):293–301.
5. Aligizakis AC, Katonis PG, Sapkas G, Papagelopoulos PJ, Galanakis I, Hadjipavlou A. Gertzbein and load sharing classifications for unstable thoracolumbar fractures. Clin Orthop Relat Res. 2003;411:77–85.
6. Kose KC, Inanmaz ME, Isik C, Basar H, Caliskan I, Bal E. Short segment pedicle screw instrumentation with an index level screw and cantilevered hyperlordotic reduction in the treatment of type-A fractures of the thoracolumbar spine. Bone Joint J. 2014;96-B(4):541–7.
7. Scholl BM, Theiss SM, Kirkpatrick JS. Short segment fixation of thoracolumbar burst fractures. Orthopedics. 2006;29(8):703–8.
8. Yurac R, Marré B, Urzua A, Munjin M, Lecaros MA. Residual mobility of instrumented and non-fused segments in thoracolumbar spine fractures. Eur Spine J. 2006;15(6):864–75.
9. Liljenqvist U, Mommsen U. Surgical treatment of thoracolumbar spinal fractures with internal fixator and transpedicular spongiosa-plasty. Unfallchirurgie. 1995;21(1):30–9.
10. Defino HL, Scarparo P. Fractures of thoracolumbar spine: monosegmental fixation. Injury. 2005;36 Suppl 2:B90–97.
11. Liu S, Li H, Liang C, Long H, Yu B, Chen B, Han G, Zhang X, Li F, Wei F. Monosegmental transpedicular fixation for selected patients with thoracolumbar burst fractures. J Spinal Disord Tech. 2009;22(1):38–44.
12. Wei FX, Liu SY, Liang CX, Li HM, Long HQ, Yu BS, Chen BL, Chen KB. Transpedicular fixation in management of thoracolumbar burst fractures monosegmental fixation versus short-segment instrumentation. Spine (Phila Pa 1976). 2010;35(15):E714–720.
13. Wilke HJ, Geppert J, Kienle A. Biomechanical in vitro evaluation of the complete porcine spine in comparison with data of the human spine. Eur Spine J. 2011;20(11):1859–68.
14. Wilke HJ, Wenger K, Claes L. Testing criteria for spinal implants: recommendations for the standardization of in vitro stability testing of spinal implants. Eur Spine J. 1998;7(2):148–54.
15. Lu WW, Luk KD, Ruan DK, Fei ZQ, Leong JC. Stability of the whole lumbar spine after multilevel fenestration and discectomy. Spine (Phila Pa 1976). 1999;24(13):1277–82.

16. Mermelstein LE, McLain RF, Yerby SA. Reinforcement of thoracolumbar burst fractures with calcium phosphate cement. A biomechanical study. Spine (Phila Pa 1976). 1998;23(6):664–70.

17. Rommens PM, Weyns F, Van Calenbergh F, Goffin J, Broos PL. Mechanical performance of the Dick internal fixator: a clinical study of 75 patients. Eur Spine J. 1995;4(2):104–9.

18. Stauff MP, Freedman BA, Kim JH, Hamasaki T, Yoon ST, Hutton WC. The effect of pedicle screw redirection after lateral wall breach–a biomechanical study using human lumbar vertebrae. Spine J. 2014;14(1):98–103.

19. Zhu Q, Ouyang J, Lu W, Lu H, Li Z, Guo X, Zhong S. Traumatic instabilities of the cervical spine caused by high-speed axial compression in a human model. An in vitro biomechanical study. Spine (Phila Pa 1976). 1999;24(5):440–4.

20. Panjabi MM. Biomechanical evaluation of spinal fixation devices: I. A conceptual framework. Spine (Phila Pa 1976). 1988;13(10):1129–34.

21. Yamamoto I, Panjabi MM, Crisco T, Oxland T. Three-dimensional movements of the whole lumbar spine and lumbosacral joint. Spine (Phila Pa 1976). 1989;14(11):1256–60.

22. Crawford NR, Peles JD, Dickman CA. The spinal lax zone and neutral zone: measurement techniques and parameter comparisons. J Spinal Disord. 1998;11(5):416–29.

23. Wood KB, Li W, Lebl DS, Ploumis A. Management of thoracolumbar spine fractures. Spine J. 2014;14(1):145–64.

24. Khare S, Sharma V. Surgical outcome of posterior short segment trans-pedicle screw fixation for thoracolumbar fractures. J Orthop. 2013;10(4):162–7.

25. Dai LY, Jiang LS, Jiang SD. Posterior short-segment fixation with or without fusion for thoracolumbar burst fractures. a five to seven-year prospective randomized study. J Bone Joint Surg Am. 2009;91(5):1033–41.

26. Pellisé F, Barastegui D, Hernandez-Fernandez A, Barrera-Ochoa S, Bagó J, Issa-Benítez D, Cáceres E, Villanueva C. Viability and long-term survival of short-segment posterior fixation in thoracolumbar burst fractures. Spine J. In press.

27. Junge A, Gotzen L, von Garrel T, Ziring E, Giannadakis K. Monosegmental internal fixator instrumentation and fusion in treatment of fractures of the thoracolumbar spine. Indications, technique and results. Unfallchirurg. 1997;100(11):880–7.

28. Yu BS, Zhuang XM, Zheng ZM, Zhang JF, Li ZM, Lu WW. Biomechanical comparison of 4 fixation techniques of sacral pedicle screw in osteoporotic condition. J Spinal Disord Tech. 2010;23(6):404–9.

29. Zheng ZM, Zhang KB, Zhang JF, Yu BS, Liu H, Zhuang XM. The effect of screw length and bone cement augmentation on the fixation strength of iliac screws: a biomechanical study. J Spinal Disord Tech. 2009;22(8):545–50.

30. Zhu Q, Lu WW, Holmes AD, Zheng Y, Zhong S, Leong JC. The effects of cyclic loading on pull-out strength of sacral screw fixation: an in vitro biomechanical study. Spine (Phila Pa 1976). 2000;25(9):1065–9.

31. McLain RF. The biomechanics of long versus short fixation for thoracolumbar spine fractures. Spine (Phila Pa 1976). 2006;31(11 Suppl):S70–79.

32. Dai LY, Jin WJ. Interobserver and intraobserver reliability in the load sharing classification of the assessment of thoracolumbar burst fractures. Spine (Phila Pa 1976). 2005;30(3):354–8.

33. McCormack T, Karaikovic E, Gaines RW. The load sharing classification of spine fractures. Spine (Phila Pa 1976). 1994;19(15):1741–4.

34. Suk SI, Lee CK, Kim WJ, Chung YJ, Park YB. Segmental pedicle screw fixation in the treatment of thoracic idiopathic scoliosis. Spine (Phila Pa 1976). 1995;20(12):1399–405.

35. Zindrick MR. The role of transpedicular fixation systems for stabilization of the lumbar spine. Orthop Clin North Am. 1991;22(2):333–44.

36. Brasiliense LB, Lazaro BC, Reyes PM, Newcomb AG, Turner JL, Crandall DG, Crawford NR. Characteristics of immediate and fatigue strength of a dual-threaded pedicle screw in cadaveric spines. Spine J. 2013;13(8):947–56.

37. Sheng SR, Wang XY, Xu HZ, Zhu GQ, Zhou YF. Anatomy of large animal spines and its comparison to the human spine: a systematic review. Eur Spine J. 2010;19(1):46–56.

38. Yu BS. Biomechanical comparison of the posterolateral fusion and posterior lumbar interbody fusion using pedicle screw fixation system for unstable lumbar spine. Hokkaido Igaky Zasshi. 2003;78(3):211–8.

Ultrasonographic findings in cows with left displacement of abomasum, before and after reposition surgery

Xin-Wei Li[1†], Qiu-Shi Xu[1†], Ren-He Zhang[1], Wei Yang[2], Yu Li[3], Yu-Ming Zhang[1], Yu Tian[1], Min Zhang[1], Zhe Wang[1], Guo-wen Liu[1], Cheng Xia[2] and Xiao-Bing Li[1*]

Abstract

Background: The natural incidence of left displacement of abomasum (LDA) in dairy cows was high. The diagnosis of LDA usually relies on characteristic physical exam findings but that transabdominal ultrasound is a useful technique that has been applied to the diagnosis of gastrointestinal diseases of dairy cows in equivocal cases.

Methods: Forty dairy cows with LDA were clinically and ultrasonographically examined to determine the position and the echogenic property of the abomasum. The cows were examined ultrasonographically on the left side, from the 9th intercostal space (ICS) to the 12th ICS as well as the ventral left abdomen before and after reposition surgery.

Results: The vital signs were within normal range in most of the cows and the 'pinging' were clearly heard in 37 cows. The abomasal gas cap was visualized from the 9th to 12th ICS in 37 cows and characterized by reverberation artifacts. The abomasal ingesta appeared as homogeneous hypoechoic fluid with scattered hyperechoic foci and were mainly visible in the median region and ventral region of the 9th to 11th ICS in 35 cows. The pyloric canal was detected from the ventral left abdomen wall in 30 cows and appeared as a loop with hypoechogenic wall and echogenic luminal contents in cross section.

Conclusion: These typical ultrasonograms, including reverberation artifacts, homogenous hypoechoic structures, are important diagnostic feature in ultrasonography of LDA. Furthermore, the circular acoustic image structure of the pyloric canal is an important characteristic of LDA, so it can be used as an important diagnostic basis of LDA.

Keywords: Cows, Diagnosis, Left displacement of abomasum, Ultrasonography

Background

Since the first case was reported in 1950s [1], left displacement of abomasum (LDA) has become an important disease in dairy cows. LDA is a multifactorial disease that the abomasum partially or completely displaces between the left abdominal wall and rumen. Reduction of milk yield and risk of adhesions make it necessary to diagnose LDA early and precisely. Auscultation and simultaneous percussion or ballottement on the left mid-flank area is a traditional diagnostic method. In most LDA cases, an area of high-pitched 'pinging' will be heard. Although a diagnosis usually can be made directly by the specific 'pinging', some intensive methods such as rectal examination, blowing air into the rumen through a stomach tube or abomasocentesis are required to differentiate rumen collapse syndrome, rumen tympany and peritonitis pneumoperitoneum from LDA [2]. Furthermore, laparoscopic exploratory, an invasive procedure, is also recommended to make definite diagnosis in borderline cases [3].

In recent times, the use of transabdominal ultrasound has become more widespread over the past 20 years to diagnosed abdominal disorders in cattle [4, 5]. Some studies about ultrasonographic findings of abomasum in healthy cows or LDA cows have been published [6, 7].

* Correspondence: xbli@jlu.edu.cn
†Equal contributors
[1]Key Laboratory of Zoonosis, Ministry of Education, College of Veterinary Medicine, Jilin University, 5333 Xi'an Road, Changchun, Jilin 130062, China
Full list of author information is available at the end of the article

According to these studies, the abomasum can be seen well through ultrasonography in both normal and displaced state. These studies indicated that ultrasound is a helpful tool to diagnose the LDA. However, the interpreting of the ultrasonogram is still not easy to undertake. The present study was designed to ultrasonographically examine the left abdomen of LDA cows before and after reposition surgery, in order to obtain more useful differentiating features of LDA.

Methods
Animals
Forty Holstein cows (2–7 years old; 5 ± 1.6 years) were selected by experienced veterinarians depending on auscultations and percussion in a 10,000-cow dairy farm in Changchun, China. All these cows were finally confirmed to be LDA via exploratory laparotomy and underwent an abomasum reposition surgery. The study protocol was approved by the Ethics Committee on the Use and Care of Animals, Jilin University (Changchun, China). During the experimental work, the cows were housed in a climate-controlled barn in individual tie stalls to reduce environmental effects.

Clinical examination
Simultaneous auscultation and percussion were performed over the left flank of the cows as Richmond described [8]. The heart rate, respiratory rate and rectal temperature of these cows were recorded.

Ultrasonographic examination
The ultrasonographic examination was performed using a lightweight real-time B-mode scanner with a 3.5 MHz low-frequency curvilinear transducer (Shantou Institute of Ultrasonic Instruments Co., Ltd., Shantou, China; Model: CTS-7700V). The penetration depth of transducer was 15 cm. The procedure was performed according to the study of Braun et al., [6]. The cows were unsedated and standing during the examination. The hair was clipped over the left 9~12th intercostal spaces and the left ventral abdominal wall. After the application of transmission gel (ULT0250, Health & Beyond), these intercostal space was scanned, beginning dorsally and progressing ventrally with the transducer held parallel to the ribs (Fig. 1). The ventral left abdomen was scanned with the transducer held parallel to the long axis of the cows (Fig. 1). The 9~12th intercostal spaces were divided into three regions: Dorsal (Ds), Median (Md), and Ventral (Vt) (Fig. 1), and in each region the presence of abomasal characteristics such as abomasal ingesta, abomasal gas cap, and abomasal folds was noted. The same area was examined again immediately after reposition surgery of abomasum.

Treatment
A right flank laparotomy was performed in all the cows to confirm the diagnosis and then a right flank pyloropexy was adopted to immobilize the abomasum (Mueller [2]).

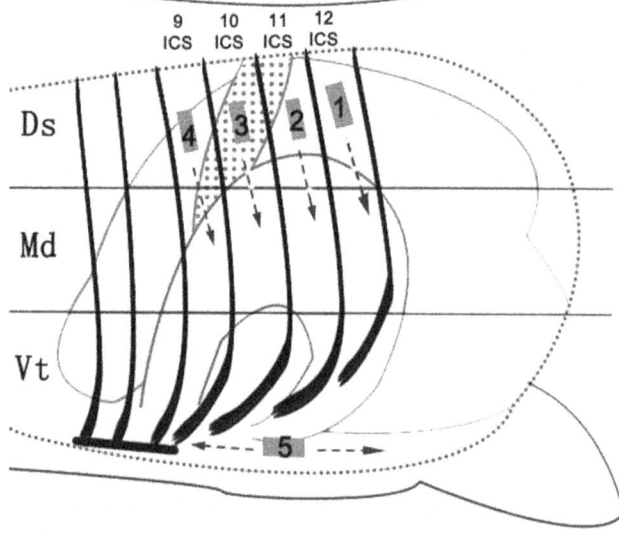

Fig. 1 Examination routes. Routes 1–5: Ultrasonographic routes which the transducer followed systematically. The rib cage was divided into three regions: Dorsal (Ds), Median (Md), and Ventral (Vt). The presence of abomasal ultrasonographic characteristics in each region was respectively noted. ICS: intercostal space

Results

Clinical findings

The vital signs were within normal range in the cows, except for five cows with concurrent disease (two with endometritis, three with mastitis). The heart rate was 64 to 110 (81 ± 12) beats/min, the respiratory rate was 15 to 50 (23 ± 8) breaths/min and the rectal temperature ranged from 38.5 to 40.1 (38.8 ± 0.3). Simultaneous auscultation and percussion over the left flank revealed different degrees of 'pinging' in the cows. In 24 cows, the 'pinging' could be heard distinctly on the dorsal third of the 11th, 12th and 13th rib. In 13 cows, the 'pinging' could be heard only as high as the middle third of the rib cage. Three of the cows had only vague or intermittent 'pinging' to be heard.

Ultrasonographic findings

Before the reposition surgery, the abomasum could be visualized in all of the left 9th, 10th, 11th, 12th intercostal space (ICS) of 37 cows, and could be only identified in the left ventral abdomen region in three cows. The ultrasonographic findings were similar in nearly all cows with LDA consisting of a dorsal gas cap, echogenic luminal ingesta and visualization of the pyloric canal. (Table 1). Reverberation artifact was observed while the transducer was put on the dorsal part of the examined ICSs in all the cows (Fig. 2).

Abomasal ingesta came into view, while the transducer was placed on the median or ventral part of the ICSs. These ingesta were visualized from the 9th to the 11th ICS of 29 cows and in 9th–12th ICS of eight cows. Abomasal ingesta mostly appeared as homogenous hypoechoic structures with echogenic spots (Fig. 3); however there were some cows ($n = 5$) whose abomasal ingesta

Table 1 Ultrasonographic findings of 40 cows with LDA

Exploratory area	Findings	Number of animals
Dorsal part of rib cage	Reverberation artifacts	40
Median part of rib cage	Reverberation artifacts	37
	Homogenous hypoechoic structure	23
Ventral part of rib cage	Reverberation artifacts	14
	Homogenous hypoechoic structure	32
	Heterogeneous echogenic structure	5
	Wavy or sickle shaped echogenic strips	26
Left ventral abdomen region	Homogenous hypoechoic structure	3
	Wavy or sickle shaped echogenic strips	2
	Echogenic loop	30

appeared messy (Fig. 3). There was an interface between the gas cap and the ingesta beneath which reverberation artifacts disappeared abruptly and the echogenic ingesta appeared clearly (Fig. 4). The abomasal ingesta depth was usually beyond the maximal penetration depth (15 cm) of the transducer at start (Fig. 4) and only when the transducer moved ventrally, the ruminal wall which immediately contacted with the left abdominal wall in healthy cows could be visible medial to the abomasum as a thick, smooth echogenic band (Fig. 3). The left longitudinal groove of the rumen was identified medial to the abomasum as a typical notch in ventral part of 11th intercostal space in one cow (Fig. 5). Some abomasal folds were usually observed within the abomasal ingesta as wavy or sickle shaped echogenic strips in 30 cows (Fig. 3).

After the reposition surgery, the abomasal characteristic findings mentioned above left no trace in the same exploring area in all the cows, except that some reverberation artifacts was still observed in the dorsal region of the ICSs (Fig. 6). The ultrasound examination of the left abdomen became uncomplicated and the rumen and spleen returned to their normal position.

Exploratory laparotomy findings

The diagnosis of LDA was confirmed in all the cows via exporatory laparotomy. The abomasum could be felt reclining on the dorsal rumen and distended in 37 of the cows, when the hand advanced over the dorsal rumen across to the dorsal left side of the abdomen. In the other three cows, the abomasum could be palpated only when the hand went under the rumen across to the ventral left side of the abdomen.

Discussion

In dairy farms, diagnostic ultrasound is mainly used to the diagnosis and management of reproductive conditions. However, more and more studies have indicated that ultrasonography is useful to the diagnosis of some nonreproductive diseases of cows, especial gastrointestinal diseases [8]. In the present study, we showed that the abomasum of the cows with LDA could be generally ultrasonographically identified in the left abdominal cavity. The ultrasonograms probing from the left 9th to 12th ICS and the left ventral abdomen were considerably different before and after reposition surgery in the cows with LDA.

In healthy adult dairy cows, the abomasum could be imaged in ventral abdominal region approximately 8–15 cm caudal to the xiphoid process from the ventral midline, and that more of the abomasum was situated to the right of the ventral midline than to the left. The position of the abomasum depends on the degree of ruminal filling and the stage of pregnancy. Abomasal dimensions, position, and volume change markedly during the last

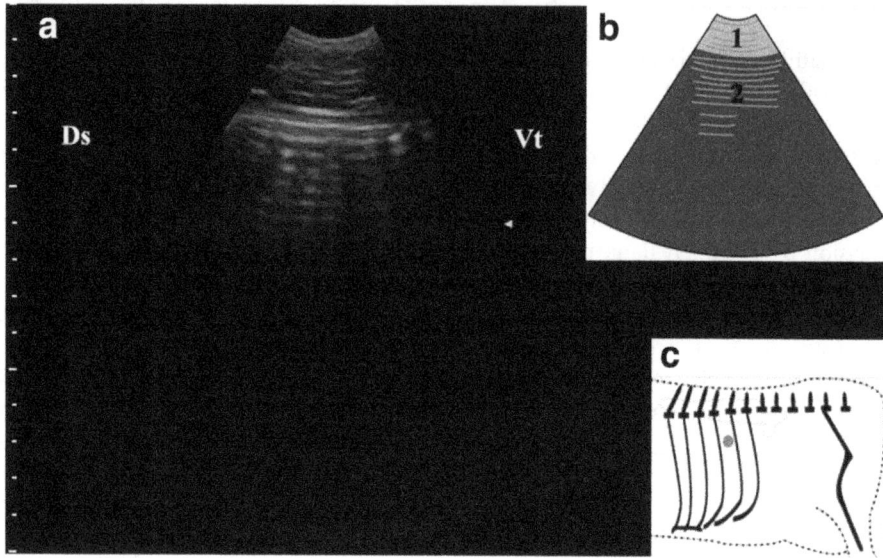

Fig. 2 Ultrasonogram of abomasal gas cap (**a**), schematic diagram (**b**) and position of transducer (**c**). A 3.5 MHz low-frequency curvilinear transducer was placed in the left dorsal part of 11th ICS of a cow with LDA, some reverberation artifacts produced by abomasal gas cap appeared as parallel lines. 1-thoracic wall; 2-Reverberation artifacts; Ds-dorsal; Vt-ventral; Grey spot-position of transducer

3 months of gestation and first 3 months of lactation [11]. In cows with LDA, because of gases accumulation, the abomasum enlarges and slides leftwards beneath the ruminal atrium and ventralruminal sac, ultimately rising (like a balloon) between the rumen and the abdominal wall [9]. The abomasal gas cap as a trait of the distended abomasum can produce reverberation artifacts owing to the reflection of the ultrasound beam backwards and forwards between the transducer and the highly reflective surface of gas-filled abomasum [10]. In the present study, reverberation artifacts appeared in most regions of the 9th to 12th ICS in 37 cows with LDA. However, it disappeared largely after the reposition surgery and only a little remained in the dorsal region. According to the previous studies [11–13], the remaining artifacts in the dorsal region resulted from the exploratory laparotomy obscured examination of the dorsal abdomen for at least 24 h after surgery.

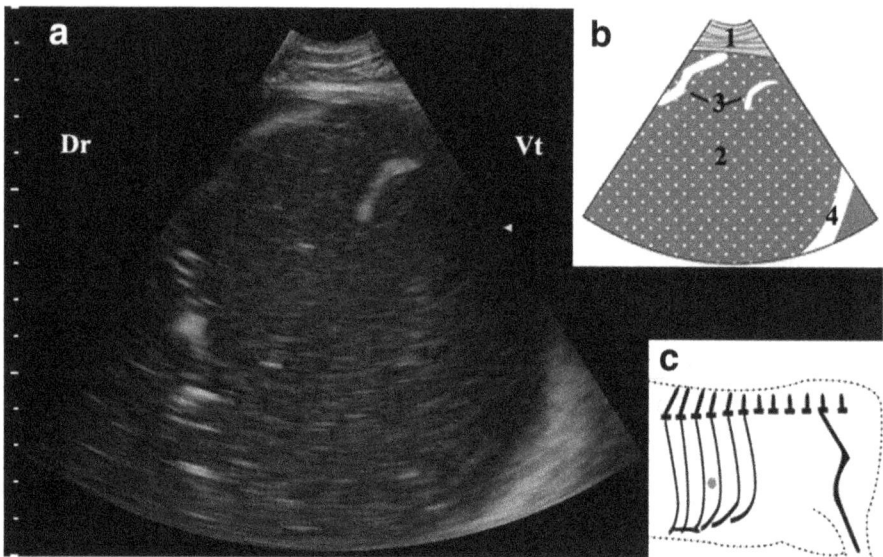

Fig. 3 Ultrasonogram of abomasal ingesta (**a**), schematic diagram (**b**) and position of transducer (**c**). A 3.5 MHz low-frequency curvilinear transducer was placed on the ventral part in 10th ICS on the left side of a cow with LDA, homogenous hypoechoic structures with echogenic spots produced by abomasal ingesta appeared. 1-thoracic wall; 2-abomasal ingesta; 3-abomasal fold; 4-ruminal wall; Ds-dorsal; Vt-ventral; Grey spot-position of transducer

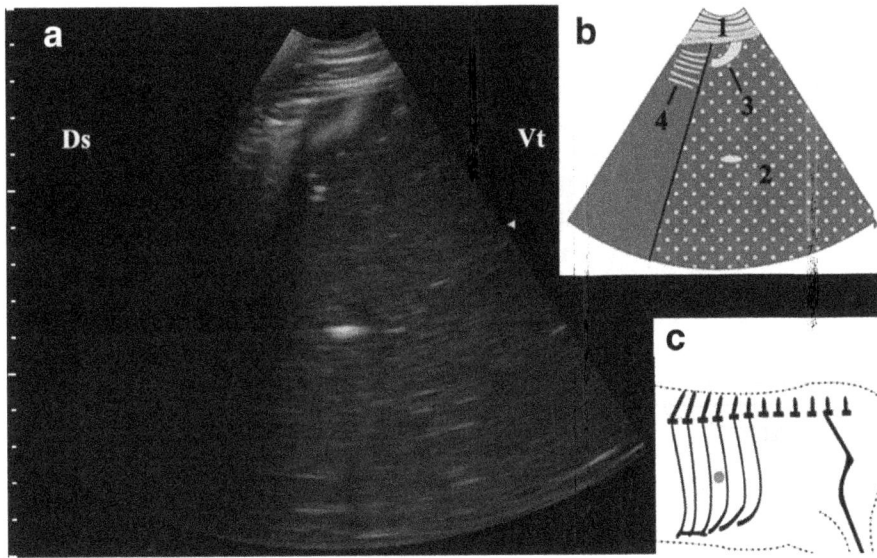

Fig. 4 Ultrasonogram of interface between abomasal gas and ingesta (**a**), schematic diagram (**b**) and position of transducer (**c**). A 3.5 MHz low-frequency curvilinear transducer was placed in the median part of 10th ICS on the left side of a cow with LDA, an interface between the gas cap and the ingesta appeared. 1-thoracic wall; 2-abomasal ingesta; 3-abomasal fold; 4-Reverberation artifacts; Ds-dorsal; Vt-ventral; Grey spot-position of transducer

Homogenous hypoechoic structures with echogenic spots could be viewed from the ventral or median part of the left 9th to the 12th ICS in most of the cows in the present study. As stated by previous studies [6, 7, 14], these structures were produced by the abomasal ingesta and could not be viewed from the same region in normal cows or other diseased cows. The vanishment of these structures in the cows, after the reposition surgery, further clarified this conclusion. The

abomasal folds were recognized in 28 (70%) of the cows with LDA. In contrast with healthy cows, cows with displaced abomasum have more chances to show the abomasl folds [14].

Earlier research about the ultrasonography of LDA mainly described the findings probed from the left 10th to the 12th ICS [6, 7, 11]. In the present study, we extended the examining area to the ventral left abdomen and some interesting ultrasonograms were found. The

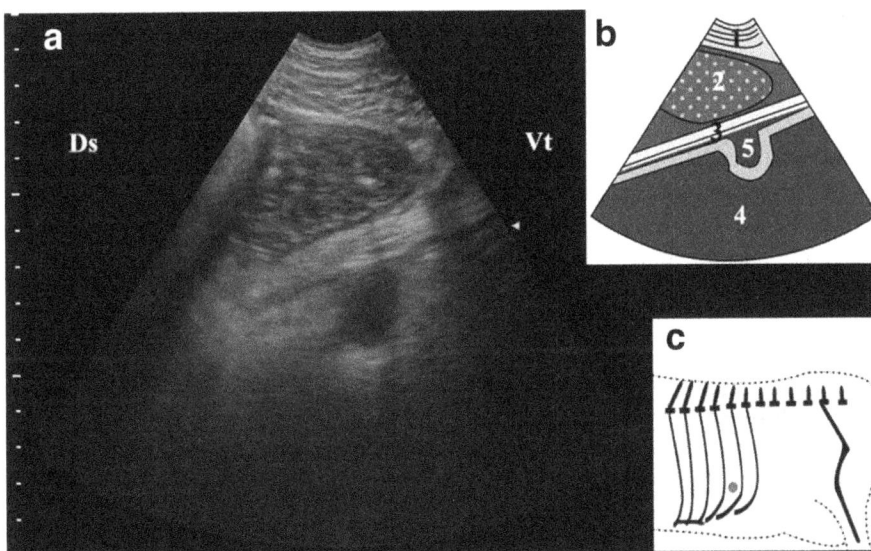

Fig. 5 Ultrasonogram of the left longitudinal groove of the rumen median to abomasum (**a**), schematic diagram (**b**) and position of transducer (**c**). A 3.5 MHz low-frequency curvilinear transducer was placed in the ventral part of 11th ICS on the left side of a cow with LDA, the left longitudinal groove of the rumen appeared as a typical notch median to the abomasum. 1-thoracic wall; 2-abomasal ingesta; 3-greater omentum; 4-rumen; 5-left longitudinal groove of the rumen; Ds-dorsal; Vt-ventral; Grey spot-position of transducer

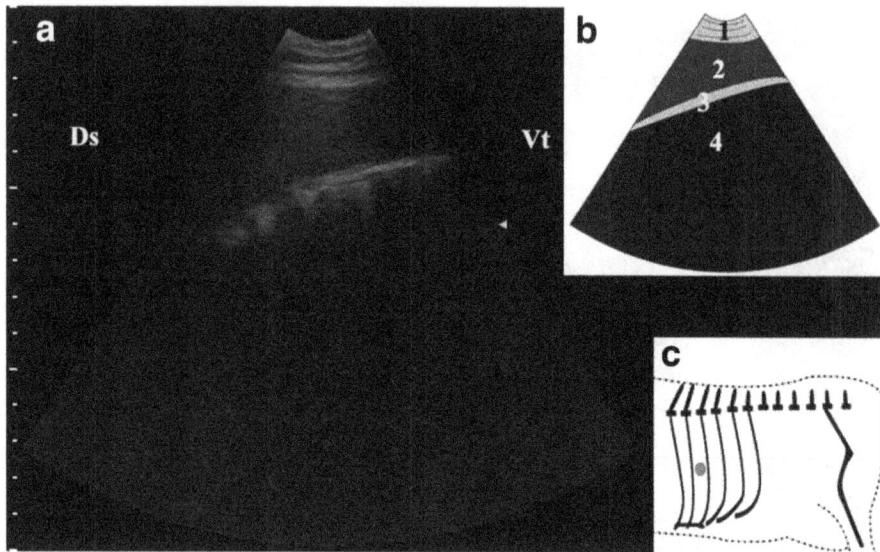

Fig. 6 Ultrasonogram of spleen (**a**), schematic diagram (**b**) and position of transducer (**c**). A 3.5 MHz low-frequency curvilinear transducer was placed in the median part of 9th ICS on the left side of a cow just after abomasum reposition surgery, the spleen appeared as homogenous hypoechoic structures. 1-thoracic wall; 2-spleen; 3-ruminal wall; 4-rumen; Ds-dorsal; Vt-ventral; Grey spot-position of transducer

pyloric canal was visualized from the ventral left abdomen in 30 (75%) of the cows with LDA. Ultrasonographic description related to LDA about pyloric canal in cows is rare and one study reported that the pylorus was positively visible from the right 10th ICS in one healthy cow [6]. The pyloric canal, as part of the abomasum, has a unique circular structure in the ultrasonography. However, the ultrasonographic image of pyloric canal is often confused with small intestine, so it is difficult to observe in normal cattle. Our findings could be explained by that when the body of the abomasum displaced to the left abdomen and trapped, the pylorus canal was also dragged to the left abdomen cavity but placed more ventrally as the result described in the study of Itoh et al. [15]. The pylorus canal is an important characteristic of LDA, so it is worthy to put some attention on the left ventral abdomen when one proposes to examine a suspected cow ultrasonographically. The characteristic circular acoustic image structure of the pyloric cross section is easier to be identified than the ultrasonographic ingesta, so it can be used as an important diagnostic basis of LDA.

It is enough to make a diagnosis, depending on the findings mentioned above; however things are not always consistent. Just as the typical clinical features like 'pinging' usually do not exist in the cows with lesser displacement of abomasum, these ultrasonographic features of abomasum may not be detected in mild cases. In the present study, there were three cows whose abomasum could only be visualized from the ventral left abdominal wall and neither the median or ventral reverberation artifacts nor the pyloric canal ultrasonogram could be found; the abomasal ingesta was looming and less deep

but more echogenic. The exploratory laparotomy proved that the abomasum of the three cows was lying ventral to the rumen. Since displacement tends to start in the reticulorumen groove, the abomasum of mild cases usually place near the reticulorumen groove [2]. Therefore extending examining region to the area under the left 9th to 10th costal arches is warranted.

Conclusions

We conclude that ultrasonography is a useful tool for the diagnosis of LDA. The self-controlled method adopted in our study showed that the characteristic findings such as homogenous hypoechoic structures described by previous studies were produced by LDA. In addition, the abnormal position of pyloric canal found in our study is an important diagnostic feature in ultrasonography of LDA. These characteristics make significant difference between LDA cows and healthy cows, so one can depend on them to diagnose LDA easily.

Abbreviations
ICS: Intercostal space; LDA: Left displacement of abomasum

Acknowledgements
This work was supported by the National key research and development program (Beijing, China; grant no. 2016YFD0501007-3 and 2016YFD0501206), National Natural Science Foundation of China (Beijing, China; grant nos. 31572581, 31472247, 31402265 and 31772810), Jilin province Science Foundation for Youths (Changchun, China; grant no. 20160520063JH) and Natural Science Foundation of Jilin Province (Changchun, China, Grant No. 20170101148JC).

Authors' contributions

XWL, YL, CX and XBL conceived and designed the experiments; QSX, RHZ, WY, CX, YL, YMZ YT MZ and ZW performed the experiments; ZW, XWL, RHZ, WY, YMZ and QSX carried out the ultrasound examinations and drafted the paper; GWL, XBL, YT, MZ and CX shared in discussing the results; and RHZ and XWL wrote the paper; GWL and XBL edited the final manuscript. All authors read and approved the final manuscript.

Consent for publication

Not applicable.

Competing interests

The authors declare that they have no competing interests.

Author details

[1]Key Laboratory of Zoonosis, Ministry of Education, College of Veterinary Medicine, Jilin University, 5333 Xi'an Road, Changchun, Jilin 130062, China. [2]College of animal science and veterinary medicine, Heilongjiang Bayi Agricultural University, Daqing 163319, Heilongjiang, China. [3]College of Animal Science and Technology, Anhui Agricultural University, 130 West Changjiang Road, Hefei 230036, Anhui, China.

References

1. Begg H. Diseases of the stomach of the adult ruminant. Vet Rec. 1950; 62(51):797–808.
2. Mueller K. Diagnosis, treatment and control of left displaced abomasum in cattle. Practice. 2011;33(9):470–81.
3. Wilson AD, Ferguson JG. Use of a flexible fiberoptic laparoscope as a diagnostic aid in cattle. Can Vet J. 1984;25(6):229–34.
4. Braun U. Ultrasonography in gastrointestinal disease in cattle. Vet J. 2003; 166(2):112–24.
5. Toholj B, Cincović M, Stevančević M, Spasojevic J, Ivetić V, Potkonjak A. Evaluation of ultrasonography for measuring solar soft tissue thickness as a predictor of sole ulcer formation in Holstein-Friesian dairy cows. Vet J. 2014; 199(2):290–4.
6. Braun U, Wild K, Guscetti F. Ultrasonographic examination of the abomasum of 50 cows. Vet Rec. 1997;140(4):93–8.
7. Ok M, Arican M, Turgut K. Ultrasonographic findings in cows with left and right displacement of abomasum. Rev Med Vet. 2002;153(1):15–8.
8. Richmond DH. The use of percussion and auscultation as a diagnostic aid in abomasal displacement of dairy cows. Can Vet J. 1964;5(1):5
9. Streeter RN, Step DL. Diagnostic ultrasonography in ruminants. Veterinary clinics of North America food animal. Practice. 2007;23(3):541–74.
10. Doll K, Sickinger M, Seeger T. New aspects in the pathogenesis of abomasal displacement. Vet J. 2009;181(2):90.
11. Braun U, Pusterla N, Schonmann M. Ultrasonographic findings in cows with left displacement of the abomasum. Vet Rec. 1997;141(13):331–5.
12. Tschuor A, Clauss M. Investigations on the stratification of forestomach contents in ruminants: an ultrasonographic approach. Eur J Wildl Res. 2008; 54(4):627–33.
13. Imran S, Kumar A, Tyagi SP, Kumar A, Sharma S. Ultrasonographic examination of the rumen in healthy cows. Vet Med Int. 2011,2011:840629
14. Braun U, Schweizer A, Trösch L. Ultrasonography of the rumen of dairy cows. BMC Vet Res. 2013;9(1):44.
15. Braun U, Feller. Ultrasonographic findings in cows with right displacement of the abomasum and abomasal volvulus. Vet Rec J Br Vet Assoc. 2008;162(10):311–5.

Comparative measurements of bone mineral density and bone contrast values in canine femora using dual-energy X-ray absorptiometry and conventional digital radiography

K. Lucas[1], I. Nolte[1*], V. Galindo-Zamora[2], M. Lerch[3], C. Stukenborg-Colsman[3], B. A. Behrens[4], A. Bouguecha[4], S. Betancur[4], A. Almohallami[4] and P. Wefstaedt[1]

Abstract

Background: Aseptic loosening due to bone remodelling processes after total hip replacement is one common cause for revision surgery. In human medicine, dual-energy X-ray absorptiometry (DEXA) is the gold standard for quantitative evaluation of bone mineral density, whereas in veterinary medicine conventional radiography is used for follow-up studies. Recently, a method has been described using digital X-ray images for quantitative assessment of grey scale values of bone contrast. Therefore, the aim of the present study was to evaluate the correlation of bone mineral density (BMD) measured by DEXA with grey scale values (GV) measured in digital X-ray images (RX50, RX66) ex vivo.

Results: The measured GV in the chosen X-ray settings showed on average a good correlation ($r = 0.61$) to the measured BMD with DEXA. Correlation between the two X-ray settings was very good ($r = 0.81$). For comparisons among regions of interests (ROIs) a difference of 8.2% was found to be statistically significant, whereas in the case of RX50 and RX66 differences of 5.3% and 4.1% were found to be statistically significant.

Conclusions: Results indicate that measuring absolute changes in bone mineral density might be possible using digital radiography. Not all significant differences between ROIs detectable with DEXA can be displayed in the X-ray images because of the lower sensitivity of the radiographs. However, direct comparison of grey scale values of the periprosthetic femur in one individual patient during the follow-up period, in order to predict bone remodelling processes, should be possible, but with a lesser sensitivity than with DEXA. It is important that the same X-ray settings are chosen for each patient for follow-up studies.

Keywords: Bone mineral density, DEXA, Digital radiography, Canine, Femur, Bone remodelling

* Correspondence: ingo.nolte@tiho-hannover.de
[1]Small Animal Hospital, University of Veterinary Medicine Hannover, Foundation, Bünteweg 9, D-30559 Hannover, Germany
Full list of author information is available at the end of the article

Background

In humans and dogs, severe damage of the hip joint is usually treated with total hip replacement (THR) [1]. Different prosthetic devices exist on the market. These include cemented, cementless and hybrid implants [2–8]. Complications following THR are luxation, infection, aseptic or septic loosening, femoral fracture and sciatic neurapraxia [9, 10]. Aseptic loosening is one common cause for revision surgery [10, 11]. Different reasons for aseptic loosening processes are assumed, including particle disease, micromotion and stress shielding [12]. Stress shielding is due to different load transfer because of the higher modulus (E) of the prosthesis compared to bone which leads to loss of bone mineral density. It is of utmost importance to diagnose loosening processes in good time in order to minimise patients' pain and distress. Therefore, it is necessary to detect as soon as possible the amount and localisation of bone loss around the prosthesis, which is reflected in changes in bone mineral density [13].

According to the World Health Organisation (WHO), dual-energy X-ray absorptiometry (DEXA) is the gold standard for quantitative measurements of bone mineral density in human medicine [14, 15]. DEXA measurements are performed in the spine and in the hip for diagnosing osteoporosis [16]. To measure bone mineral density in the periprosthetic femur, the proximal part of the femur surrounding the prosthesis is usually divided into 7 regions of interest called Gruen zones in human medicine, according to the description of Gruen et al.[17].

However, DEXA devices are not commonly available in veterinary medicine and are therefore rarely used for follow-up studies after THR in dogs. Conventional radiography is usually applied in veterinary medicine to predict the clinical outcome. Usually, X-ray images are used to evaluate parameters such as femoral cortical thickening/atrophy, signs of fissure/fracture, radiolucent lines, thickness of the cement mantle, position of the implant parts and subluxation [4, 7, 10, 18]. To the authors' knowledge, the question if bone remodelling processes around femoral implants are reliably detected with digital radiography in dogs has not been answered yet. One study examined these processes after THR in dogs using X-ray images from digital radiography for evaluating grey scale values (GV) [19]. For evaluating bone remodelling processes in the canine femur, Gruen zones were adapted and reduced to five region of interests (ROIs) [19, 20]. Another study reported a correlation of mean grey value in digitalised and digital images of conventional and digital radiography of bovine and equine bone specimens with BMD assessed with DEXA of 0.910 and 0.937, respectively [21]. These results indicate that also differences in bone mineral density as found in the different regions of the canine femur should be detectable with digital radiography. To the authors' knowledge, no comparable study exists in dogs. Therefore, the aim of this study was to compare BMD from DEXA measurements with GV in digital radiography and to evaluate the influence of different X-ray settings on the mean GV in canine carcass femora.

Methods

Material

Bones were obtained from cadavers of 15 dogs (mean body weight = 26.4 kg; SD = 5.6 kg; 3 Alsatians, 3 mixed breeds, 2 Golden Retrievers, 2 Small Muensterlaenders, 2 Irish Setters, 2 English Bulldogs, 1 Border Collie) that were euthanised due to medical reasons not related to this study and ceded for use for research purposes either to the Institute of Anatomy or the Small Animal Hospital of the University of Veterinary Medicine Hannover, Foundation. Written owner consent was obtained by the Small Animal Hospital of the University of Veterinary Medicine Hannover, Foundation. Both explanted femora from all 15 dogs were measured using DEXA and conventional X-ray for quantitative analysis of bone mineral density (DEXA) and grey scale values (X-ray) as well. Up to the time of examination, the femora were wrapped in cloth, soaked with 0.9% saline solution and frozen at –20 °C.

DEXA measurements

DEXA measurements were performed with the scanning mode "metal hip removal" of a Hologic Discovery A S/N 80600 device (Hologic Inc., Waltham, MA, USA). The afore-mentioned mode was chosen to create data that are comparable with studies investigating patients after total hip replacement although the bones in this study did not include a metal implant. Two different anterior-posterior positions were chosen to evaluate whether there is an influence of different rotations of the respective femur. For the anterior-posterior positioning 1 (Fig. 1, ap1), the femur was rotated medially about 20° in order to prevent the femoral neck from superimposing with the femoral head. This is the standard position for human patients. The conventional anterior-posterior positioning (Fig. 1, ap2) is commonly used for evaluating hip dysplasia. Additionally, two measurements were carried out in mediolateral projection (ml1 and ml2) with the femur laterally rotated 90° to ap1 and ap2, respectively (see online Additional file 1: ml1_ml2.tif). Evaluation of DEXA images was performed using the integrated software of the afore-mentioned DEXA device (Hologic Inc., Waltham, MA, USA).

X-ray examination

For digital X-ray examination (S/N 09000024; Philips Medical Systems DMC GmbH; Hamburg; Germany), the

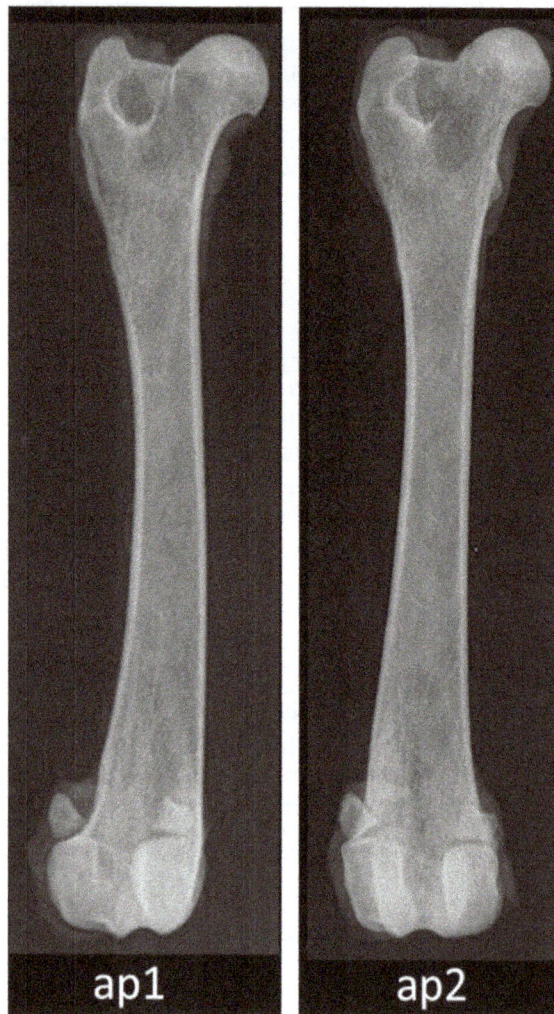

Fig. 1 Anterior-posterior positions ap1 and ap2. X-ray of patient no. 8 (Alsatian, 24 kg) right femur in anterior-posterior positions (ap1, ap2). ap1: anterior-posterior position, femur rotated medially about 20°; ap2: conventional anterior-posterior position like for HD diagnosis

femora were positioned the same way as for the DEXA measurements. Two different X-ray settings (RX50 = 50 kV/6.3 mAs and RX66 = 66 kV/8 mAs) commonly used for X-ray imaging of the hind limb in living dogs were applied. After data export as *.jpeg, radiographs were analysed using the freely available image processing software ImageJ (Rasband, W.S., ImageJ, U. S. National Institutes of Health, Bethesda, Maryland, USA, http://imagej.nih.gov/ij/).

Zonal classification

For analyses of DEXA images as well as of X-ray images, Gruen Zones [17] were adapted to the canine femur and reduced to 5 regions of interest (ROIs) as described previously (Figs. 2 and 3) [19, 20]. For defining ROI sizes within X-ray data sets by means of ImageJ, a virtual

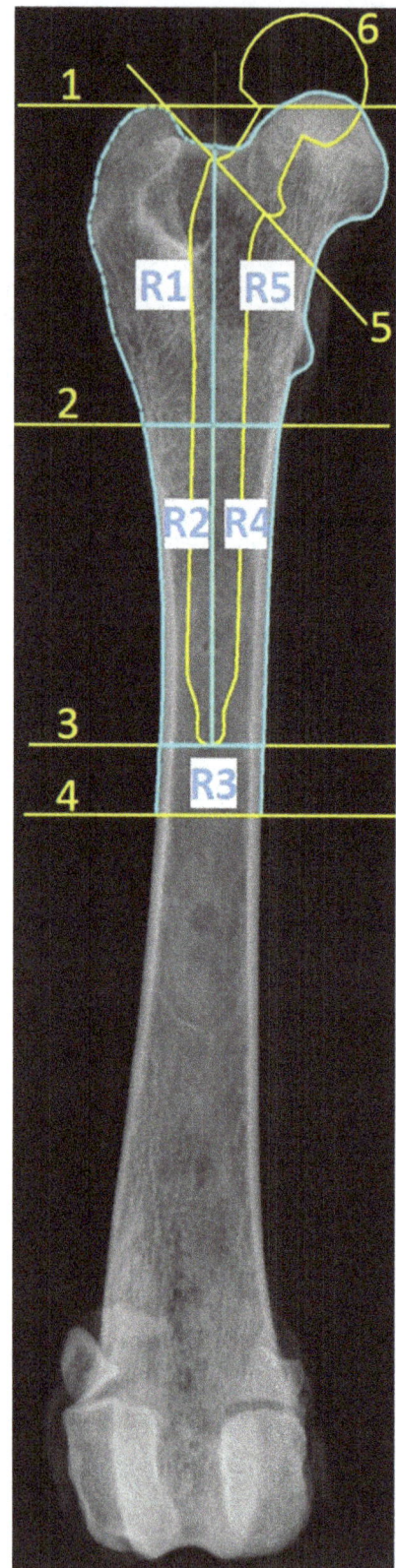

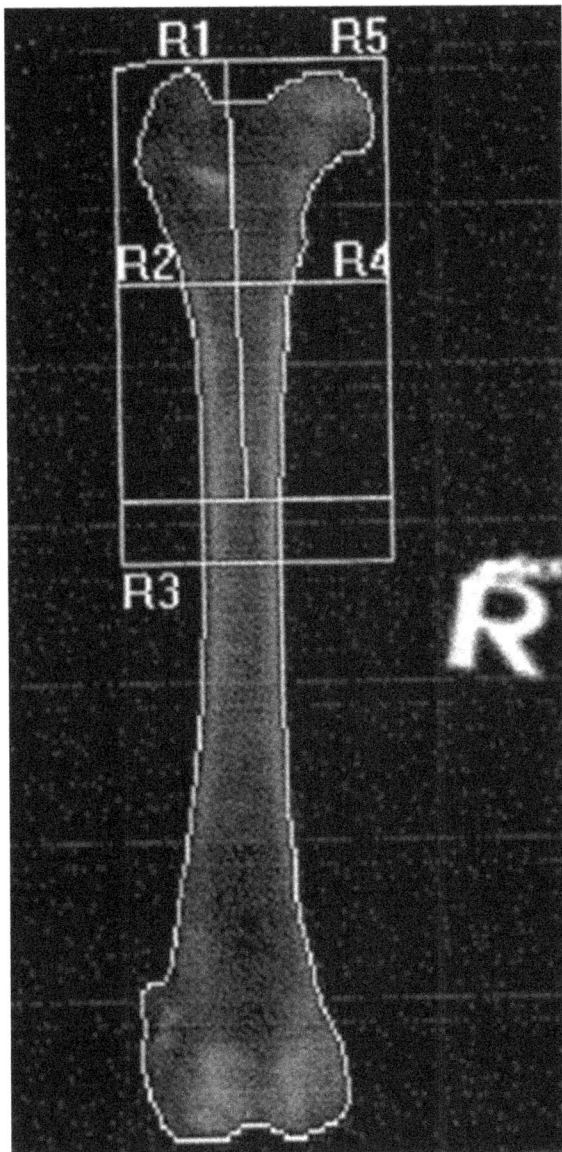

Fig. 3 DEXA scan ap2. DEXA scan in anterior-posterior position ap2 (Hologic Discovery A S/N 80600), right femur of patient no 8 (Alsatian, 24 kg) as an example. R1 – R5 = Region of Interest 1–5

Fig. 2 Definition of ROIs. X-ray image (66 kV, 8mAs) in anterior-posterior position ap2, right femur of patient no. 8 (Alsatian, 24 kg) as an example. R1 – R5 = Region of Interest 1–5; 1: greater trochanter line, 2: bisector line, 3: tip of prosthesis, 4: 1 cm distal tip of prosthesis, 5: femoral head dissection line, 6: template of a prosthesis

the greater trochanter (Fig. 2; 1). By halving the shaft lengthwise, ROI1 and ROI2 (lateral) as well as ROI4 and ROI5 (medial) were generated in the proximal femur. ROI3, with a fixed height of 1 cm (distance between line 3 and line 4, Fig. 2), was located directly distal of the tip of the virtual prosthesis. These 5 ROIs were determined separately for every femur. The location and dimension of every ROI was exactly measured and also applied for DEXA analysis to ensure the evaluation of the same area in the two different modalities.

Statistical analysis

Statistical analysis was performed with SPSS® (SPSS Inc. Chicago, IL, USA). Pearson's correlation coefficient between DEXA and RX50, between DEXA and RX66 and between RX50 and RX66 was calculated for each position and every ROI. Correlation was considered as follows: $r = 0 \rightarrow$ no correlation; $0 < r \leq 0.2 \rightarrow$ very poor; $0.2 < r \leq 0.4 \rightarrow$ poor; $0.4 < r \leq 0.6 \rightarrow$ moderate; $0.6 < r \leq 0.8 \rightarrow$ good; $0.8 < r < 1 \rightarrow$ very good; $r = 1$ perfect. One-way ANOVA followed by a Tukey post hoc test was performed to analyse differences between the different ROIs for DEXA, RX50 and RX66 and for each positioning.

Results

Measured bone mineral density (DEXA) and grey scale values (X-ray) for all ROIs in both ap1 and ap2 are displayed in Tables 1 and 2 (mean value (M) ± standard deviation (SD), coefficient of variation [CV]). Results of the measurements in mediolateral positioning ml1 and ml2 are presented in the online supplements (Additional file 2: BMD_GV_ml1_ml2.docx, Additional file 3: Boxplots_ml1.tif, Additional file 4: Boxplots_ml2.tif, Additional file 1: ml1_ml2.tif).

Correlation between DEXA and X-ray

For ap1, correlation between DEXA and RX50 was good in ROI3 (r = 0.8) and in ROI1 (r = 0.6), moderate in ROI4 (r = 0.5) and ROI5 (r = 0.54) and poor in ROI2 (r = 0.34). Correlation between DEXA and RX66 in ap1 was good in ROI3 (r = 0.72), moderate in ROI1 (r = 0.49), ROI4 (r = 0.49) and ROI5 (r = 0.47) and poor in ROI2 (r = 0.34).

For ap2, correlation between DEXA and RX50 was good in ROI3 (r = 0.8) and in ROI4 (r = 0.62) and moderate in ROI1 (r = 0.56), ROI2 (r = 0.58) and ROI5 (r = 0.57). Correlation between DEXA and RX66 for ap2 showed slightly better results than ap1, being good in

prosthesis template of appropriate size was generated and positioned as an overlay on the respective femur image (Fig. 2). The axis of the virtual prosthesis was aligned to the femoral axis. Approximately 2–3 mm space for a cement mantle was left free between the prosthesis and the inner border of the compacta. The prosthesis was inserted into the femur until the neck closed up with a line where the femoral head was virtually dissected (Fig. 2; 5). A horizontal line perpendicular to the femur axis was inserted to mark the tip of the virtual prosthesis (Fig. 2; 3). A bisector line (Fig. 2; 2) was drawn in the middle between the tip of the prosthesis and a second line positioned at the proximal margin of

Table 1 Measured bone mineral density (DEXA) and grey scale values (X-ray) for the regions of interest 1–5 (ROI1 – ROI5) in ap1: mean value (M) ± standard deviation (SD), coefficient of variation [CV]

Region of Interest	Anterior-posterior position ap1		
	DEXA (g/cm^2)	RX50 (grey scale value)	RX66 (grey scale value)
ROI1	0.62 ± 0.04 [0.07]	123.28 ± 9.65 [0.08]	118.78 ± 7.25 [0.06]
ROI2	0.74 ± 0.06 [0.08]	127.84 ± 7.07 [0.05]	122.24 ± 4.93 [0.04]
ROI3	0.79 ± 0.10 [0.13]	125.64 ± 7.51 [0.06]	119.09 ± 6.64 [0.05]
ROI4	0.79 ± 0.07 [0.09]	128.58 ± 6.53 [0.05]	122.49 ± 4.97 [0.04]
ROI5	0.73 ± 0.05 [0.07]	129.81 ± 9.97 [0.08]	125.23 ± 7.78 [0.06]

ROI1 (r = 0.61), ROI2 (r = 0.66), ROI3 (r = 0.79) and ROI4 (r = 0.69) and moderate in ROI5 (r = 0.58). All correlations were highly significant ($p < 0.01$). Only in ap1 ROI2, where the correlation was poor for both DEXA – RX50 and RX66, respectively, were the results not significant (p > 0.05).

Correlation between the different X-ray settings
Correlation between RX50 and RX66 was very good in ap1 ROI1 (r = 0.83) and ROI5 (r = 0.86), in ap2 ROI1 (r = 0.85) and ROI5 (r = 0.88). Correlation between RX50 and RX66 was good in ap1 ROI2 (r = 0.78), ROI3 (r = 0.66) and ROI4 (r = 0.63), in ap2 ROI2 (r = 0.78), ROI3 (r = 0.79) and ROI4 (r = 0.79). All correlations were highly significant ($p < 0.01$).

Differences between ROIs
Statistically significant differences are shown in Figs. 4 and 5 (* - *** = $p < 0.05 – p < 0.001$).

In ap1 statistically significant differences could be detected in the case of DEXA measurements for ROI1 compared to all other ROIs, whereas in RX50 and RX66 this was only the case between ROI1 and ROI5. The significance of differences when comparing ROI3 to ROI5 and ROI4 to ROI5 as seen in ap1 in DEXA could not be detected in RX50. RX66 detected differences between ROI3 and ROI5 as seen with DEXA, but not between ROI4 and ROI5.

For ap2, DEXA detected significant differences between ROI1 and all other ROIs and between all ROIs

except for ROI1 compared to ROI5. Values measured in ROI2, ROI3 and ROI4 did not differ significantly. Similar to ap1, also in ap2 RX66 detected more significant differences than RX50. For ap2, differences in RX50 could be observed between ROI1 compared to ROI2, ROI1 compared to ROI4 and ROI1 compared to ROI5. The same holds true for RX66 ap2, and additionally differences between ROI2 compared to ROI3 were observed in RX66 ap2.

Discussion
Both modalities used in this study (digital radiography and DEXA) are based on X-radiation and produce a 2-dimensional image of a 3-dimensional object. The produced image is the result of the radiation absorption of the respective tissue which depends on its density and thickness [22]. The higher the density and thickness of the tissue, the greater is the absorption. Depending on how much radiation reaches the detector, every pixel of the image is assigned a grey value depending on the attenuation value [22]. The difference between conventional radiography and DEXA is that the latter uses two different X-ray voltages from different sources at the same time (100 kV and 140 kV in this study). In contrast, conventional radiography only uses one source of energy (in this study 50 kV for RX50 or otherwise 66 kV for RX66). Thus, in DEXA every pixel includes two different attenuation values. This information is automatically converted to Bone Mineral Density (BMD) by the DEXA software (in g/cm^2).

Table 2 Measured bone mineral density (DEXA) and grey scale values (X-ray) for the regions of interest 1–5 (ROI1 – ROI5) in ap2: mean value (M) ± standard deviation (SD), coefficient of variation [CV]

Region of Interest	Anterior-posterior position ap2		
	DEXA (g/cm^2)	RX50 (grey scale value)	RX66 (grey scale value)
ROI1	0.63 ± 0.04 [0.07]	122.73 ± 8.37 [0.07]	118.56 ± 7.11 [0.06]
ROI2	0.80 ± 0.07 [0.09]	132.10 ± 6.34 [0.05]	127.61 ± 5.21 [0.04]
ROI3	0.82 ± 0.11 [0.13]	127.39 ± 7.37 [0.06]	122.56 ± 7.42 [0.06]
ROI4	0.80 ± 0.07 [0.09]	129.42 ± 6.55 [0.05]	124.68 ± 5.99 [0.05]
ROI5	0.72 ± 0.06 [0.08]	129.20 ± 7.66 [0.06]	125.16 ± 6.43 [0.05]

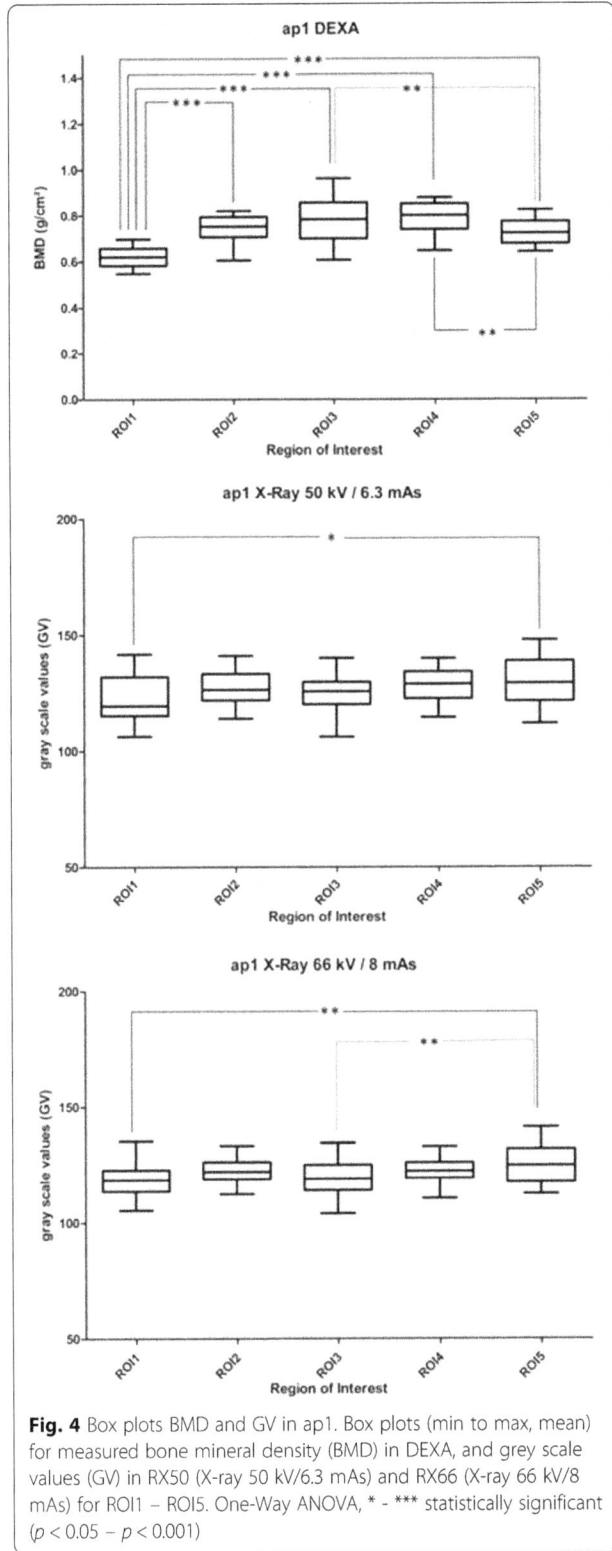

Fig. 4 Box plots BMD and GV in ap1. Box plots (min to max, mean) for measured bone mineral density (BMD) in DEXA, and grey scale values (GV) in RX50 (X-ray 50 kV/6.3 mAs) and RX66 (X-ray 66 kV/8 mAs) for ROI1 – ROI5. One-Way ANOVA, * - *** statistically significant ($p < 0.05 – p < 0.001$)

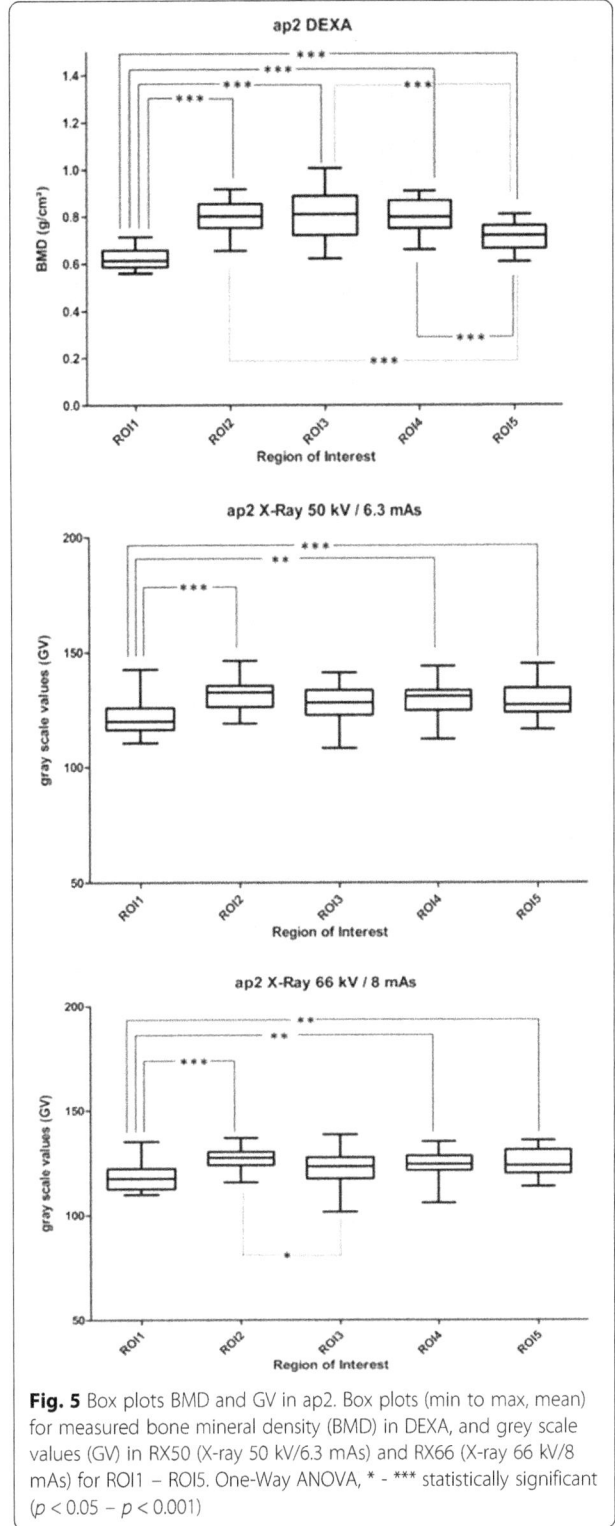

Fig. 5 Box plots BMD and GV in ap2. Box plots (min to max, mean) for measured bone mineral density (BMD) in DEXA, and grey scale values (GV) in RX50 (X-ray 50 kV/6.3 mAs) and RX66 (X-ray 66 kV/8 mAs) for ROI1 – ROI5. One-Way ANOVA, * - *** statistically significant ($p < 0.05 – p < 0.001$)

In the literature, the influence of the rotation of DEXA results is reported from −10.5% to + 2.8% and in individual cases up to 60% [23]. Although the positioning of the femora for the X-ray and DEXA examinations was performed with utmost care, it might be possible that the degree of rotation of the femur was not 100% the same between DEXA and X-ray due to the manual positioning. A positioning guide should be used in further studies to reduce bias particularly when examining living patients where correct positioning is more challenging due to the soft tissue covering the bone. Another methodical limitation of the study was that the definition of ROI geometry and position was based on the X-ray examinations. This setup was transferred to the DEXA images which could have led to small differences in the examined areas. For ap1 and ap2, both X-ray settings detected fewer significant differences between ROIs than DEXA. In veterinary medicine, the anterior-posterior position ap1, which is equivalent to the hip dysplasia examination, is the most common position used for follow-up studies. Variance of DEXA measurements were slightly higher (CV = 0.07–0.13) than in RX50 (CV = 0.05–0.08) or RX66 (CV = 0.04–0.08). The minimal detectable difference of BMD with DEXA amounted to 8.2% (ap1: ROI3 – ROI5 and ROI4 – ROI5). For RX50, the minimal difference was 5.3% (ap1: ROI1 – ROI5), whereas RX66 was able to detect changes in grey values with a difference of 4.1% (ap2: ROI2 – ROI3). In follow-up studies using DEXA after THR, statistically significant differences in BMD between ROIs after 6 months, 12 months and 2 years to baseline value 1 week postoperatively were detected between −11.54 and +10.6% [13, 24]. The only previous study evaluating grey scale values in follow-up radiography after THR in dogs detected a statistical significant difference at 10.74% 4 months after surgery [19]. Our results therefore show a clinical relevance for follow-up studies aiming to investigate changes in grey scale values of bone X-rays over time. However, this technique is of course less sensitive than DEXA. The chosen X-ray setting has an influence on the grey scale values. Lower X-ray current and voltage revealed slightly higher grey scale values in the same ROIs. Nevertheless, there is a very good correlation between the two chosen X-ray settings (r = 0.81). For the evaluation of bone mineral density with digital radiography in the canine femur, e.g., for follow-up studies after THR, our results indicate the importance of always choosing the same X-ray setting for one patient. Both chosen settings showed on average a good (r = 0.61) correlation with the BMD measured with DEXA. However, our correlation results differ remarkably from a previous study reporting correlation results of 0.937 between mean grey values obtained from digital radiography and BMD (DEXA) in equine bone specimens [21]. One reason for these differing results could be that in the reported study femora specimens with an overall low variability of BMD were used to calculate the correlation between DEXA and digital radiography. In contrast, our study aimed to investigate the correlation between both methods using different areas of canine femora with varying BMDs. Thus, the higher variability of BMD in our

study could have been the reason for the overall lower correlation than reported by Vaccaro et al. [21] for equine bone specimens. Furthermore, it is unclear how ROI positioning was done in this specific study [21].

One factor known to influence the absorption of X-rays is the tissue surrounding the femur [22]. The surrounding tissue increases the absorption of radiation. Thus, less radiation reaches the detector and the affected pixel is given a higher grey scale value. For example, Mostafa et al. [19] measured on average 161.9–188.8 GV immediately postoperative, and 146.2–188.1 GV 4 months postoperative compared to 114.22–154.62 GV measured in our study, where femora were examined without surrounding tissues. Further studies are needed to evaluate influences of surrounding tissues. Another limitation of the study is that the influence of a total hip prosthesis on measurement results in the adjacent bone was not evaluated. Further studies are needed to investigate if the same correlations between GV (X-Ray) and BMD (DEXA) measurement like in the present study are to be found when examining canine femora with THR.

The evaluated ROIs in uncemented THR after 4 months revealed greater grey scale values than the ROIs in this study. One reason is that, due to the implanted uncemented prosthesis, the evaluated area in the study of Mostafa et al. was smaller and mainly contained compacta, while in the ROIs in this study both compacta and spongiosa were evaluated together. The other reason for differences in grey scale values is that in the study of Mostafa et al. the dogs were alive. Therefore, the radiographs were taken from the whole leg and not only from the bone. Further studies on whole legs with and without total hip implants are necessary to evaluate the influence of surrounding tissue and the metal implant (e.g., uberschwinger artefact [25]) on the measurements of GV.

Conclusions

Results indicate that measuring absolute changes in bone mineral density in canine femoras is not possible using digital radiography due to technical limitations. Nevertheless, differences in grey scale values of the bone can be identified using digital radiography. Not all significant differences between ROIs detectable with DEXA can be displayed in the X-ray images because of the lower sensitivity of the radiographs. However, further studies are necessery to evaluate whether direct comparison of grey scale values of the periprosthetic femur in individual patients over time is possible,keeping in mind that X-rays have a lower sensitivity than DEXA. It is important that the same X-ray settings are chosen for each patient for follow-up studies.

Additional files

Additional file 1: ml1_ml2.tif. Anterior-posterior positions ml1 and ml2. X-ray of patient no. 8 (Alsatian, 24 kg) right femur in mediolateral positions (ml1, ml2). ml1: mediolateral position, femur rotated 90° to ap1; ml2: femur rotated 90° to ap2.

Additional file 2: BMD_GV_ml1_ml2.docx. Results BMD and GV. Measured bone mineral content (DEXA) and gray scale values (X-ray) for the regions of interest 1–5 (ROI1 – ROI5) in ml1 and ml2: mean value (M) ± standard deviation (SD), coefficient of variation [CV].

Additional file 3: Boxplots_ml1.tif. Box plots BMD and GV in ml1. Box plots (min to max, mean) for measured bone mineral density (BMD) in DEXA, and grey scale values (GV) in RX50 (X-ray 50 kV/6.3 mAs) and RX66 (X-ray 66 kV/8 mAs) for ROI1 – ROI5. One-Way ANOVA, * - *** statistically significant ($p < 0.05 – p < 0.001$).

Additional file 4: Boxplots_ml2.tif. Box plots BMD and GV in ml2. Box plots (min to max, mean) for measured bone mineral density (BMD) in DEXA, and grey scale values (GV) in RX50 (X-ray 50 kV/6.3 mAs) and RX66 (X-ray 66 kV/8 mAs) for ROI1 – ROI5. One-Way ANOVA, * - *** statistically significant ($p < 0.05 – p < 0.001$).

Abbreviations

Ap: Anterior-posterior; BMD: Bone mineral density; DEXA: Dual-energy X-ray absorptiometry; E: Modulus; GV: Grey scale value; ml: Mediolateral; ROI: Region of interest; RX50: X-ray image with 50 kV and 6.3 mAs; RX66: X-ray image with 66 kV and 8.0 mAs; SD: Standard deviation; THR: Total hip replacement; WHO: World Health Organisation

Acknowledgement

The authors wish to thank Prof. Dr. C. Pfarrer and O. Stünkel from the Institute of Anatomy, University of Veterinary Medicine Hannover, Foundation, Bischofsholer Damm 15, D-30173 Hannover, Germany, for helping to acquire dog cadavers. Furthermore, the authors thank Frances Sherwood-Brock for proofreading the translation.

Funding

This study was performed in association with the subproject D6 of the collaborative research center 599: "Sustainable degradable and permanent implants out of metallic and ceramic materials". The authors wish to thank the German Research Foundation (DFG) for its financial support.

Authors' contribution

KL, IN, VGZ, ML, CSC, BAB, AB, SB, AA, PW: Made substantial contributions to conception and design of the study and interpretion of data. KL: Performed X-ray measurements and statistical analysis. KL, ML, CSC: Performed DEXA measurements. KL: Analysed DEXA and X-ray data. KL, IN VGZ, PW drafted the manuscript. AB, SB, AA, CSC, BAB: Gave technical support. All authors read and approved the final manuscript. All authors agreed to be accountable for all aspects of the work in ensuring that questions related to the accuracy or integrity of any part of the work are appropriately investigated and resolved.

Competing interests

The authors declare that they have no competing interests.

Consent to publication

Not applicable.

Author details

[1]Small Animal Hospital, University of Veterinary Medicine Hannover, Foundation, Bünteweg 9, D-30559 Hannover, Germany. [2]Small Animal Clinic, Faculty of Veterinary Medicine, National University of Colombia, Bogotá, Colombia. [3]Department of Orthopaedic Surgery, Hannover Medical School, Hanover, Germany. [4]Institute of Forming Technology and Machines, Leibniz University Hannover, Hannover, Germany.

References

1. Allen MJ. Advances in total joint replacement in small animals. J Small Anim Pract. 2012;53(9):495–506.
2. Guerrero TG, Montavon PM. Zurich cementless total hip replacement: retrospective evaluation of 2nd generation implants in 60 dogs. Vet Surg. 2009;38(1):70–80.
3. Torres BT, Budsberg SC. Revision of cemented total hip arthroplasty with cementless components in three dogs. Vet Surg. 2009;38(1):81–6.
4. Ganz SM, Jackson J, VanEnkevort B. Risk factors for femoral fracture after canine press-fit cementless total hip arthroplasty. Vet Surg. 2010;39(6):688–95.
5. Hummel DW, Lanz OI, Werre SR. Complications of cementless total hip replacement. A retrospective study of 163 cases. Vet Comp Orthop Traumatol. 2010;23(6):424–32.
6. Yates GD, Wasik SM, Edwards GA. Femoral component failure in canine cemented total hip replacement: a report of two cases. Aust Vet J. 2010; 88(6):225–30.
7. Gemmill TJ, Pink J, Renwick A, Oxley B, Downes C, Roch S, McKee WM. Hybrid cemented/cementless total hip replacement in dogs: seventy-eight consecutive joint replacements. Vet Surg. 2011;40(5):621–30.
8. Minto BW, Brandão CVS, Pereira GJ, Campagnol D, Mamprim MJ, Padovani CR, Ranzani JJ. Modular hybrid total hip arthroplasty. Experimental study in dogs. Acta Vet Scand. 2011;53(1):46.
9. Olmstead ML, Hohn RB, Turner TM. A five-year study of 221 total hip replacements in the dog. J Am Vet Med Assoc. 1983;183(2):191–4.
10. Bergh MS, Gilley RS, Shofer FS, Kapatkin AS. Complications and radiographic findings following cemented total hip replacement: a retrospective evaluation of 97 dogs. Vet Comp Orthop Traumatol. 2006;19(3):172–9.
11. VanEnkevort BA, Markel MD, Manley PA. Alterations in bone remodeling in the femur after medullary reaming and cemented hip arthroplasty in dogs. Am J Vet Res. 1999;60(8):922–8.
12. Sundfeldt M, Carlsson LV, Johansson CB, Thomsen P, Gretzer C. Aseptic loosening, not only a question of wear: a review of different theories. Acta Orthop. 2006;77(2):177–97.
13. Lerch M, von der Haar-Tran A, Windhagen H, Behrens BA, Wefstaedt P, Stukenborg-Colsman CM. Bone remodelling around the Metha short stem in total hip arthroplasty: a prospective dual-energy X-ray absorptiometry study. Int Orthop. 2011;36(3):533–8.
14. Blake GM, Fogelman I. Technical principles of dual energy x-ray absorptiometry. Semin Nucl Med. 1997;27(3):210–28.
15. 921 WTRS. Prevention and management of osteoporosis. Geneva: World Health Organisation; 2003.
16. Chun KJ. Bone densitometry. Semin Nucl Med. 2011;41(3):220–8.
17. Gruen TA, McNeice GM, Amstutz HC. "Modes of failure" of cemented stem-type femoral components: a radiographic analysis of loosening. Clin Orthop Relat Res. 1979;141:17–27.
18. Fitzpatrick N, Law AY, Bielecki M, Girling S. Cementless total hip replacement in 20 juveniles using BFX arthroplasty. Vet Surg. 2014;43(6): 715–25.
19. Mostafa AA, Druen S, Nolte I, Wefstaedt P. Radiographic evaluation of early periprosthetic femoral bone contrast and prosthetic stem alignment after uncemented and cemented total hip replacement in dogs. Vet Surg. 2011; 41(1):69–77.
20. Marcellin-Little DJ, DeYoung BA, Doyens DH, DeYoung DJ. Canine uncemented porous-coated anatomic total hip arthroplasty: results of a long-term prospective evaluation of 50 consecutive cases. Vet Surg. 1999; 28(1):10–20.
21. Vaccaro C, Busetto R, Bernardini D, Anselmi C, Zotti A. Accuracy and precision of computer-assisted analysis of bone density via conventional and digital radiography in relation to dual-energy x-ray absorptiometry. Am J Vet Res. 2012;73(3):381–4.

22. Barr FJ, Kirberger RM. BSAVA Handbuch Bildgebende Diagnostik des muskuloskelettalen Systems bei Hund und Katze. 2009.
23. Martini F, Lebherz C, Mayer F, Leichtle U, Kremling E, Sell S. Precision of the measurements of periprosthetic bone mineral density in hips with a custom-made femoral stem. J Bone Joint Surg (Br). 2000;82(7):1065–71.
24. Lerch M, Kurtz A, Stukenborg-Colsman C, Nolte I, Weigel N, Bouguecha A, Behrens BA. Bone remodeling after total hip arthroplasty with a short stemmed metaphyseal loading implant: finite element analysis validated by a prospective DEXA investigation. J Orthop Res. 2012;30(11):1822–9.
25. Drost WT, Reese DJ, Hornof WJ. Digital radiography artifacts. Vet Radiol Ultrasound. 2008;49(s1):S48–56.

Skin asepsis protocols as a preventive measure of surgical site infections in dogs: chlorhexidine–alcohol versus povidone–iodine

Luís Belo[†], Isa Serrano[†], Eva Cunha, Carla Carneiro, Luis Tavares, L. Miguel Carreira and Manuela Oliveira[*] [iD]

Abstract

Background: Most of surgical site infections (SSI) are caused by commensal and pathogenic agents from the patient's microbiota, which may include antibiotic resistant strains. Pre-surgical asepsis of the skin is one of the preventive measures performed to reduce SSI incidence and also antibiotic resistance dissemination. However, in veterinary medicine there is no agreement on which biocide is the most effective.

The aim of this study was to evaluate the effectiveness of two pre-surgical skin asepsis protocols in dogs. A total of 46 animals were randomly assigned for an asepsis protocol with an aqueous solution of 7.5% povidone-iodine or with an alcoholic solution of 2% chlorhexidine. For each dog, two skin swab samples were collected at pre-asepsis and post-asepsis, for bacterial quantification by conventional techniques and isolation of methicillin-resistant species.

Results: Most samples collected at the post-asepsis did not present bacterial growth, both for the animals subjected to the povidone-iodine (74%) or to the chlorhexidine (70%) protocols. In only 9% of the cases a significant bacterial logarithmic reduction was not observed, indicating possible resistance to these agents. Also, the logarithmic reduction of the bacterial quantification from pre- and post-asepsis time, was not statistically different for povidone-iodine (6.51 ± 1.94 log10) and chlorhexidine (6.46 ± 2.62 log10) protocol.

From the 39% pre-asepsis swabs which showed bacterial growth in MRSA modified chromogenic agar medium, only one isolate was identified as *Staphylococcus aureus* and one as *S. epidermidis*. False positives were mainly other staphylococci species, as well as Enterobacteriaceae.

Conclusions: Pre-surgical skin asepsis protocols with povidone-iodine or chlorhexidine showed similar efficacy in the elimination of methicillin resistant bacteria and preventing surgical site infections in dogs undergoing surgery.

Keywords: Asepsis, Antimicrobial resistance, Chlorhexidine, Dogs, Povidone-iodine, Skin infection, *Staphylococci*, MRSA, MRSP, Pre-surgery

Background

Surgical site infections (SSI) are the most common type of medical-related infection in developing countries, and the second most frequent type in Europe and the United States [1]. These infections remain a significant cause of morbidity and mortality worldwide, being responsible for significant healthcare costs [1, 2]. Since most SSI are caused by microorganisms from the commensal microbiota of the patient, it is important to perform and ensure efficient pre-surgical skin asepsis [3]. With the aim of standardize pre-, intra- and post- surgical procedures to prevent surgical site infections in human medicine, some guidelines were recently developed [1, 2]. The World Health Organization (WHO) as well The Center for Disease Control and Prevention (CDC) recommended the use of alcohol-based agents for the skin asepsis of patients undergoing surgery [1, 2].

* Correspondence: moliveira@fmv.ulisboa.pt

[†]Equal contributors

Centre for Interdisciplinary Research in Animal Health (CIISA) / Faculty of Veterinary Medicine, University of Lisbon, Avenida da Universidade Técnica, 1300-477 Lisbon, Portugal

In veterinary medicine there is no agreement on which biocide has the greatest efficacy in reducing the skin microbiota, aiming at preventing SSI development [4–6]. In addition, different skin asepsis protocols may be adopted according to the location of surgery in dogs [7–9]. For instance, in bitches undergoing ovariohysterectomy, 0.3% stabilized glutaraldehyde and alcohol (SG + A), 0.3% SG and water, and 4% chlorhexidine gluconate tincture revealed to be equally effective [8].

Due to their commensal and opportunistic nature, staphylococci are the main bacterial agents isolated from surgical site infections in dogs [10], being *Staphylococcus pseudintermedius* the most frequent [11]. *S. pseudintermedius* is commensal in dogs, whereas *S. aureus* is commensal in humans, and the presence of *S. aureus* on dogs have a human origin. It is also important to refer that in the last decade there has been a rapid emergence of infections by methicillin-resistant *S. pseudintermedius* (MRSP) in dogs and cats [3]. There is a great concern about MRSP, which is the main cause of surgical site infections in some regions and its treatment is greatly hampered by the high levels of antimicrobial resistance [12]. Due to its high resistance levels, the incidence of MRSP is an even more relevant problem than methicillin-resistant *S. aureus* (MRSA) [10]. Also, although *S. aureus* is also isolated from SSI, its occurrence is less frequent [10].

To date, studies comparing different pre-surgical skin asepsis protocols with application in veterinary medicine are scarce. Therefore, it is vital to clarify which is the most efficient protocol for preventing bacterial growth and the dissemination of multiresistant pathogenic bacteria, such as MRSP and MRSA.

The aim of this study was to evaluate two pre-surgical skin asepsis protocols as a preventive measure of SSI in dogs, namely an aqueous solution of 7.5% povidone-iodine or an alcoholic solution of 2% chlorhexidine. Povidone-iodine has an excellent immediate antimicrobial effect [13], whereas chlorhexidine is the most used biocide in antiseptic products, being more effective against gram-positive bacteria than gram-negative bacteria, fungi and viruses [14].

Methods
Samples
A total of 46 dogs presented for orthopedic or soft tissues surgery in several anatomical regions were included in this study. The group comprised 17 males and 29 females, aged between 7 months and 16.3 years (average ($\overline{X}$) ± standard deviation (δ) = 6.6 ± 4.3 years), and weights ranging between 1.8 kg and 38.2 kg (median ± interquartile range = 15.6 ± 13.0). All dogs included in the study performed pre-surgical exams, and those which laboratory standard tests results deviated from the reference values

were automatically excluded. Of the 46 canids, 23 were selected randomly and blindly for the evaluation of the 7.5% povidone-iodine asepsis protocol, and the remaining 23 for the evaluation of the 2% chlorhexidine. From each canid, one skin swab sample was collected before asepsis (t0), and the second post-asepsis (t1).

Post-surgical evaluation of all dogs was performed at 24 h and at day 30 (no implants applied) by the veterinary surgeon, to access the presence of SSI signs.

Pre-surgical skin asepsis protocols
With the patient already anesthetized with Propofol in lipid emulsion at 10 mg/mL (1–4 mg / kg i.v.), an area of 10 × 10 cm was delimited for sampling using a sterile dressing, after which the hair removal and removal of dirt from the surgical site were performed. The first sample (t0) was collected, performing a skin smear of the previously delimited area, with the aid of a swab (swabs with Amies transport medium) (VWR, Alfragide, Portugal). Subsequently, the biocide selected for the group to which the animal was allocated was applied over the area, using sterile 10 × 10 cm compresses.

A group of 23 animals was submitted to the asepsis protocol with an aqueous solution of 7.5% povidone-iodine (Braunol®) (B. Braun Medical, Lda, Queluz de Baixo, Portugal), followed by the application of Braunol® spray, and the other 23 animals were submitted to an asepsis protocol with an alcohol solution of 2% chlorhexidine gluconate (Desinclor® 2%) (Laboratorios Vaza, Madrid, Spain), followed by the application of 70% isopropyl alcohol spray. One minute after application of the biocide, a second smear of the delimited area (t1) was performed.

All swabs collected at the pre-asepsis were placed in test tubes with 1 mL of sterile saline, vortexed, and diluted (10 to 10^{-5}). From each dilution, 100 μL were collected and plated on Brain Heart Infusion agar (VWR, Alfragide, Portugal), a nonspecific enrichment culture medium, and incubated at 37 °C for 48 h. From the initial suspension, 100 μL were also plated on MRSA agar (CONDA laboratories - pronadisa, Madrid, Spain), a selective and differential chromogenic agar medium supplemented with cefoxitin, for the isolation of *S. aureus* and *S. epidermidis* after a 24–48 h incubation at 35 ± 2 °C.

Skin swabs collected at post-asepsis were also placed in test tubes with 1 mL of sterile saline, vortexed, and plated on BHI and MRSA agar.

After incubation, bacterial quantification was performed by determining the colony forming units in BHI agar at 24 h and 48 h, and also at 72 h in in the MRSA medium.

Colonies grown in MRSA agar were isolated on Columbia agar medium + 5% sheep blood (Biomérieux, Linda-a-Velha, Portugal) before microscopic observation after Gram staining and identification. Gram-positive cocci were further evaluated by catalase and potassium hydroxide (KOH) tests, and catalase-positive isolates were identified by API® Staph biochemical galleries (Biomérieux, Linda-a-Velha, Portugal). Gram-positive bacilli were evaluated by catalase and KOH tests (VWR, Lisbon, Portugal), and catalase-positive isolates were identified using API® Coryne. Gram-negative bacilli were submitted to the oxidase (VWR, Lisbon, Portugal) and KOH tests, and oxidase-negative isolates were identified through API® 20E galleries. Finally, gram-positive coccobacillus was plated onto Edwards and Slanetz and Bartley agar medium (VWR, Lisbon, Portugal) for presumptive identification of *Enterococcu*s spp.

Statistical analysis

The analysis of variance was performed using ANOVA with repeated measures. For statistical purposes, microbial quantifications in BHI culture medium were subsequently converted to base 10 logarithms, using the formula log10(CFU/mL + 1), allowing to include in the analysis all null quantifications at the post-asepsis time. Plates where quantification proved to be uncountable were considered as $> 10^9$ CFU / mL (> 9 log10).

Results

Distribution of dogs in the two groups subjected to the different pre-surgical skin asepsis protocols was similar regarding sex, age and weight, type of surgery, and previous exposure to antibiotic therapy and immunosuppressants (Table 1).

All surgically created wounds were clean, according to surgical wound classifications identified by CDC [15].

Bacterial quantification in BHI agar

Only 26% (6/23) of the animals submitted to the asepsis protocol with povidone-iodine, and 30% (7/23) of the ones submitted to the chlorhexidine protocol presented positive bacterial growth after incubation of the skin swab collected at post-asepsis.

Regarding bacterial load reduction between pre- and post-asepsis, only 4.3% (1/23) of the animals subjected

to povidone-iodine and 13% (3/23) subjected to chlorhexidine did not present a significant logarithmic reduction in bacterial quantification.

For the povidone-iodine protocol, the mean bacterial quantification at pre-asepsis was 8.03×10^7 CFU/mL and the log mean was 7.47 log10. The mean bacterial quantification at post-asepsis was 4.35×10^7 CFU/mL and the log mean was 0.95 log10. There was a decrease of $3.68X10^7$ CFU/mL between pre-asepsis and post-asepsis quantifications, and the logarithmic reduction was 6.51 ± 1.94 log10 (mean ± standard deviation) (Fig. 1).

For the chlorhexidine protocol, the mean bacterial quantification at pre-asepsis was 4.0×10^8 CFU/mL, and baseline log mean was 7.51 log10. The mean bacterial quantification at post-asepsis was 4.42×10^7 CFU/mL, and the log mean was 1.05 log10. There was a decrease of $3.56X10^8$ CFU/mL between pre-asepsis and post-asepsis quantifications, and the logarithmic reduction was 6.46 ± 2.62 log10 (Fig. 1).

Bacterial quantification in MRSA agar

Approximately 39% (18/46) of the samples corresponding to the pre-asepsis swabs showed bacterial growth in MRSA medium. Also, none of the swabs harvested at post-asepsis after the two protocols showed bacterial growth in this medium. Subsequently, isolates were identified, being observed that only one isolate was confirmed to be *S. aureus* and one isolate as *S. epidermidis*. The false positive cultures corresponded to other members of the genus *Staphylococcus* (*S. capitis*, *S. saprophyticus*, *S. xylosus* and *S. sciuri*) and of the Enterobacteriaceae family (*Enterobacter cloacae*, *Proteus* sp., *Klebsiella* sp., *Klebsiella pneumoniae* and *Serratia*

Table 1 Distribution of the animals included in this study ($n = 46$)

Canids features	A	B
Males (n)	8	9
Females (n)	15	14
Age (average in years)	6.62	6.65
Weight (average in Kg)	16.23	15.75
Orthopedic Surgery	5	5
Abdominal Surgery	15	9
Non-abdominal Surgery	3	9
Prophylactic antibiotic therapy	23	23

Animals distributed according to gender, age and weight average, type of surgery, prophylactic antibiotic therapy, between the two groups A (pre-asepsis protocol with povidone-iodine) and B (pre-asepsis protocol with chlorhexidine)

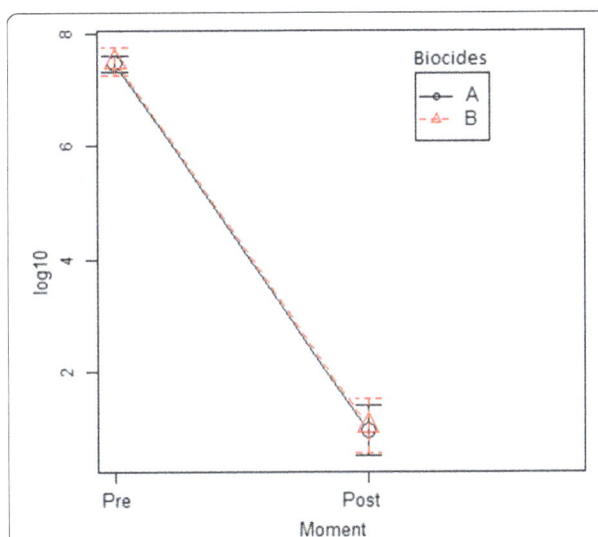

Fig. 1 Logarithmic reduction of the bacterial quantification at pre-asepsis and post-asepsis: The log reduction of the bacterial quantification between samples collected at pre-asepsis and post-asepsis using povidone-iodine (A) and chlorhexidine protocols (B)

sp.). *Corynebacterium pseudodiphteriticum*, *Cellulomonas* sp. and *Enterococcus* sp. were also found, and filamentous fungi were detected in one sample.

Statistics

Statistical analysis using ANOVA test with repeated measures showed that there was no significant difference between the logarithmic reduction of bacterial quantification relative to the pre- and post-asepsis in both groups (p value > 0.05) (Fig. 1), and the distribution curve of the log reductions was very similar for both agents (Fig. 2).

Discussion

A SSI is defined as a post-surgery infection in the incisional superficial or deep tissue, including organs, which occurs in the first 30 days after the procedure [15]. According to WHO, SSI are directly related with extended hospitalization and higher healthcare costs, as well as with increased morbidity and mortality rates, in both human and veterinary medicines [16, 17]. These infections can be a result of surgical bacterial contamination, with the animals' immune system and the bacteria virulence potential playing important roles in SSI development and severity [15]. In a surgical context, skin asepsis is one of the most important preventive measures of SSI, targeting the elimination or a major reduction of the skin transient microbiota, preventing its multiplication in the short term (i.e. hours) [6, 18].

In this study, the clear majority of the samples evaluated did not present positive bacterial growth, both for the swabs collected at post-asepsis either with povidone-iodine (74%) or with chlorhexidine (70%), evidencing that both protocols were generally efficient. It is known that the currently

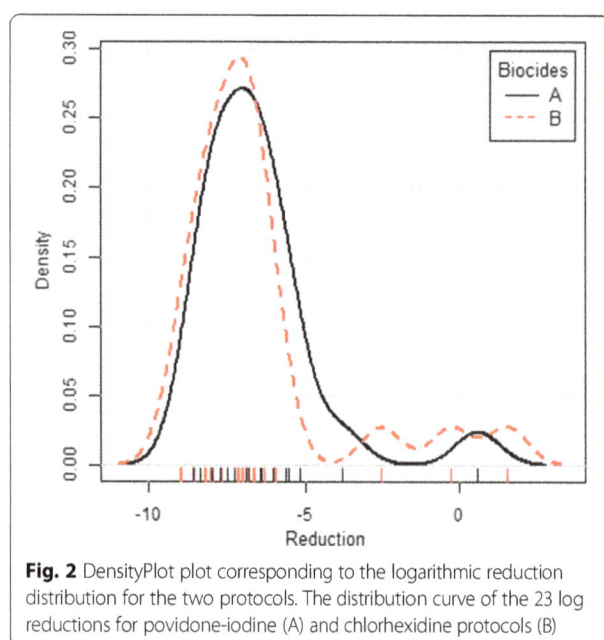

Fig. 2 DensityPlot plot corresponding to the logarithmic reduction distribution for the two protocols. The distribution curve of the 23 log reductions for povidone-iodine (A) and chlorhexidine protocols (B)

available antiseptic products cannot eliminate all the microorganisms present in the skin, and approximately 20% of the skin microbiota of small animals' remains protected in deeper strata and follicles, regardless of the asepsis protocol adopted [6]. As such, Food and Drug Administration (FDA) defines a skin disinfectant as a fast-acting agent with a broad spectrum of action and with persistent antiseptic power, capable of significantly reduce the number of microorganisms on intact skin [16].

Only approximately 9% of the samples did not present a significant logarithmic reduction relative to the bacterial quantification before and after asepsis, which may indicate resistance to antiseptic agents. These bacteria were isolated and cryopreserved for future characterization. To preserve the role of antiseptic agents in the control of infections, it is essential to prevent the emergence of bacteria resistant to these compounds, as well as cross resistance, promoting the appropriate use of these antimicrobial compounds [19].

Most pre-asepsis swabs (approximately 61%, 28/46 animals) and all post-asepsis swabs did not show bacterial growth in MRSA medium. Surprisingly, from the ones which allowed bacteria isolation, none of the isolate was identified as *S. pseudintermedius*, the most prevalent agent isolated from surgical site infections in dogs, and thus none MRSP was detected. Only one *S. aureus* and one *S. epidermidis* were detected in MRSA medium (4.3%, 2/46 animals). Therefore, only 4.3% animals had methicillin-resistant species. Chromogenic agar media are selective for MRSA and are widely used, since they are easy to interpret, although they may present false-positive results. Different authors have concluded that most false positives in MRSA media are staphylococci [20–22], but other microorganisms can be found, such as *Proteus*, *Corynebacterium* and *Micrococcus* [22]. Filamentous filaments fungi can also be isolated in chromogenic medium ChromID MRSA [20]. In accordance, in our study other bacterial species resistant to methicillin have grown in MRSA medium (34.8%, 16/46 animals), mainly other staphylococci as well as Enterobacteriaceae. According to Michael et al., 2015 [21], the use of a selective chromogenic agar medium was shown to be non-specific for the presumptive diagnosis of the presence of MRSA in canine skin. As such, the combined use of two selective media for MRSA or the combined use of other methods for identifying these agents should be performed, aiming at increasing detection specificity [21]. In the present study, Chapman agar was not used because our aim was studying the effect of biocides in methicillin-resistant species from clinical samples, and not in staphylococci in general. The use of blood agar was not considered for the same reason, and the use of MacConkey agar was discarded as staphylococci do not grow in this medium. MRSA medium results were confirmed by PCR, by detection of the *mecA* gene in all staphylococci performed as previously described [23], confirming the absence of methicillin-resistant bacterial species.

Although the sample size in this study is not high (46 dogs), it should not be neglected. No statistically significant differences ($p > 0.05$) were observed in the logarithmic reduction of the bacterial quantification between samples collected at pre-asepsis and post-asepsis times in both protocols (Figs. 1 and 2), allowing to conclude that the efficacy of both antiseptic solutions tested were similar. These results are in line with the ones of Osuna et al., 1990 [5], which compared three pre-surgical skin preparation protocols of dogs using povidone-iodine, 4% chlorhexidine gluconate with saline and 70% isopropyl alcohol rinse, and concluded that they were equally effective.

The combination of alcohol and chlorhexidine gluconate allows to combine the immediate antimicrobial effect of the alcohol to the effect of chlorhexidine, resulting in a superior antiseptic efficacy [24]. Likewise, the combination of isopropyl alcohol with an iodophor allows to obtain a product with immediate effectiveness, requiring a shorter application period when compared to the iodophors individually [25]. Although an alcoholic solution of povidone-iodine was not evaluated in this study, a previous work by Gibson et al., 1997 [4] had already concluded that a one-step iodophor skin preparation solution (0.7% available iodine in isopropyl alcohol - DuraPrep) was as effective in pre-surgical skin antisepsis as chlorhexidine gluconate solution followed by alcohol.

According to Cronquist et al., 2001 [26], the log means of bacteria on the skin of humans varies significantly between anatomical regions, being much lower than the one from the skin of canids. The differences in the bacterial load on the skin of dogs and humans may explain why in our study the mean log reduction in the skin bacterial load after application of either protocol is above that the one specified by the Tentative Final Monograph published by the FDA in 1994.

The higher mean of bacterial quantification in dogs' skin appears to be a greater challenge when compared to humans, since dogs have thicker coating, low hygiene frequency and contact with a more contaminated environment. Therefore, it is understandable that the techniques that are effective in humans may be less efficient in animals [4]. In fact, our results differ from the ones observed in human medicine, where it was concluded that alcoholic solutions of chlorhexidine had superior efficacy then povidone-iodine [27, 28], in accordance to WHO and CDC guidelines for human medicine [1, 2]. The different efficiency between biocides in human and veterinary settings allows to hypothesize that there is probably a limiting bacterial load, from which the presence of alcohol in skin asepsis protocols will not improve its efficacy for application to dogs.

Regarding SSI development, all animals in our study were examined by the veterinary surgeon 24 h and 30 days after surgery. Despite being previously stated that there is a high risk for SSI development if the skin

bacterial load at the surgery region is higher than 10^5 CFU/mL [15], in our study none of the animals developed SSI, revealing the efficiency of the prophylactic therapeutic protocols performed.

Conclusions

Studies on pre-surgical skin asepsis protocols with application in veterinary medicine are scarce, and the available protocols using povidone-iodine or chlorhexidine biocides are the two most frequently used in both human and veterinary surgery. According to our study, the use of 7.5% povidone-iodine or an alcoholic solution of 2% chlorhexidine appears to have similar efficacy in reducing the total load of skin bacteria, including methicillin-resistant bacterial species present on the skin and preventing surgical site infections in dogs undergoing surgery.

Abbreviations
CDC: Center for Disease Control and Prevention; FDA: Food and Drug Administration; MRSA: Methicillin-resistant *S. aureus*; MRSP: Methicillin-resistant *S. pseudintermedius*; SSI: Surgical site infections; WHO: World Health Organization

Acknowledgments
The authors want to thank to FCT and the CIISA - Centre for Interdisciplinary Research in AnimalHealth, Faculty of Veterinary Medicine, University of Lisbon, Portugal, for supporting this work, and to Veterinarian Surgeons from Anjos of Assis Veterinary Medicine Centre (CMVAA), Barreiro, Portugal, for the samples used in the present study. The authors would like to acknowledge Professor Telmo Nunes for his valuable help in the statistical analysis of the results.

Funding
This study was financed by the Fundação para a Ciência e a Tecnologia (FCT), Portugal (Project UID/CVT/00276/2013; Fellowship SFRH/BD/131384/2017), and CIISA - Centre for Interdisciplinary Research in Animal Health, Faculty of Veterinary Medicine, University of Lisbon, Portugal. The funding bodies had no role in the design of the study or collection, analysis, and interpretation of data or in writing the manuscript.

Authors' contributions
LB performed the experiments and analyzed the data. IS wrote the manuscript. EC participated in the experiments and helped to analyze the data. CC participated in the experiments. LT contributed to the analysis and interpretation of data and helped to draft and revise the manuscript. LC and MO conceived the study and participated in its coordination, helped to draft the manuscript and supervision throughout. All authors read and approved the final manuscript.

Author's information
LB – DVM. IS – MSc, PhD, Researcher at FMV. EC - DVM, Researcher at FMV. CC – MSc. LT - DVM, PhD, Full Professor at FMV. LC - DVM, PhD, Assistant Professor at FMV. MO – MSc, DVM, PhD, Assistant Professor at FMV.

Ethics approval and consent to participate
All animals were cared for according to the rules given by the current EU (Directive 2010/63/EC) and national (DL 113/2013) legislation and by the competent authority (Direção Geral de Alimentação e Veterinária, DGAV, www.dgv.min-agricultura.pt/portal/page/portal/DGV) in Portugal. Only non-invasive samples were collected during routine procedures with consent of owners, and no ethics committee approval was needed. Trained veterinarians obtained all the samples, following standard routine procedures. No animal experiment has been performed in the scope of this research. Verbal informed consent was obtained from all the owners. As some of the participants in the study are unaccustomed to deal with forms, all the necessary

information about the study was provided to all the participants before obtaining their consent.

Consent for publication
Not applicable.

Competing interests
The authors declare that they have no competing interests.

References
1. World Health Organization. In: *Global Guidelines for the Prevention of Surgical Site Infection.* edn. Geneva; 2016.
2. Berrios-Torres SI, Umscheid CA, Bratzler DW, Leas B, Stone EC, Kelz RR, Reinke CE, Morgan S, Solomkin JS, Mazuski JE, et al. Centers for disease control and prevention guideline for the prevention of surgical site infection, 2017. JAMA Surg. 2017;152(8):784–91.
3. Singh A, Walker M, Rousseau J, Weese JS. Characterization of the biofilm forming ability of *Staphylococcus pseudintermedius* from dogs. BMC Vet Res. 2013;9:93.
4. Gibson KL, Donald AW, Hariharan H, McCarville C. Comparison of two pre-surgical skin preparation techniques. Can J Vet Res. 1997;61(2):154–6.
5. Osuna DJ, DeYoung DJ, Walker RL. Comparison of three skin preparation techniques. Part 2: clinical trial in 100 dogs. Vet Surg. 1990;19(1):20–3.
6. Renberg WC. Preparation of the patient, operating team, and operating room for surgery. In: Tobias KM, Johnston SA, editors. Veterinary surgery small animal. St. Louis, USA: Elsevier Saunders; 2011. p. 164–9.
7. Neihaus SA, Hathcock TL, Boothe DM, Goring RL. Presurgical antiseptic efficacy of chlorhexidine diacetate and providone-iodine in the canine preputial cavity. J Am Anim Hosp Assoc. 2011;47(6):406–12.
8. Lambrechts NE, Hurter K, Picard JA, Goldin JP, Thompson PN. A prospective comparison between stabilized glutaraldehyde and chlorhexidine gluconate for preoperative skin antisepsis in dogs. Vet Surg. 2004;33(6):636–43.
9. Stubbs WP, Bellah JR, Vermaas-Hekman D, Purich B, Kubilis PS. Chlorhexidine gluconate versus chloroxylenol for preoperative skin preparation in dogs. Vet Surg. 1996;25(6):487–94.
10. Verwilghen D, Singh A. Fighting surgical site infections in small animals: are we getting anywhere? Vet Clin North Am Small Anim Pract. 2015;45(2):243–76.
11. Sasaki T, Kikuchi K, Tanaka Y, Takahashi N, Kamata S, Hiramatsu K. Reclassification of phenotypically identified *Staphylococcus intermedius* strains. J Clin Microbiol. 2007;45(9):2770–8.
12. Stull JW, Weese JS. Hospital-associated infections in small animal practice. Vet Clin North Am Small Anim Pract. 2015;45(2):217–33.
13. Capriotti K, Capriotti JA. Topical iodophor preparations: chemistry, microbiology, and clinical utility. Dermatol Online J. 2012;18(11):1.
14. Karpinski TM, Szkaradkiewicz AK. Chlorhexidine-pharmaco-biological activity and application. Eur Rev Med Pharmacol Sci. 2015;19(7):1321–6.
15. Mangram AJ, Horan TC, Pearson ML, Silver LC, Jarvis WR. Guideline for Prevention of Surgical Site Infection, 1999. Centers for Disease Control and Prevention (CDC) hospital infection control practices advisory committee. Am J Infect Control. 1999;27(2):97–132. quiz 133-134; discussion 196
16. World Health Organization. In: *WHO Guidelines for Safe Surgery* 2009: Safe Surgery Saves Lives edn Geneva; 2009.
17. Turk R, Singh A, Weese JS. Prospective surgical site infection surveillance in dogs. Vet Surg. 2015;44(1):2–8.
18. Anderson ME, Foster BA, Weese JS. Observational study of patient and surgeon preoperative preparation in ten companion animal clinics in Ontario, Canada. BMC Vet Res. 2013;9:194.
19. European Commission: Scientific committee on emerging and newly identified health risks. Assessment of the Antibiotic Resistance Effects of Biocides 2009. http://ec.europa.eu/health/ph_risk/committees/04_scenihr/docs/scenihr_o_021.pdf
20. Van Hoecke F, Deloof N, Claeys G. Performance evaluation of a modified chromogenic medium, ChromID MRSA new, for the detection of
21. methicillin-resistant *Staphylococcus aureus* from clinical specimens. Eur J Clin Microbiol Infect Dis. 2011;30(12):1595–8.
22. Micheel V, Hogan B, Koller T, Warnke P, Crusius S, Hinz R, Hagen RM, Schwarz NG, Frickmann H. Screening agars for MRSA: evaluation of a stepwise diagnostic approach with two different selective agars for the screening for methicillin-resistant *Staphylococcus aureus* (MRSA). Mil Med Res. 2015;2:18.
23. Nahimana I, Francioli P, Blanc DS. Evaluation of three chromogenic media (MRSA-ID, MRSA-select and CHROMagar MRSA) and ORSAB for surveillance cultures of methicillin-resistant *Staphylococcus aureus*. Clin Microbiol Infect. 2006;12(12):1168–74.
24. Mottola C, Semedo-Lemsaddek T, Mendes JJ, Melo-Cristino J, Tavares L, Cavaco-Silva P, Oliveira M. Molecular typing, virulence traits and antimicrobial resistance of diabetic foot staphylococci. J Biomed Sci. 2016;23:33.
25. Paulson, D.S.: Introduction to topical antimicrobials and their applications. In: Handbook of topical antimicrobials: Industrial applications in consumer products and pharmaceuticals D S Paulson (Ed) New York, USA: Marcel Dekker, Inc Segal & Anderson; 2002: 11–27.
26. Segal CG, Anderson JJ. Preoperative skin preparation of cardiac patients. AORN J. 2002;76(5):821–8.
27. Cronquist AB, Jakob K, Lai L, Della Latta P, Larson EL. Relationship between skin microbial counts and surgical site infection after neurosurgery. Clin Infect Dis. 2001;33(8):1302–8.
28. Darouiche RO, Wall MJ Jr, Itani KM, Otterson MF, Webb AL, Carrick MM, Miller HJ, Awad SS, Crosby CT, Mosier MC, et al. Chlorhexidine-alcohol versus povidone-iodine for surgical-site antisepsis. N Engl J Med. 2010;362(1):18–26.
29. Hibbard JS. Analyses comparing the antimicrobial activity and safety of current antiseptic agents: a review. J Infus Nurs. 2005;28(3):194–207.

Diagnosis and surgical management of malignant ovarian teratoma in a green iguana (*Iguana iguana*)

Lucia Bel[1], Marco Tecilla[2], Gabriel Borza[3], Cosmin Pestean[4], Robert Purdoiu[5], Ciprian Ober[6*], Liviu Oana[6] and Marian Taulescu[3]

Abstract

Background: Ovarian tumors in reptiles are uncommonly reported in the literature and for green iguanas previously reported cases include teratomas, one adenocarcinoma and one papillary cystadenocarcinoma. The present report is the first of a malignant ovarian teratoma in a green iguana. Complete and detailed pathological features, differential diagnosis and surgical management of malignant ovarian teratoma are discussed in this paper.

Case Presentation: A 9-year-old intact female green iguana (*Iguana iguana*) with a clinical history of persistent anorexia and progressive abdominal distension was referred to the surgery department. On physical examination, a presumptive diagnosis of follicular stasis was established. Radiographic evaluation showed a large radioopaque mass within the abdomen, which was visible both in latero-lateral and ventro-dorsal exposures. Abdominal ultrasonography showed a large intra-abdominal mass, with numerous cyst-like structures filled with liquid and a heterogeneous aspect with hypoechoic areas. Exploratory laparatomy was thus suggested and the mass was removed surgically. The histologic findings of the neoplasm were consistent with those of ovarian malignant teratoma. Surgical excision of the mass in our case was considered curative and after a follow-up period of 6 months the animal has recovered completely.

Conclusions: A malignant ovarian teratoma has not been previously reported in green iguana and should be included in the list of differential diagnosis of ovarian tumors in this species. This report will contribute to a better understanding of the pathology of this rare tumor in green iguanas.

Keywords: Green iguana, Ovarian malignant teratoma, Pathology, Reptile, Surgery

Background

In domestic mammals, primary ovarian tumors are classified into 3 different categories based on the embryological cell of origin of the predominating neoplastic cell: epithelial tumors (adenocarcinoma and adenoma), germ cell tumors (dysgerminomas and teratomas), and sex cord tumors (GCT, thecoma, granulosa-theca cell, and luteoma) [1].

Ovarian neoplasms have been reported in different species including reptiles [2–4], but among them malignant teratomas are reported as rare. Previously reported ovarian tumors in green iguanas, include teratomas [5, 6], one adenocarcinoma [7], and one papillary cystadenocarcinoma [4].

Teratoma is a gonadal germ cell tumour that predominantly occurs in the gonads: the testis and ovaries [8]. The tumor is based on primordial germ cells from the top cell layer of the blastocyst. From this arise the ectodermal, mesodermal and endodermal germ cell layers [9]. The content of teratomas is complex, reflecting their heterogeneity of germ-cell origin. Neural tissue, woven bone, hyaline cartilage, hair follicles, sebaceous and apocrine glands, respiratory epithelium and adipose tissue have all been reported in animals [10–12]. These histological elements are either seen in associations that resemble normal organs or intermingled haphazardly [13].

* Correspondence: ciprian.ober@usamvcluj.ro
[6]Department of Surgical Techniques, University of Agricultural Sciences and Veterinary Medicine, 3-5 Mănăştur Street, Cluj-Napoca 400372, Romania
Full list of author information is available at the end of the article

Teratomas are classified as benign (mature) or malignant (immature) depending on the degree of anaplasia or the presence of undifferentiated elements resembling those of the embryo [14]. Moreover, the term teratocarcinoma is used only for malignant tumors, which are malignant by virtue of the continued presence of stem cells-the embryonal carcinoma (EC) cells [15].

The current report is the first of a malignant ovarian teratoma in a green iguana. Pathological features, differential diagnosis and surgical management of malignant ovarian teratoma are also discussed in this paper.

Case Presentation

In February 2015, a 9 year old Green Iguana (*Iguana iguana*) was presented for consult with a history of 3 weeks anorexia and a distended abdomen (Fig. 1a). Prior to the consult the patient was believed to be a male and was diagnosed with coprostasis. After the initial examination, a presumptive diagnosis of follicular stasis was made, due to the fact that the patient was in fact a female. Blood was collected from the ventral coccygeal vein for hematological and biochemistry evaluation, with no significant alterations. Both a full body radiographs and an abdominal ultrasound were performed. Radiographic evaluation showed a large radiopaque intra-abdominal mass, that was visible both in latero-lateral and ventro-dorsal exposure (Fig. 1b).

The abdominal ultrasound examination was performed using a Mind Ray DC-6 ultrasound device with a linear probe of 7.5–10 MHz. The 7.5 MHz frequency was enough to highlight the abdominal modification. B-Mode abdominal ultrasonography showed a large mass into the coelomic cavity (Fig. 1c1), with numerous cyst-like structures filled with liquid. On ultrasound, the coelomic cavity was partially filled by liquid surrounding an approximatelly 2.5 × 1.5 cm (Fig. 1c2) hypoechoic mass on the lateral right side and fully formed eggs on the left side. Exploratory laparatomy was thus suggested.

Prior to surgery, meloxicam (Metacam®, Boehringer Ingelheim, Germany) at 0.2 mg/kg and butorphanol (Butomidor®, Richter Pharma ag, Austria) at 1 mg/kg were administered in the musculature of the right thoracic limb. After the intravenous induction of anesthesia with alphaxalone (Alfaxan®, Vetoquinol, France) at 15 mg/kg, the animal was intubated using a 3.5 endotracheal tube and was kept on IPPV ventilation, using Isoflurane 1–1.5 % (Anesteran®, Rompharm Company SRL, Romania) and 0.6 l/min air.

The laparatomy was performed using a paramedian craniocaudal incision. Egg yolk content was present in the coelomic cavity (Fig. 1d, e), probably due to the massages that were performed while the animal was presumably coprostatic. After a more thorough examination, a large mass was identified on the left ovary. This mass

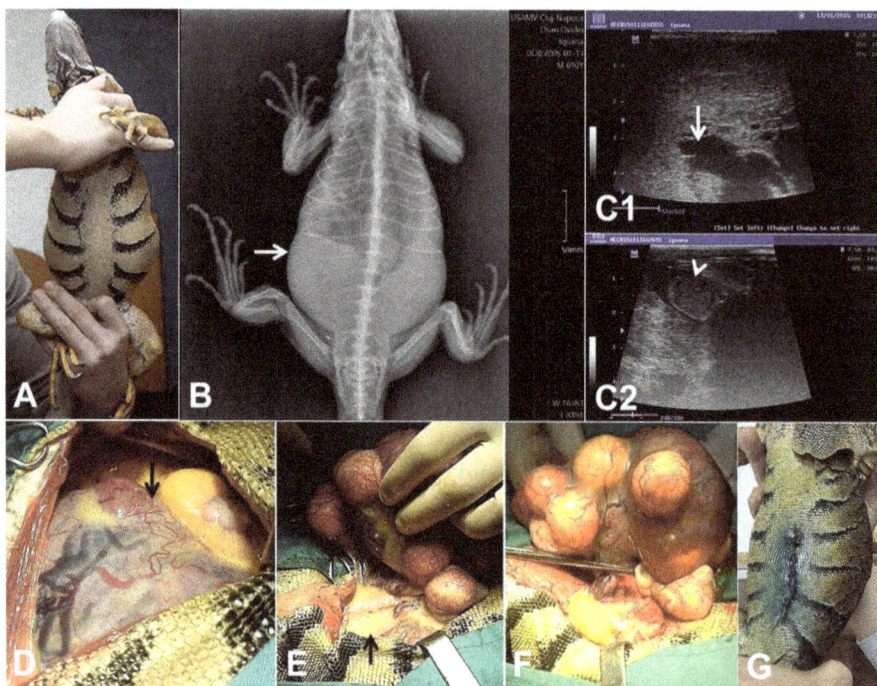

Fig. 1 Clinical aspects and surgical management of ovarian teratocarcinoma in Green Iguana. **a** The iguana presenting a marked abdominal distension. **b** Ventro-dorsal radiologic appearance. Note the distended abdomen (arrow). **c1** Ultrasonography showing a large mass inside the abdomen, with cyst like structures filled with liquid. **c2** A round hypoechoic mass of approximately 2.5/1.5 cm surrounded by liquid was identified by ultrasonography. **d** and **e**) Egg yolk content present in the coelomic cavity. **f** Excision of the left ovary. **g** Final aspect of the surgery

was then removed, after clamping (Fig. 1f) and ligating the mezovarium vessels with monofilament suture material (Polidioxanone® 3.0, BioSintex, Romania). Ovariectomy of the right ovary was then performed and both the mass and the ovary were submitted for histological analysis. Warm saline lavage was used to remove as much yolk leakage as possible and the abdominal muscles were sutured in a simple interrupted pattern using 3.0 polidioxanone. Skin was closed in a vertical pattern using 3.0 monofilament non absorbable suture material (Nylon®, BioSintex, Romania) (Fig. 1g).

Postoperative, the iguana received 20 mg/kg cephtazidime (Fortum®, GlaxoSmithKline, UK) every 72 h, 10 administrations, 0.2 mg/kg meloxicam every 48 h, 4 administration and oral fluid therapy. Several days after surgery the animal was offered food, but refused to eat, and Emeraid Herbivore® Critical Care was administered. One month after surgery a biochemical recheck was done, using Avian/Reptile profile (Abaxis, Germany) proving no significant alterations and the patient was discharged after the removal of the skin suture. 6 months after surgery, the animal has recovered completely. An abdominal ultrasound was performed, with no evidence of regrowth.

Grossly, rising from the left ovary, a well-demarcated mass expanding and compressing the surrounding vitellogenic follicles was present. The mass was 9 × 8.5cm in size, with a gray to reddish color and a weight of 340 g compared with the right ovary (203 g). The mass was surrounded by a variably thick, smooth and well vascularized capsule originating from outer layer of the ovary. On section, the neoplastic structure showed multiple necrotic and haemorrhagic areas and variably in size cystic filled cavities containing reddish to brownish fluid (Fig. 2a).

For histological examination, samples from the neoplastic mass were fixed in 10 % phosphate buffered formalin for 24 h, embedded in paraffin wax, cut into 3–5 µm sections, and stained with hematoxylin and eosin.

Histologically, the neoplasm was composed by elements of all germ cell layers (endoderm, mesoderm and ectoderm), haphazardly arranged within the mass. I) Endoderm: Two different epithelial populations were present in the sample. The first one was composed by pleomorphic epithelial cells arranged in cords and islets, multifocally circumscribing variable in size cysts filled with a pale eosinophilic and globous material (proteinaceous material) (Fig. 2b). The cells were cuboidal to polygonal or oval, 30 to 40µm in width, with indistinct cells borders and with an intermediate to high nucleocytoplasmic (N/C) ratio. The cytoplasm was moderate in amount, clear and with multiple and variable in size

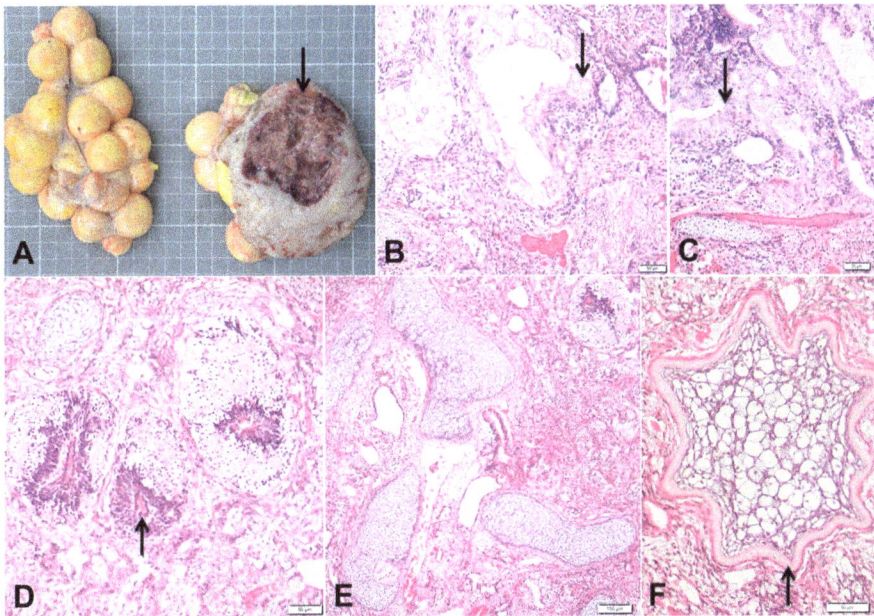

Fig. 2 Pathological features of ovarian malignant teratoma in Green Iguana. **a** The neoplastic mass showing multiple necrotic and haemorrhagic areas and variably in size cystic filled cavities containing reddish to brownish fluid. **b** Histologic section of the teratoma showing epithelial cells arranged in cords and islet, multifocally circumscribing variable in size cysts filled with a pale eosinophilic and globous material (proteinaceous material). Hematoxylin and eosin (H&E) stain. Bar = 50µm. **c** Epithelial population organized in acini and tubules lined by 1 to 7 layers of cells. H&E stain. Bar = 50µm. **d** Small and round islet of nervous tissue, characterized by a central channel surrounded by a concentric layer of epithelial cells and abundant neuropil. H&E stain. Bar = 50µm. **e** Neoplastic tissue composed by normal and mature cartilage tissue. H&E stain. Bar = 1000µm. **f** Islets of chondrocytes focally surrounded by a thin layer of mature bone tissue. H&E stain. Bar = 50µm

eosinophilic and amorphous granules. The nuclei were large, central to paracentral with a vesicular chromatin and a single nucleolus. Anisokaryosis and anysocytosis were severe with karyomegaly and moderate numbers of mitotic figures. Cytological characteristics were compatible with atypical granulosa cells. Multifocally, admixed to the neoplastic granulosa cells, numerous polygonal cells of 10–12 µm in diameter, with a pale and homogeneous eosinophilic cytoplasm and a small, round and central nucleus were identified (intermediate cells of the follicle wall).

The second epithelial population was organized in acini and tubules lined by 1 to 7 layers of cells (Fig. 2c). The cells were cuboidal to cylindrical, 10–15 µm in diameter, with indistinct cells border and with an intermediate N/C ratio. The cytoplasm was moderate, pale eosinophilic, homogeneous and with an apical brush border. The nuclei were large, round to oval with lacy reticular chromatin. Randomly, a single 2–4 µm in width, eosinophilic nucleolus was detected. Anisokaryosis and anysocytosis were moderate and mitoses were also rare. The lumen of the acini was partially filled with mucus. These epithelial structures could have corresponding to tissue from the respiratory or the genital tract. Multiple small areas of necrosis within the epithelial cell population were identified. II) Ectoderm: A lesser part of the tumor was composed by small and round islet of nervous tissue, characterized by a central channel surrounded by a concentric layer of epithelial cells (ependymal channel) and abundant neuropil (Fig. 2d). III) Mesoderm: Remaining neoplastic tissue was composed by mature hyaline cartilage (Fig. 2e), organized in variably in size islets of chondrocytes focally surrounded by a thin layer of mature bone (Fig. 2f) and scattered foci of striated muscle tissue. All mesenchymal tissues were well differentiated.

According to the largest retrospective publication to date regarding the prevalence of neoplasia in reptiles [16], the tumors are most frequently in snakes, followed by lizards, chelonians, and crocodilians.

Although most gonadal [6] and extragonadal teratomas [12] from animals are benign, malignant teratomas have also been recorded [17]. Histologically, malignant teratomas contain less well-differentiated embryonal elements in addition to mature structures, increased cellular atypia [13] and numerous mitotic figures [17]. Multicentric growth secondary to direct implantation or distant metastases represent other features of malignant teratoma [18]. In the present case, only the endodermal layer showed characteristic features of malignancy characterized by cellular atypia, anysokariosis, karyomegaly, mitoses and necrosis.

Yolk coeliomitis may be the result of yolks being released from the reproductive tract into coelomic cavity or rupture of follicles while still on the ovary [19]. In our case, yolk coeliomitis was caused by rupture of the follicles due to the pressure put on the abdomen while there was a coprostasis suspition.

Iguana ovarian tissue is diffuse and intimately associated with the vena cava and adrenal gland and this makes oophorectomy technically challenging. If the procedure is incomplete, even small remnants will regrow and folliculogenesis will develop [3]. The use of hemostatic clips and microsurgical instruments in complete ovarian removal in reptiles [20] is well known.

In this reported case the bilateral oophorectomy was performed using microsurgical instruments and monofilament absorbable suture material.

Six months later, the patient has recovered completely with no signs of ovarian regrowth.

Conclusions

To our knowledge, this is the first reported case of malignant ovarian teratoma described antemortem in green iguana (*Iguana iguana*). In our opinion the condition should be included in the list of differential diagnosis of ovarian and other intra-abdominal tumors in this species.

Abbreviations
GCT, granulosa cell tumor

Funding
This paper was published under the frame of European Social Fund, Human Resources Development Operational Programme 2007–2013, project no. POSDRU/159/1.5/S/136893.

Authors' contributions
LB performed the surgery and helped to draft the manuscript. MTe performed the data analysis and interpretation. GB and MTa carried out the histopathological data analysis and revised the manuscript. CP carried out the anesthesia. RP performed diagnostic imaging examination and participated in the manuscript design. CO participated in the design of the study and drafted the manuscript. LO helped in case surgical management and revised the manuscript. All authors read and approved the final manuscript.

Competing interests
The authors declare that they have no competing interests.

Consent for publication
Not applicable.

Author details
[1]Department of Surgery, University of Agricultural Sciences and Veterinary Medicine, 3-5 Mănăştur Street, Cluj-Napoca 400372, Romania. [2]Department of Veterinary Sciences and Public Health, University of Milan, Milan, Italy. [3]Department of Veterinary Pathology, University of Agricultural Sciences and Veterinary Medicine, 3-5 Mănăştur Street, Cluj-Napoca 400372, Romania. [4]Department of Anesthesiology and Intensive Care, University of Agricultural

Sciences and Veterinary Medicine, 3-5 Mănăştur Street, Cluj-Napoca 400372, Romania. [5]Department of Radiology, University of Agricultural Sciences and Veterinary Medicine, 3-5 Mănăştur Street, Cluj-Napoca 400372, Romania. [6]Department of Surgical Techniques, University of Agricultural Sciences and Veterinary Medicine, 3-5 Mănăştur Street, Cluj-Napoca 400372, Romania.

References

1. MacLachlan NJ, Kennedy PC. Tumors of the genital system. In: Meuten DJ, editor. Tumors in domestic animals. Ames: Iowa State Press; 2002. p. 547–75.
2. Petterino C, Bedin M, Podestá G, Ratto A. Undifferentiated tumor in the ovary of a corn snake (Elaphe guttata guttata). Vet Clin Pathol. 2006;35:95–100.
3. Cruz Cardona JA, Conley KJ, Wellehan JF, Farina LL, Origgi FC, Wamsley HL. Incomplete ovariosalpingectomy and subsequent malignant granulosa cell tumor in a female green iguana (Iguana iguana). J Am Vet Med Assoc. 2011;239:237–42.
4. Stacy BA, Vidal JD, Osofsky A, Terio K, Koski M, De Cock HE. Ovarian papillary cystadenocarcinomas in a green iguana (Iguana iguana). J Comp Pathol. 2004;130:223–8.
5. Anderson NL, Williams J, Sagartz JE, Barnewall R. Ovarian Teratoma in a Green Iguana (Iguana iguana). J Zoo Wildl Med. 1996;27:90–5.
6. Levine B. Treatment of a malignant ovarian teratoma in a green iguana (Iguana iguana). Exotic DVM. 2004;6:12–4.
7. Gibbons P, Schiller C. What's your diagnosis: ovarian adenocarcinoma in a green iguana (Iguana iguana). J Herpetol Med Surg. 2000;10:34–8.
8. Wein AJ, Kavoussi LR, Novick AC, Partin AW, Peters CA. Campbell-Walsh Urology. 10th ed. Philadelphia: Saunders; 2012.
9. Patterson-Kane JC, Schulman FY, Santiago N, McKinney L, Davis CJ. Mixed germ cell tumor in the eye of a dog. Vet Pathol. 2001;38:712–4.
10. Miyoshi N, Yasuda N, Kamimura Y, Shinozaki M, Shimizu T. Teratoma in a feline unilateral cryptorchid testis. Vet Pathol. 2001;38:729–30.
11. Sato T, Hontake S, Shibuya H, Shirai W, Yamaguchi T. A solid mature teratoma of a feline ovary. J Feline Med Surg. 2003;5:349–51.
12. Ober CA, Taulescu M, Oana L, Bel L, Cătoi C, Fărcas L, Pestean C. An unusual case of a mature teratoma on the left perineal region of a young cat: surgical treatment and pathological description. Acta Vet Scand. 2013;55:51.
13. Nielsen SW, Kennedy PC. Tumors of the genital systems. In: Moulton JE, editor. Tumors in domestic animals. 3rd ed. Los Angeles: University of California Press; 1990. p. 489–91.
14. Klein MK. Tumors of the female reproductive system. In: Withrow SJ, MacEwen EG, editors. Small animal clinical oncology. 2nd ed. Philadelphia: Saunders; 1989. p. 347–55.
15. Damjanov I. Teratocarcinoma: neoplastic lessons about normal embryogenesis. Int J Dev Biol. 1993;37:39–46.
16. Garner MM, Hernandez-Divers SM, Raymond JT. Reptile neoplasia: a retrospective study of case submissions to a specialty diagnostic service. Vet Clin North Am Exot Anim Pract. 2004;7:653–71.
17. Newman SJ, Brown CJ, Patnaik AK. Malignant ovarian teratoma in a red-eared slider (Trachemys scripta elegans). J Vet Diagn Invest. 2003;15:77–81.
18. Trasti SL, Schlafer DH. Theriogenology question of the month. Malignant teratoma of the ovary. J Am Vet Med Assoc. 1999;214:785–6.
19. Mader DR. Reptile Medicine and Surgery. 2nd ed. Philadelphia: Saunders; 2006.
20. Lock BA. Reproductive surgery in reptiles. Vet Clin North Am Exot Anim Pract. 2000;3:733–52.

Evaluation of chemical castration with calcium chloride versus surgical castration in donkeys: testosterone as an endpoint marker

Ahmed Ibrahim[1*], Magda M. Ali[1], Nasser S. Abou-Khalil[2] and Marwa F. Ali[3]

Abstract

Background: For the last few years, researchers have been interested in developing a method for chemical sterilization which may be a better alternative to surgical castration. An ideal chemical sterilant would be one that effectively arrests spermatogenesis and androgenesis as well as libido with absence of toxic or other side effects. Calcium chloride in various solutions and concentrations has been tested in many animal species, but few studies have been evaluated it in equines as a chemical sterilant. So, the objective of this study was to evaluate the clinical efficacy of chemical castration with 20 % calcium chloride dissolved in absolute ethanol in comparison with surgical castration in donkeys based on the changes in the serum testosterone level and the histopathological changes in treated testes.

Methods: Twelve clinically healthy adult male donkeys were used in this study. Donkeys were divided randomly and equally into two groups: a surgical (S) group ($n = 6$) and a chemical (C) group ($n = 6$). Animals in the (S) group were subjected to surgical castration while those in the (C) group received a single bilateral intratesticular injection of 20 % calcium chloride dissolved in absolute ethanol (20 ml/testis). Animals were kept under clinical observation for 60 days. Changes in animals' behavior and gross changes in external genitalia were monitored daily. Serum concentrations of testosterone were measured prior to treatment and at 15, 30, 45 and 60 days post-treatment. Testicles in the (C) group were examined histopathologically at the end of the experiment.

Results: Chemical castration with intratesticular calcium chloride vs. surgical castration failed to reduce serum concentrations of testosterone throughout the whole duration of the study; however it induced orchitis that was evident by focal necrotic areas in seminiferous tubules, cellular infiltration of neutrophils, proliferative intertubular fibrosis with a compensatory proliferation of Leydig cells. Donkeys tolerated the intratesticular injection of calcium chloride. There were no detectable changes in the general health status of the animals with the exception of swelling in external genitalia, scrotal ulcerations and fistulas. Food and water consumption and the gait of animals remained unaffected.

Conclusion: Intratesticular calcium chloride can't be considered an effective method for chemical castration in donkeys.

Keywords: Calcium chloride, Chemical castration, Testosterone, Donkeys

* Correspondence: elgrah38@gmail.com
[1]Department of Surgery, Anesthesiology and Radiology, Faculty of veterinary medicine, Assuit University, Assuit 70155, Egypt
Full list of author information is available at the end of the article

Background

Castration is one of the most common equine surgical procedures and is usually performed to sterilize animals unsuitable for the genetic pool and to eliminate masculine behavior. Orchitis, epididymitis, testicular neoplasia, hydrocele, varicocele, testicular damage caused by trauma, torsion of the spermatic cord, or inguinal herniation may necessitate orchidectomy [1].

For many years, surgical castration has been considered a standard gold tool for sterilization of male animals. However, several drawbacks have been associated with this procedure such as high cost, time consumption, need for postoperative care and management, risk of post-operative complications, small-scale application, the requirement of anesthesia, medical equipment, a sterile surgical suite, a trained veterinarian, recovery time, and incision site observation [2–4].

For the last few years, researchers have been interested in developing a method for chemical castration which may be a better alternative to surgical one [2]. Different agents have been used for non-surgical chemical sterilization in domestic animals. These include intratesticular injection of cadmium chloride [5], ferric chloride and ferrous sulfate [6], glycerol [7], lactic acid [8] and calcium chloride [9]. An ideal chemical sterilizing agent would be one that effectively arrests spermatogenesis and androgenesis as well as libido with absence of toxic or other side effects [7].

Advantages of chemical castration are apparent reduction in pain and stress as well as elimination of hemorrhage, hernia, infection, myiasis and other surgical sequelae. It is also suited for mass-scale sterilization, simple and inexpensive [10].

Intratesticular injection of calcium chloride has been applied to a variety of animal species including rats [3, 4], dogs [2, 11–13], cats [14], goats [15, 16] and bulls [10, 17, 18], in a variety of formulations and concentrations. Calcium chloride has been found to cause atrophy of the seminiferous tubules and reduce circulating concentrations of testosterone and sperm counts in a dose-dependent manner in male dogs [2].

The aim of the present study was to evaluate the clinical efficacy of chemical castration with intratesticular 20 % calcium chloride dissolved in absolute ethanol in comparison with surgical castration in donkeys based on changes in circulating concentrations of testosterone and histopathological changes in treated testes. We hypothesized that calcium chloride castration would be a suitable alternative to surgical one and would possess the upper hand based on the risk/benefit analysis and welfare issue.

Methods
Animals
The study was carried out in accordance with the Egyptian laws and University guidelines for the animal care. All

procedures of the current work have been approved by the National Ethical Committee of the Faculty of Veterinary Medicine, Assiut University, Egypt. The animals were selected in a minimum number required to obtain valid results [19].

Twelve clinically healthy, adult male donkeys, 2–3 years old and weighing 100 to 120 kg were used for this study. The animals were housed in a well-ventilated stable with water and food ad libitum.

Experimental protocol
Donkeys were divided randomly into two equal groups: a surgical (S) group ($n = 6$) and a chemical (C) group ($n = 6$). Animals in the (S) group were subjected to surgical castration using the scrotal ablation technique while those in the (C) group received a single bilateral intratesticular injection of 20 % calcium chloride dissolved in absolute ethanol in a dose of 20 ml/testis.

Technique of the intratesticular injection of calcium chloride solution
Under physical restraint, the animal was positioned in lateral recumbency. The scrotal area was thoroughly scrubbed. The lower testicle was injected first. The testicle was secured firmly against the skin of the scrotum. The site of injection near the tail of the epididymis was disinfected with 10 % Betadine solution. Under a complete aseptic condition, a 21G × 1.5 needle was directed from the caudoventral aspect of each testis approximately 0.5 cm from the epididymal tail towards the dorsocranial aspect of the testis. The solution was carefully deposited along the entire route by linear infiltration while withdrawing the needle from the proximal to the distal end. Necessary care was taken to prevent the seepage of solution from the injection site.

Clinical observation
All animals were kept under clinical observation for 60 days. Changes in animals' behavior, food and water consumption, gait of animals and gross changes in external genitalia were monitored daily.

Blood sampling
Blood samples were collected from the jugular vein under a complete aseptic condition at 8.30 a.m. prior to and at 15, 30, 45 and 60 days from the beginning of the experiment in both groups, (S) and (C). Serum was isolated after centrifugation at 3000 rpm for 10 min stored at−20 °C until analyzed for determination of testosterone levels.

Serum testosterone assay
It was determined by ELISA using testosterone enzyme immunoassay test kit according to the manufacturer's

instruction (BioCheck, Inc.) with a minimum detectable concentration of 0.05 ng/ml.

Histopathological examination

At the end of the experiment (60 days), the testicles of donkeys in the (C) group were removed surgically under general anesthesia (intravenous thiopental, 10 mg/kg BW) [20] for histopathological examination.

Testes were sectioned transversely and examined grossly. Representative samples from gross lesions were taken. These samples were immersed in 10 % neutral buffer formalin for 2 days after removal of tunica albicans, prepared in 1×1 cm size and dehydrated in a graded alcohol series. Histopathological sections were prepared at a thickness of 4 μ, fixed in 10 % neutral buffered formalin, cleared with methyl benzoate then embedded in paraffin wax and cleared in methyl benzoate. These sections were stained with hematoxylin-eosin and examined by light microscope [21]. Histopathological lesions of testes were scored according to Fox et al. [22].

Statistical analysis

The analysis was carried out using a standard statistical software program (SPSS version 16, SPSS Inc, Chicago, Ill). The data were expressed as means ± standard error of the mean (SEM). One-way ANOVA was used to determine the effects of each type of castration on serum testosterone levels followed by individual comparison using Tukey's post-test. The effects of treatment, time, and the interaction of treatment with time were evaluated using univariate general linear model. Differences were considered statistically significant at $P < 0.05$.

Results

Clinical observation

Donkeys in the (C) group exerted mild discomfort and irritability during the intratesticular injection of 20 % calcium chloride dissolved in absolute alcohol. By the end of the injection, testes appeared to be enlarged and firm in consistency. A painful and hot swelling in the scrotum and the prepuce was evident 24 h post-injection in all donkeys (Fig. 1a and b). The swelling increased markedly from the 2nd day post-injection reaching its peak at the 5th day post-injection (Fig. 1c). Phimosis was recorded at the 3rd day post-injection, however urination process retained unaffected. The swelling began to decay at the 6th day post injection (Fig. 1d) to be subsided completely from both, the scrotum and the prepuce by the 14th day post-injection (Fig. 1e and f).

Four out of six donkeys developed scrotal ulcerations and fistulas (Fig. 1g), which were managed surgically by evacuation, curetting and lavage with Betadine 10 % for several times. This was followed by daily dressing with Betadine 10 %.

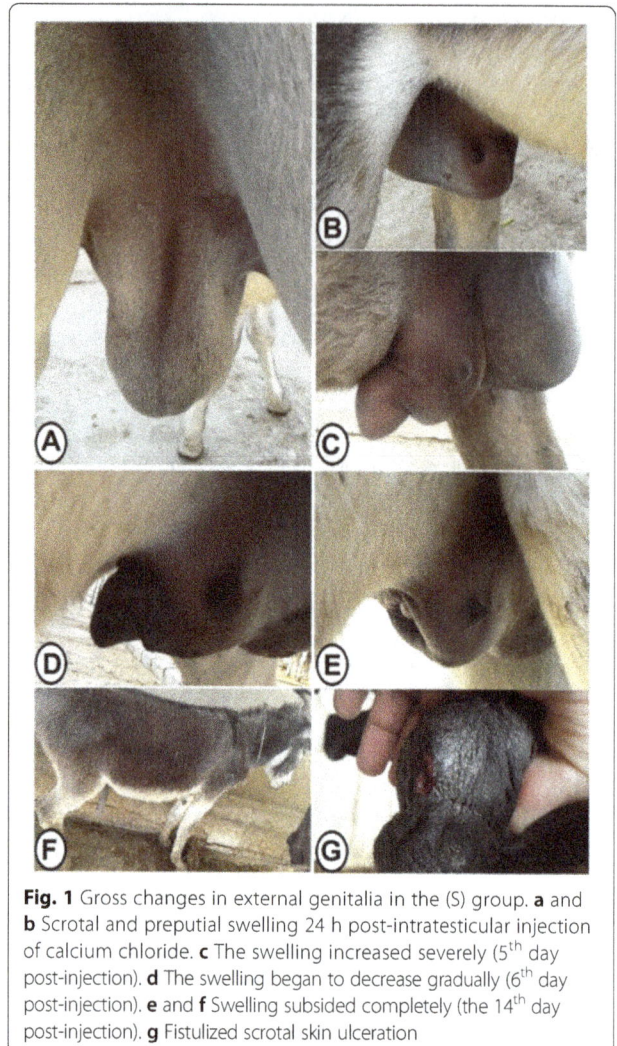

Fig. 1 Gross changes in external genitalia in the (S) group. **a** and **b** Scrotal and preputial swelling 24 h post-intratesticular injection of calcium chloride. **c** The swelling increased severely (5th day post-injection). **d** The swelling began to decrease gradually (6th day post-injection). **e** and **f** Swelling subsided completely (the 14th day post-injection). **g** Fistulized scrotal skin ulceration

There were no detectable changes in the general health status of the animals with the exception of swelling in external genitalia, scrotal ulcerations and fistulas. Food and water consumption and animal gait remained unaffected.

Donkeys in the (S) group did not record any post-surgical complications following castration by scrotal ablation technique.

Histopathological examination

Gross appearance

Grossly, the testes of donkeys in the (C) group revealed hemorrhagic areas on the parietal vaginal tunics (Fig. 2a). Orchitis presented by extensive adhesions between the visceral and parietal vaginal tunics (Fig. 2b).

Testicular cross section showed severe necrosis and sloughing in the testicular parenchyma in two animals (Fig. 2c and d). Testes in one donkey developed hemorrhagic necrosis that manifested by dark coffee discoloration with sloughed testicular parenchyma (Fig. 3a).

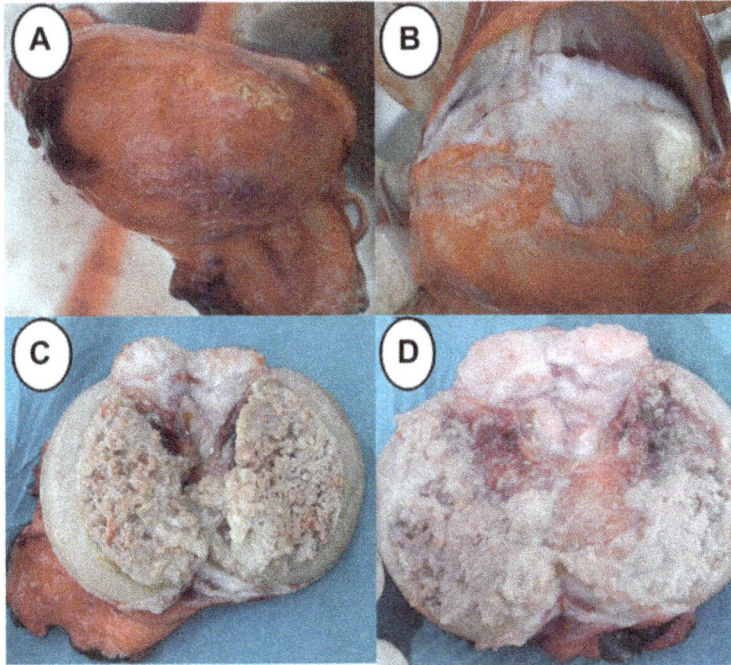

Fig. 2 Pathological gross findings in testes in the (C) group. **a** Hemorrhagic areas on the testicular membranes. **b** Severe adhesions between tunica albuginea and tunica vaginals. **c** and **d** Testes showing necrosed and sloughed tissues in the testicular parenchyma

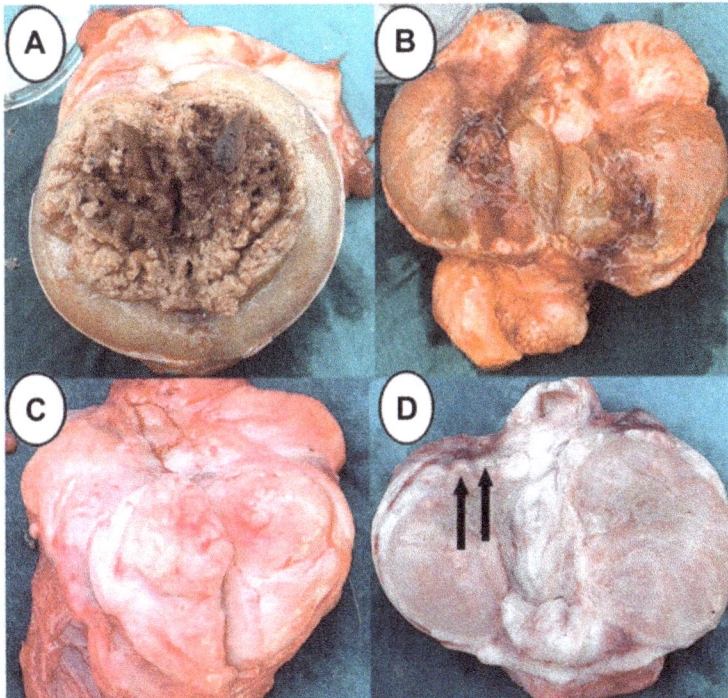

Fig. 3 Pathological gross appearance in testes in the (C) group. **a** Hemorrhagic necrosis with dark coffee discoloration. **b** Hemorrhagic areas with softness inconsistency. **c** and **d** Atrophied testes with mineralization (arrow)

Table 1 Gross pathological findings in donkeys treated with calcium chloride

Gross lesions	Case number					
	1	2	3	4	5	6
Orchitis	++	+++	++	+	–	–
Necrosis & Sloghing	++++	+++	–	–	–	–
Heamorrhagic necrosis	–	–	++	++	–	–
Atrophy of testes	–	–	–	–	++	++

The severity degree of lesions: very severe = ++++, severe = +++, moderate = ++, mild = +, no damage = –

In another animal, testes were soft in consistency with hemorrhagic areas in the testicular parenchyma (Fig. 3b). Also, there were two animals that had atrophied testes which were firm in consistency with mineralization at the periphery of the testes (Fig. 3c and d), Table 1.

Microscopic appearance

Inflammatory reaction was the main detectable finding in the histopathological examination of treated testes in the (C) group. This reaction expressed by a progressive connective tissue that was heavily infiltrated with large number of neutrophils and fewer mononuclear cellular reactions (Fig. 4a and b), Table 2. Testes from two donkeys showed a decrease in spermatogenesis which reached two or three layers of spermatogenic cells within the seminiferous tubules (Fig. 5a). Other seminiferous tubules showed diffuse tubular coagulative necrosis of germinal epithelium with necrosed tissue collected in their lumens (Fig. 5b). Most seminiferous tubules were empty, dilated with irregular basement membranes, with complete depletion of both germinal and Sertoli cells leaving only a basement membrane. Also, there were atrophied seminiferous tubules characterized by complete hyalinized scarring of the tubule with varying degrees of tubular collapse (Fig. 5c).

Proliferative intertubular stroma was infiltrated with large clusters of Leydig cells. These Leydig cells were surrounded by collagen fibers (Figs. 5d, 6a and b). Hyalinization was a prominent finding in the examined cases (Fig. 5e and f).

Vascular changes expressed by hyperplasia of endothelial cells lining blood vessels, and formation of red thrombus inside the lumen of blood vessel that consisted of RBCs and platelets (Fig. 7a and b). Dystrophic calcification was observed within large infracted areas within the testicular parenchyma and the walls of some blood vessels (Fig. 7c and d).

Serum testosterone assay

Serum testosterone levels of surgically castrated donkeys at day 15 exhibited a significantly sudden drop (2.928 ± 0.806 ng/ml) as compared with day 0 (5.135 ± 0.574 ng/ml). Similarly at day 30, 45, and 60 it significantly maintained lower levels than day 0 (2.617 ± 0.729, 2.360 ± 0.617 and 2.889 ± 0.447 ng/ml, respectively).

On the other hand, there were no significant differences between pre-sterilization testosterone levels (5.111 ± 1.052 ng/ml) relative to post-sterilization ones at all time intervals (15, 30, 45 and 60 days) when calcium chloride was used as a chemical sterilant in the (C) group (6.153 ± 1.360, 6.033 ± 1.276, 6.847 ± 0.680 and 7.400 ± 0.406 ng/ml, respectively) Fig. 8.

Discussion

The outcome of surgical castration risks versus its benefits necessitates a shift towards other non-invasive chemical approaches that should be characterized by full capability of arresting spermatogenesis, androgenesis and libido, effectiveness on a large scale, high safety profile, and irreversibility following single treatment. From this point of view, calcium chloride attracts much attention to be evaluated as an unconventional substitute for surgical castration in animals.

To our knowledge, the only published study which investigated chemical castration in donkeys was performed

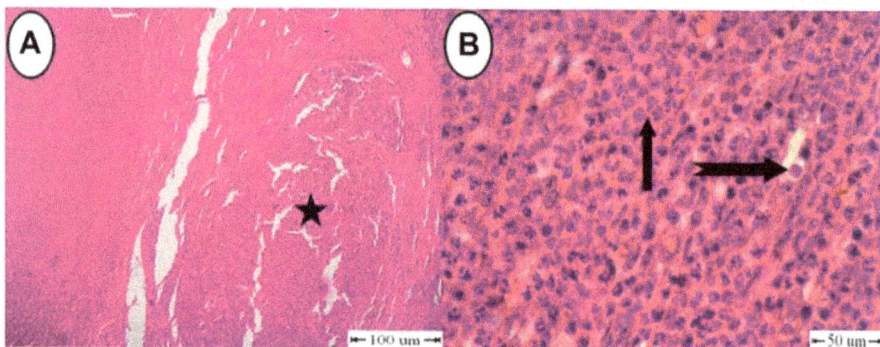

Fig. 4 Histopathological findings in testes in the (C) group. **a** Connective tissue infiltrated with neutrophils and mononuclear cellular reactions (star). **b** High power to (Fig. 4a). Connective tissue infiltrated with a large number of neutrophils (arrow) and fewer mononuclear cellular reactions (notched arrow)

Table 2 Histopathological findings in donkeys treated with calcium chloride

Histopathological lesions	Case number					
	1	2	3	4	5	6
-Inflammatory reaction	++	++	+++	+	–	–
-Fibrosis	–	–	–	++++	+++	+++
-Decrease in layers of seminiferous tubules	–	–	–	–	+++	++
-Coagulative necrosis of germinal epithelium	–	–	–	+++	++	++++
-Empty dilated seminiferous tubules	++++	++++	+++	–	–	–
-Atrophy of seminiferous tubules	+++	++	–	–	–	–
-Heamorrhage	–	–	++	+	++	–
-Thrombosis	–	–	++	–	++	–
-Dystrophic calcification	–	–	–	–	++	+

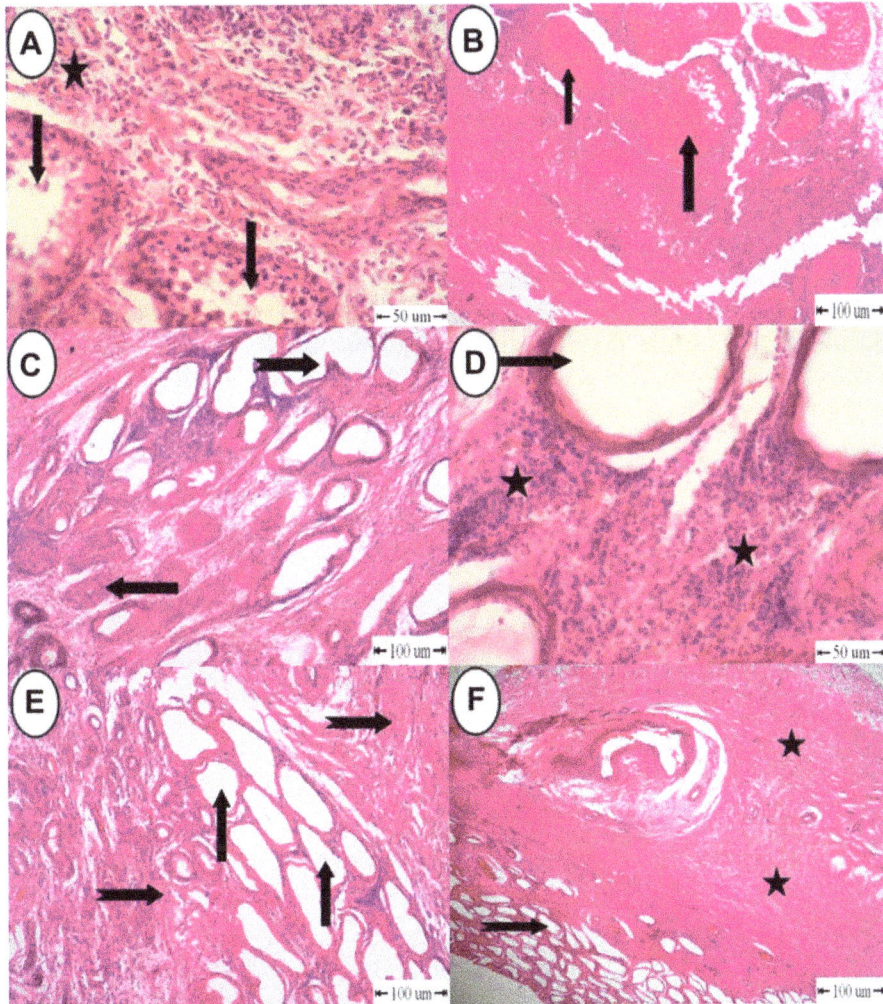

Fig. 5 Histopathological findings in testes in the (C) group. **a** Testes showing a cross section of one seminiferous tubule with a decrease in spermatogenesis to two or three layers (arrow) and thickening of intertubular stroma (star) infiltrated with interstitial cells. **b** Testes showing coagulative necrosis of germinal epithelium and necrosed tissue collected in the lumen (arrow). **c** Testes showing empty, irregular (notched arrow) and atrophied (arrow) seminiferous tubules. **d** High power showing empty seminiferous tubules (arrow) and presence of clusters of Leydig cells. **e** Testes showing empty seminiferous tubules (arrow) and intertubular fibrosis (notched arrow). **f** Testes showing intertubular fibrosis and hyalinization (star) and presence of empty seminiferous tubules (notched arrow)

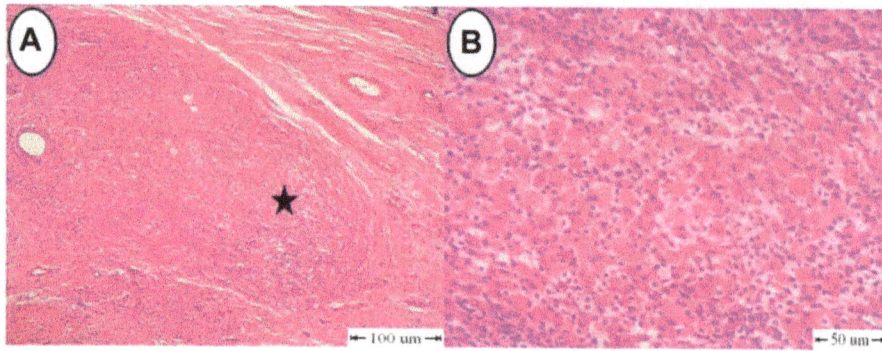

Fig. 6 Histopathological findings in testes in the (C) group. **a** Testes showing large clusters of Leydig cells surrounded by collagen fibers (star). **b** High power showing large clusters of Leydig cells

by Ali et al., [23]. They estimated the efficacy of chemical castration with intratesticular injection of calcium chloride dissolved in distilled water in concentrations of 25, 50 and 70 % by the presence or absence of sperms in testicular smears. Unfortunately, they neglected to consider its effect on serum testosterone levels, which provided the premise for this current study.

The major finding of the current study was the ineffectiveness of 20 % calcium chloride for chemical castration in donkeys. This was evident by the absence of significant changes in serum testosterone levels associated with a compensatory proliferation of Leydig cells in the histopathological sections, even so germinal epithelium and vascular endothelium are specifically targeted by calcium chloride.

We decided to apply calcium chloride in a concentration of 20 % as higher concentrations (30 % or more) were reported to have higher risk of abscessiation [18, 24], however in our study ulcerations with fistulas had been recorded between animals in the (C) group (4 donkeys). This may be attributed to absolute ethanol, as it appears to produce its effect by necrosis and infarction leading to fibrosis and sloughing of tissue [25].

In our study, the choice of absolute ethanol as a base provides the optimal formulation for calcium chloride. It has an anesthetic effect, less inflammatory reaction, fewer complications, besides high effectiveness [10, 11, 24].

Blood samples for the serum testosterone assay were taken at a fixed time at 8.30 a.m. as the highest serum

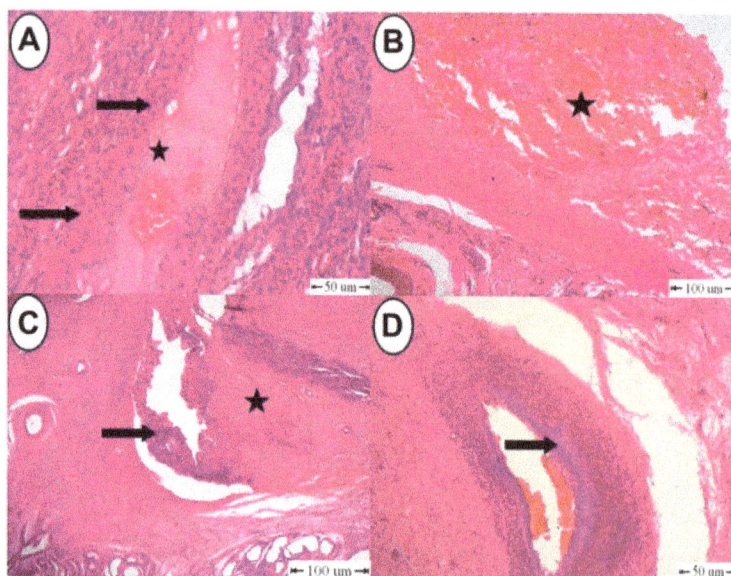

Fig. 7 Histopathological findings in testes in the (C) group. **a** Testes showing hyperplasia of endothelial cells (arrow) and presence of a red thrombus (star). **b** Testes showing hemorrhage (star). **c** Necrosis of testicular parenchyma (star) undergoes dystrophic calcification (arrow). **d** Testes showing dystrophic calcification on the wall of blood vessels (arrow)

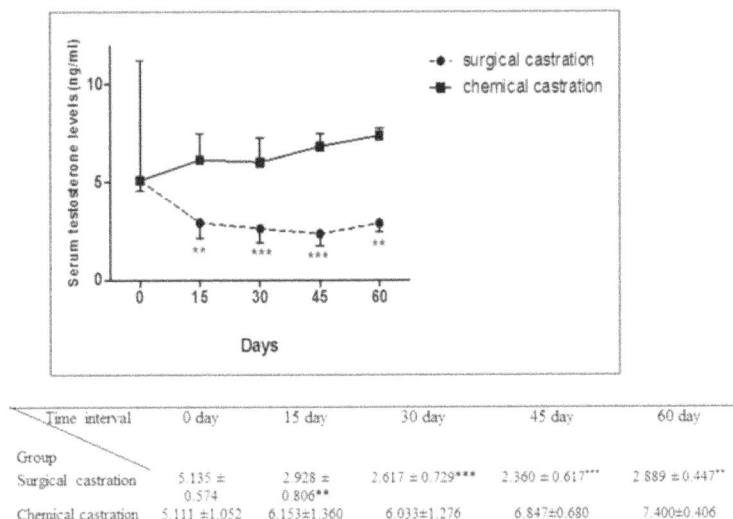

Time interval	0 day	15 day	30 day	45 day	60 day
Group					
Surgical castration	5.135 ± 0.574	2.928 ± 0.806**	2.617 ± 0.729***	2.360 ± 0.617***	2.889 ± 0.447**
Chemical castration	5.111 ±1.052	6.153±1.360	6.033±1.276	6.847±0.680	7.400±0.406

Fig. 8 Serum concentrations of testosterone in both (S) and (C) groups. Graphic representation of changes in serum testosterone levels of donkeys at day 0 (pre-castration) vs. days 15, 30, 45, and 60 following surgical or chemical castration. Values are expressed as means ± SEM, $n = 6$ animals per group. Mean values are significantly different by repeated measures ANOVA followed by Tukey post-test. **$P < 0.01$ vs. day 0; ***$P < 0.001$ vs. day 0

testosterone levels were observed between 6.00 and 10.00 a.m. [26].

Surgical castration was supported by a significant reduction in post-castration levels of serum testosterone at all time points against pre-castration ones. This is exactly what happened in previous studies [27, 28]. This provides confirmation for the fact that testes act as a primary source of male sex hormones [29].

On the other hand, chemical castration with calcium chloride failed to induce any significant changes in serum concentrations of testosterone as approved histopathologically by the presence of proliferative Leydig cells. This was in line with the findings of Leoci [12] but contradicts others [2–4, 14, 15].

Confirming to our results, even the highest effective dose reported in literatures (60 % solution of calcium chloride) decreased testosterone levels to only near its lower limit of physiological range, and concentration up to 30 % was not enough to induce complete testicular fibrosis, whereas testosterone levels return to normal within 12-month time point by the current dose [12, 30].

Intratesticular administration of calcium chloride in donkeys produced inflammation that has been confirmed by testicular gross and histopathological changes. This inflammatory reaction was supposed to be the mechanism of calcium chloride by its irritating effect on testicular tissues [25].

The severe fibrosis in the interstitial spaces was associated with chronic inflammation. Similar findings were reported by Jana and Samanta [2]. Hyperplasia of the endothelial cells lining the blood vessels as well as thromboses of blood vessels led to ischemia resulted in swelling, firmness, and atrophy of the testicular tissues [18, 31].

Over the course of treatment, calcium chloride caused damage to the spermatogonial stem cells that may lead to filling with necrotic germ cells. Thus, it could not reinitiate spermatogenesis in these seminiferous tubules [4]. The complete hyalinized scarring of the seminiferous tubules with varying degrees of a tubular collapse was associated with inflammation induced by calcium chloride [32].

Leydig cell proliferation is likely to be a compensatory mechanism to increase testicular steroidogenesis stimulated by testosterone insufficiency [33–35]. However, our results were in disagreement with Jana and Samanta [14] who reported that there was no sign of regeneration in Leydig cells.

Conclusion

Single bilateral intratesticular injection of 20 % calcium chloride dissolved in absolute ethanol failed to significantly reduce the serum levels of testosterone within 60 days of treatment in donkeys. It is unlikely to modify the male-like behavior of donkeys and cannot be accepted as an alternative method to the surgical castration. Further studies are warranted to explore other chemical sterilants in other solvents to achieve the highest efficacy with less adverse impacts.

Competing interests
The authors declare that they have no competing of interests.

Authors' contribution
AI designed the experiment, AI and MMA performed the surgical and chemical castration and monitored the animals post-operatively, NA measured the serum concentrations of testosterone and carried out the statistical analysis, MFA helped with the histopathological examination. All authors wrote, read and approved the final manuscript.

Author details

[1]Department of Surgery, Anesthesiology and Radiology, Faculty of veterinary medicine, Assuit University, Assuit 70155, Egypt. [2]Department of Medical physiology, Faculty of medicine, Assuit University, Assuit, Egypt. [3]Department of Pathology and clinical pathology, Faculty of veterinary medicine, Assuit University, Assuit, Egypt.

References

1. Auer JA, Stick JA. Reproductive system in equine surgery. In: Auer JA, Stick JA, editors. Equine surgery. 3rd ed. USA: Saunders Elsevier; 2006.
2. Jana K, Samanta PK. Sterilization of male stray dogs with a single intratesticular injection of calcium chloride: a dose-dependent study. Contraception. 2007;75(5):390–400.
3. Jana K, Samanta PK. Evaluation of single intratesticular injection of calcium chloride for nonsurgical sterilization in adult albino rats. Contraception. 2006;73(3):289–300.
4. Jana K, Samanta PK, Ghosh D. Dose-dependent response to an intratesticular injection of calcium chloride for induction of chemosterilization in adult albino rats. Vet Res Commun. 2002;26(8):651–73.
5. Kar AB. Chemical sterilization of male rhesus monkeys. Endocrinology. 1961; 69:1116–9.
6. Kar AB, Kamboj VP, Goswami A. Sterilization of male rhesus monkeys by iron salts. J Reprod Fertil. 1965;9:115–7.
7. Wiebe JP, Barr KJ, Buckingham KD. Sustained azoospermia in squirrel monkey, saimiri sciureus, resulting from a single intratesticular glycerol injection. Contraception. 1989;39(4):447–57.
8. Fordyce G, Hodge PB, Beaman NJ, Laing AR, Campero C, Shepherd RK. An evaluation of calf castration by intra-testicular injection of a lactic acid solution. Aust Vet J. 1989;66(9):272–6.
9. Samanta PK. Chemosterilization of stray dogs. Ind J Anim Health. 1998;37:61–2.
10. Koger LM. Calcium chloride castration. Mod Vet Pract. 1978;59(2):119–21.
11. Leoci R, Aiudi G, Silvestre F, Lissner EA, Lacalandra GM. Alcohol diluent provides the optimal formulation for calcium chloride non-surgical sterilization in dogs. Acta Vet Scand. 2014;56(1):62.
12. Leoci R, Aiudi G, Silvestre F, Lissner EA, Marino F, Lacalandra GM. A dose-finding, long-term study on the use of calcium chloride in saline solution as a method of nonsurgical sterilization in dogs: evaluation of the most effective concentration with the lowest risk. Acta Vet Scand. 2014;56(1):63.
13. Vanderstichel R, Forzan MJ, Perez GE, Serpell JA, Garde E. Changes in blood testosterone concentrations after surgical and chemical sterilization of male free-roaming dogs in southern Chile. Theriogenology. 2015;83(6):1021–7.
14. Jana K, Samanta PK. Clinical evaluation of non-surgical sterilization of male cats with single intra-testicular injection of calcium chloride. BMC Vet Res. 2011;7:39.
15. Jana K, Samanta PK, Ghosh D. Evaluation of single intratesticular injection of calcium chloride for nonsurgical sterilization of male black Bengal goats (Capra hircus): a dose-dependent study. Anim Reprod Sci. 2005;86(1–2):89–108.
16. Mohammed A, James FO. Chemical castration by a single bilateral intra-testicular injection of chlorhexidine gluconate and cetrimide in bucks. Sokoto J Vet Sci. 2013;11:62–5.
17. Mitra B, Samanta PK. Testicular degeneration of scrub bulls by calcium chloride. Ind J Vet Surg. 2000;21:37–8.
18. Canapolat I, Bulut S, Eröksüz H, Gür S. An evaluation of the outcome of bull castration by intra-testicular injection of ethanol and calcium. Rev Med Vet (Toulouse). 2006;8–9:420–5.
19. Office of Laboratory Animal Welfare. A: institutional animal care and use committee guidebook. Maryland: Office of Laboratory Animal Welfare, National Institutes of Health, Department of Health and Human Services Bethesda; 2002.
20. Hall LW, Clarke KW, Trim CM. Veterinary anaesthesia. 9th ed. London: WB Saunders; 2001.
21. Lillie R. Histopathologic technic and practical histochemistry. 3rd ed. New York: McGraw-Hill Book Co; 1965.
22. Fox KA, Diamond B, Sun F, Clavijo A, Sneed L, Kitchen DN, Wolfe LL. Testicular lesions and antler abnormalities in Colorado, USA mule deer (odocoileus hemionus): a possible role for epizootic hemorrhagic disease virus. J Wildl Dis. 2015;51(1):166–76.
23. Ali MA, Selem MA, Makady FM, Shehata SH. Calcium chloride castration in donkeys (an experimental study). Assiut Vet Med J. 1991;25(49):196–202.
24. Leoci R. Calcium chloride dehydrate nonsurgical sterilization in 81 dogs: dose, formulation and best practices implications for maximal effectiveness and minimal complications, from the first large study outside of India. In: The 1st International Conference on Dog Population Management. Italy: University of Bari; 2012.
25. Zvara P, Karpman E, Stoppacher R, Esenler AC, Plante MK. Ablation of canine prostate using transurethral intraprostatic absolute ethanol injection. Urology. 1999;54(3):411–5.
26. Diver MJ, Imtiaz KE, Ahmad AM, Vora JP, Fraser WD. Diurnal rhythms of serum total, free and bioavailable testosterone and of SHBG in middle-aged men compared with those in young men. Clin Endocrinol (Oxf). 2003;58(6):710–7.
27. Cai Z, Zhang L, Jiang X, Sheng Y, Xu N. Differential miRNA expression profiles in the longissimus dorsi muscle between intact and castrated male pigs. Res Vet Sci. 2015;99:99–104.
28. Sosic-Jurjevic B, Filipovic B, Renko K, Ajdzanovic V, Manojlovic-Stojanoski M, Milosevic V, Kohrle J. Orchidectomy of middle-aged rats decreases liver deiodinase 1 and pituitary deiodinase 2 activity. J Endocrinol. 2012;215(2):247–56.
29. Starr C, Taggart R, Evers C. Animal structure and function biology. The unity & diversity of life. 13th ed. UK: Cengage Learning; 2012.
30. Martins LT, Gonçalves MC, Tavares KC, Gaudêncio S, Santos Neto PC, Dias AL, Gava A, Saito ME, Oliveira CA, Mezzalira A et al. Castration methods do not affect weight gain and have diverse impacts on the welfare of water buffalo males. Livest Sci. 2011;140(1–3):171–6.
31. Al-Asadi RN, Al-Kadi KK. Non-surgical castration in bucks a comparative study between chemical castration and external ligation of the spermatic cord. AL-Qadisiya J Vet Med Sci. 2012;11:1.
32. Shigeru H, Touichiro T, Yutaka K. Focal atrophy of the seminefrous tubule in the human testis. Pathol Int. 1979;29:901–10.
33. Mylchreest E, Sar M, Wallace DG, Foster PM. Fetal testosterone insufficiency and abnormal proliferation of Leydig cells and gonocytes in rats exposed to di(n-butyl) phthalate. Reprod Toxicol. 2002;16(1):19–28.
34. Teerds KJ. Regeneration of Leydig cells after depletion by EDS: a model for postnatal Leydig cell renewal.In: Payne AH, Hardy MP, Russell LD (eds.), The Leydig Cell. Vienna, IL: Cache River Press; 1996: 203-220.
35. Fagundes AK, Oliveira EC, Tenorio BM, Melo CC, Nery LT, Santos FA, et al. Injection of a chemical castration agent, zinc gluconate, into the testes of cats results in the impairment of spermatogenesis: a potentially irreversible contraceptive approach for this species? Theriogenology. 2014;81(2):230–9.

Prospective clinical study to evaluate an oscillometric blood pressure monitor in pet rabbits

Luca Bellini[1]* [iD], Irene A. Veladiano[2], Magdalena Schrank[2], Matteo Candaten[1] and Antonio Mollo[2]

Abstract

Background: Rabbits are particularly sensitive to develop hypotension during sedation or anaesthesia. Values of systolic or mean non-invasive arterial blood pressure below 80 or 60 mmHg respectively are common under anaesthesia despite an ongoing surgery. A reliable method of monitoring arterial blood pressure is extremely important, although invasive technique is not always possible due to the anatomy and dimension of the artery. The aim of this study was to evaluate the agreement between a new oscillometric device for non-invasive arterial blood pressure measurement and the invasive method. Moreover the trending ability of the device, ability to identify changes in the same direction with the invasive methods, was evaluated as well as the sensibility of the device in identifying hypotension arbitrarily defined as invasive arterial blood pressure below 80 or 60 mmHg.

Results: Bland-Altman analysis for repeated measurements showed a poor agreement between the two methods; the oscillometric device overestimated the invasive arterial blood pressure, particularly at high arterial pressure values. The same analysis repeated considering oscillometric measurement that match invasive mean pressure lower or equal to 60 mmHg showed a decrease in biases and limits of agreement between methods. The trending ability of the device, evaluated with both the 4-quadrant plot and the polar plot was poor. Concordance rate of mean arterial blood pressure was higher than systolic and diastolic pressure although inferior to 90%. The sensibility of the device in detecting hypotension defined as systolic or mean invasive arterial blood pressure lower than 80 or 60 mmHg was superior for mean oscillometric pressure rather than systolic. A sensitivity of 92% was achieved with an oscillometric measurement for mean pressure below 65 mmHg instead of 60 mmHg. Non-invasive systolic blood pressure is less sensitive as indicator of hypotension regardless of the cutoff limit considered.

Conclusions: Although mean invasive arterial blood pressure is overestimated by the device, the sensitivity of this non-invasive oscillometric monitor in detecting invasive mean pressure below 60 mmHg is acceptable but a cutoff value of 65 mmHg needs to be used.

Keywords: Rabbits, Arterial blood pressure, Oscillometric method, Isoflurane, Trending ability

Background

Anaesthesia related mortality at 48 h post-procedure is higher in rabbits than in dogs and cats [1]. Rabbits often suffer from subclinical cardiopulmonary diseases that may be undetected before anaesthesia [1]. Moreover sedatives and anaesthetics may cause cardiovascular depression [2–4] that may lead to hypotension with organ hypoperfusion and ischemic injuries that may precipitate subclinical diseases. Harvey et al. observed that almost 92% of rabbits showed systolic or mean arterial blood pressure lower than 80 or 60 mmHg respectively at a surgical plane of anaesthesia [4].

Direct invasive arterial blood pressure (IBP) measurement is considered the "gold standard" for arterial blood pressure measurement. This technique requires an arterial catheterization that may be technically difficult in small animals and it may lead to blood extravasation with haematoma and risk of ear necrosis [5]. The central auricular artery is often used for IBP measurement although the size of some breeds of pet rabbits limits the

* Correspondence: luca.bellini@unipd.it
[1]Veterinary Teaching Hospital, University of Padua, Viale dell'Università 16, 35020 Legnaro, PD, Italy
Full list of author information is available at the end of the article

placement of a catheter in that artery. Non-invasive arterial blood pressure (NIBP) measurement methods may overcome some of these limitations and the agreement between these methods has been evaluated.

The Doppler technique showed good agreement with systolic IBP measurements and it can be used to monitor arterial pressure [3, 4], but does not provide information of mean and diastolic blood pressure. Moreover to improve the signal quality, often the skin over the metatarsal artery is clipped and this can predispose to skin irritation and pododermatitis [6].

Traditional oscillometric techniques that use equipment designed for human use becomes inaccurate at fast pulse rate or with pulse oscillation of small magnitude during hypotension or with alpha-2 agonist sedatives [5, 7]. Moreover the same authors suggested a low accuracy of such a devices in animal weighing lower than 5–7 kg [5]. The size of the cuff is critical and may add a source of error during oscillometric and Doppler methods. The width of the cuff should be approximately 40% of limb circumference but in small rabbits may not be available [4, 5]. Additionally, specific algorithm are introduced by manufacturers of NIBP devices to estimate SAP and DAP and they may be not accurate in all species, haemodynamic conditions and cuff location [7–9].

Recently, a new oscillometric device has become available for arterial blood pressure monitoring in dogs and cats. The device is provided with a ruler to allow selection of the most appropriate cuff size for the particular animal.

The aim of this study is to compare the new NIBP oscillometric device with the IBP measured from the auricular artery in anesthetized rabbits undergoing elective neutering. A secondary aim was to study the trending ability of the device and its sensitivity and specificity in detecting systolic and mean IBP lower than 80 and 60 mmHg respectively.

Methods

Internal institutional ethics committee approved the study and owner's consent was obtained before each procedure. Nineteen ASA 1–2 cross-breed pet rabbits of both sexes (7 male, 12 female) weighing between 2.5 and 4.6 kg, older than 6 months undergoing elective neutering were enrolled in a prospective clinical study.

Anaesthesia

The animals were considered healthy based on the medical history and pre-anaesthetic clinical exam. Rabbits had free access to water and food until a combination of dexmedetomidine 50 µg/kg (Dexdomitor; Orion Corporation, Espoo, Finland) and midazolam (Midazolam-hameln; Hospira Italia, Naples, Italy) 0.6 mg/kg was administered into the lumbar muscles (total volume 0.22 ml/kg) to obtain sedation. As the rabbits lost the righting reflex the external pinnae of the left ear and the dorsal aspect of the right foreleg were clipped. A 24-gauge over-the-needle intravenous (IV) catheter was aseptically inserted in the cephalic vein. After IV access was achieved, 0.05 mg/kg of buprenorphine (Buprenodale 0.3 mg/ml; Dechra Ltd., Skipton, UK) was administered together with a subcutaneous injection of 1 mg/kg of meloxicam (Metacam; Boehringer Ingelheim, Milan, Italy) and 5 mg/kg of enrofloxacin (Baytril 25 mg/ml injection solution; Bayer Spa, Milan, Italy). Anaesthesia was induced with IV propofol (Vetofol 10 mg/ml, Norbrook Laboratories Ltd., Monaghan, Northern Ireland) and airways were secured either with an endotracheal tube or a laryngeal mask in 9 and 10 rabbits respectively. The animals were placed in dorsal recumbency and anaesthesia was maintained with isoflurane (Isoflo, Abbott Laboratories Ltd., Maidenhead, UK) in a mixture of oxygen and air (FiO$_2$ = 0.5) via a circle breathing system with paediatric tubes. The end-tidal concentration of isoflurane was adjusted to maintain an adequate surgical plane of anaesthesia while minimizing the detrimental cardiovascular effects of volatile agent. To maintain a normothermic range between 38° and 39 °C an electric heating pad (Pet-Mat; Dale Ecotech Pty Ltd., Milsons Point, Australia) was placed under the rabbits. Pulse rate, pulse oximetry, IBP, respiratory rate, end-tidal concentration of isoflurane and carbon dioxide were monitored with a portable pulseoximeter (EDAN VE-H100B, Edan USA; San Diego, CA, USA) and a multiparameter monitor (Datex S/5; GE Healthcare; Helsinki, Finland); a mixture of 50:50 lactate Ringer's solution and 5% dextrose was infused at 5 ml/kg/h IV. After surgery all monitoring devices were removed and the rabbits received subcutaneously 0.5 mg/kg of atipamezole (Antisedan, Orion Corporation, Espoo, Finland). Heart rate, respiratory rate and signs of pain were evaluated in the recovery period until discharge.

Invasive arterial blood pressure measurement

To measure the invasive arterial blood pressure a 24-gauge Teflon catheter (Delta Ven 1; DeltaMed Spa, Viadana, Italy) was inserted aseptically in the median portion of central auricular artery and it was secured with tape. If the artery was not catheterized at the first attempt the animal was removed from the study and arterial blood pressure was recorded by a Doppler ultrasound method as previously reported (Bellini et al. [3]). The arterial catheter was connected to a pressure transducer by a 150 cm long non-compliant tubing (TruWave™ pressure monitoring set; Edwards Lifesciences, Irvine, CA, USA) filled with heparinized saline (5 IU/ml) and connected to the multiparameter monitor and a pressurized (300 mmHg) bag containing saline solution. The

IBP was calibrated against a bourdon manometer (Tycos TR-2 Hand Aneroids, Welsh Allyn Ltd., Aston Abbotts, UK) at the beginning of each day. The transducer was zeroed at the level of the manubrium of the sternum once the rabbit was placed in dorsal recumbency. Dynamic response test was performed at the beginning of each procedure. Damping coefficient and natural frequency were measured according to the formula reported in literature [10].

Oscillometric arterial blood pressure measurement

A new oscillometric device (PetTrust Blood Pressure Monitor, BioCare, Aster Electrical Co. Ltd., Taiwan) was evaluated. The cuff was placed on the anterior forelimb proximal to the carpus once the animal was in dorsal recumbency; the correct size of the cuff was obtained by the ruler provided by the manufacturer and the inflation cuff line was orientated toward the distal part of the forelimb. The legs were loosely tied with a bandage role. Every 5 min 2 consecutive readings were taken and if the variability was less than 20% the data were averaged otherwise a third reading was done and the values that had the small variance were used [11].

Statistical analysis

Mean bias, precision defined as standard deviation (SD) of the bias and limits of agreement (mean bias $\pm$ 1.96 $\times$ SD) for systolic, diastolic and mean arterial blood pressure measured with IBP and NIBP was assessed by the method proposed by Bland and Altman for multiple observations per individual [12]. Analysis was performed on all paired measurements and repeated including only pair measurements matching non-invasive SAP and MAP lower than 90 and 65 mmHg respectively. An acceptable agreement between the two methods was considered achieved with a mean bias of less than 10 mmHg and a precision of less than 15 mmHg, that represent one of the criteria proposed by ACVIM Hypertension Consensus and Veterinary Blood Pressure Society, to validate a blood pressure device in dogs and cats [11]. The goodness of agreement between methods was also evaluated based on the standard of the Association for the Advancement of Medical Instrumentation (AAMI), which requires a mean bias less than 5 mmHg and a precision of less than 10 mmHg.

The "trending ability" of the oscillometric method in tracking dependable changes with the invasive method was evaluated with a four-quadrant plot and a polar plot as reported previously [13]. Both analysis were repeated for SAP, DAP and MAP; the concordance rate was calculated as the percentage of data points outside the exclusion zone representing 5% or 10% changes in arterial blood pressure, in the upper right and lower left quadrant over the data points in all quadrants. Data points, which lay in an exclusion zone of 5 and 10%, are suggesting small variations in arterial blood pressure, depending rather on the precision of the device than being a reflection of real changes in haemodynamics [14]. A concordance rate over 90% was judged indicative of good trending ability [13, 15]. The polar plot was used to quantify the trending ability that was considered adequate if mean polar angle and radial limit of agreement were lower than 5° and $\pm$ 30° respectively [13–15].

Intraoperative hypotension was arbitrary defined as invasive SAP or MAP lower than 80 and/or 60 mmHg respectively [4]. Sensitivity, specificity, positive predictive value and negative predictive value of the device in detecting hypotension were calculated considering different cutoff values. Criteria to define hypotension were non-invasive SAP of 80 or 90 mmHg and/or non-invasive MAP of 60 or 65 mmHg. Sensitivity was calculated as the number of true hypotension measurements detected with the oscillometric methods divided by the number of all hypotensive measurements obtained with the invasive method. Specificity was calculated as the number of true non-hypotension measurements detected with the oscillometric method divided by the number of all non-hypotensive measurement obtained with the invasive method. The positive predictive value was calculated as the number of true hypotensive measurements obtained with the non-invasive method divided by the number of all hypotensive measurements obtained with the non-invasive method. The negative predictive value was calculated as the number of true non-hypotension measurements detected with the oscillometric method divided by the number of all non-hypotensive measurements obtained with the invasive method.

The number of animals used was estimated on the base of the criteria proposed by ACVIM Hypertension Consensus and Veterinary Blood Pressure Society [11]. To obtain a minimum of 150 readings, at least 15 rabbits would be necessary with at least 10 matched blood pressure measurements; to cover potential missed readings due to equipment failure or dropout animals due to unsuccessful artery catheterization, 19 rabbits were enrolled.

Graphpad (GraphPad Software, La Jolla, CA, USA), Matlab R2017a (The MathWorks Inc., Natick, MA, USA), MedCalc v12 (MedCalc Software bvba, Ostend, Belgium) and Microsoft Office Excel 2011 (Microsoft Corporation, Redmond, WA, USA) were used for the statistical analysis and to plot the data. Data normally distributed are expressed as mean $\pm$ SD otherwise as median (min-max).

Results

One rabbit was excluded because arterial catheter insertion was unsuccessful; in the remaining 18 rabbits, 172-paired measurements were collected and analysed. None of the rabbits presented postoperative complication due to arterial catheterization. The dose of propofol was 1.2 (0.0–6.0) mg and anaesthesia time was between 30 and 60 min. Natural frequency and damping coefficient were 29 ± 7 Hz and 0.28 ± 0.08 respectively and an adequate dynamic response was obtained for all rabbits. The normothermic range was maintained in all animals, with a mean rectal temperature at recovery of 38.5 ± 0.9 °C.

Results of Bland-Altman analysis of matched values for IBP over NIBP are shown in Table 1 and Fig. 1. Considering the overall values IBP was overestimated by the NIBP with a negative slope and a wide limits of agreement of approximately 50 mmHg for MAP and DAP. Repeating the analysis with pairs that included invasive SAP and MAP lower or equal to 80 and 60 mmHg respectively, resulted in a reduction of bias, standard deviation and limit of agreements compare to the previous analysis only for the mean arterial pressure (Fig. 1b and d). Both MAP and DAP met the requirements to define good agreement based on the limit of the ACVIM standard. Considering the AAMI standard instead, only pair measurements matching non-invasive MAP lower than 65 mmHg, showed good agreement. Agreement between methods was not adequate for SAP.

The analysis of the trending ability is reported in Table 2. The changes in the oscillometric device poorly reflect the direction of changes of IBP. Independent of the exclusion

zone the concordance rate for MAP, although lower than 90%, was higher than that of SAP and DAP (Table 2). The polar plot analysis showed a suboptimal trending ability with mean polar angles higher than 5° and a radial limits of agreement wider than ± 30° (Table 2 and Fig. 2).

Sensitivity of the device to identify hypotension was higher if the cutoff for the corresponding non-invasive pressure limits were set at 90 and 65 mmHg respectively. Considering those cutoff values the specificity decreased. Positive predictive value for systolic pressure was higher than that of mean blood pressure while the opposite was observed for the negative predictive value (Table 3).

Discussion

According to the criteria set at priori with mean bias lower than 10 mmHg and precision of 15 mmHg, only non-invasive MAP and DAP showed an acceptable agreement with the IBP technique. If the more restrictive criteria of AAMI standard were assessed, non-invasive MAP met the requirements of the analysis that included only animals with invasive MAP lower than 60 mmHg. The oscillometric device evaluated in this study showed a sensitivity of almost 92% in detecting values of mean IBP below 60 mmHg if the cutoff for the mean NIBP was set at 65 mmHg but specificity was 61%. Non-invasive SAP below 80 or 90 mmHg have a limited ability to identify systolic IBP lower than 80 mmHg. The trending ability of the NIBP device is poor considering the four-quadrant and the polar plot analysis and the concordance rate was below 90% for all the measured pressures.

The mean bias was decreased and the limit of agreement was smaller if data points for mean IBP below 60 mmHg were analysed rather than consider the overall values. The evaluation of this subgroup was performed to detect the accuracy of the NIBP monitor in a situation of low arterial blood pressure commonly referred as clinical relevant hypotension requiring a treatment. The bias for MAP in our study is smaller than SAP similarly to the results achieved by Barter and Epstein whom compare an oscillometric device with the carotid artery IBP [2]. Oscillometric method measure MAP as the pressure recorded at the point of maximal oscillation while SAP is usually estimated [9]. The bias for systolic blood pressure was lower if only invasive SAP values below 80 mmHg were considered and this may reflect an inadequacy of the device algorithm at high SAP values. Bias between NIBP and IBP measurements for DAP are almost identical as observed in other oscillometric device by Barter & Epstein [2].

Bland-Altman analysis, although widely used to evaluate the agreement between a monitoring device with a reference technique, does not provide any information on the ability of a new technology in detecting changes

Table 1 Statistical summary and results of Bland-Altman analysis for multiple observations in 19 anaesthetized rabbits

	Systolic	Mean	Diastolic
IBP (mmHg)	74 ± 10	59 ± 10	52 ± 11
NIBP (mmHg)	87 ± 19	64 ± 18	52 ± 18
Bland-Altman agreement analysis			
Mean bias (mmHg)			
Overall	−13.8	−4.5	−0.3
Hypotension	−13.9	−1.5	–
Precision (mmHg)			
Overall	16.7	12.5	13.0
Hypotension	15.1	8.1	–
Limits of agreement (mmHg)			
Overall	−46.5 to 18.9	−29.0 to 20.0	− 25.8 to 25.3
Hypotension	− 43.5 to 15.8	−14.4 to 17.3	–

Systolic, mean and diastolic arterial pressure measured with an oscillometric method were compared to an arterial blood pressure measured invasively by central ear artery cannulation. Overall pair include all the value measured while the hypotension subgroup include all the pair measurements that had a systolic or mean invasive arterial blood pressure lower than 80 and 60 mmHg respectively. IBP invasive arterial blood pressure; NIBP non-invasive arterial blood pressure. Values are expressed as mean ± standard deviation

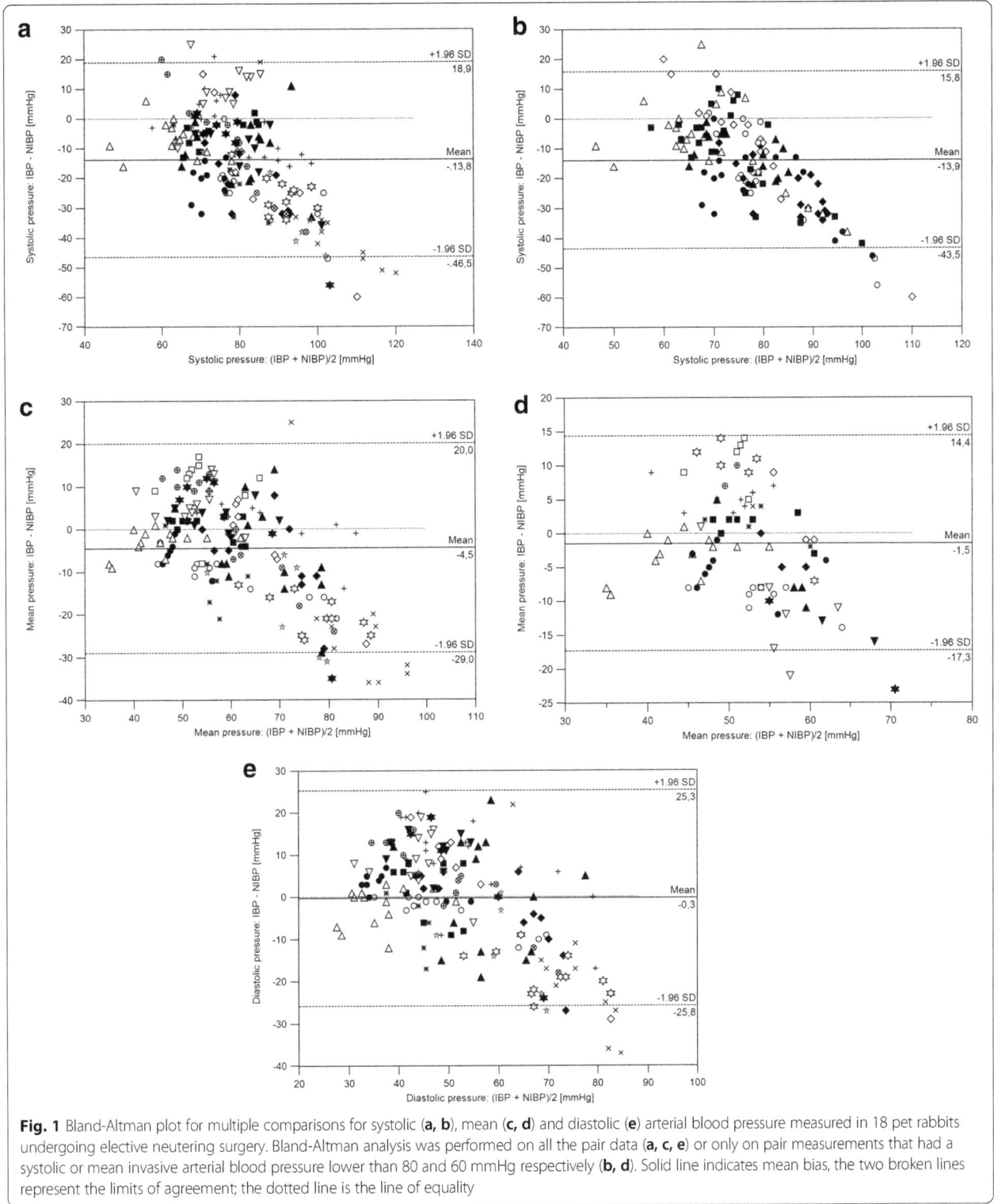

Fig. 1 Bland-Altman plot for multiple comparisons for systolic (**a, b**), mean (**c, d**) and diastolic (**e**) arterial blood pressure measured in 18 pet rabbits undergoing elective neutering surgery. Bland-Altman analysis was performed on all the pair data (**a, c, e**) or only on pair measurements that had a systolic or mean invasive arterial blood pressure lower than 80 and 60 mmHg respectively (**b, d**). Solid line indicates mean bias, the two broken lines represent the limits of agreement; the dotted line is the line of equality

consistent with those measured by the "gold standard" technique. This characteristic is known as trending ability of a device. Recently an analytical method was introduced to assess the trending ability of new devices for cardiac output measurement and the same analysis was applied to arterial blood pressure monitoring [13–15]. The trending ability in our study resulted poor with a concordance rate below 90% for SAP, DAP and MAP. However no published studies define a limit for good trending ability for blood pressure monitors either for

Table 2 Trending ability with concordance and polar plot data for 18 anaesthetized rabbits

	Systolic	Mean	Diastolic
Concordance rate			
Exclusion zone 5%	67%	84%	67%
Exclusion zone 10%	65%	87%	72%
Polar plot analysis (n)	82	100	90
Mean polar angle			
Exclusion zone 5%	−13.7°	−9.5°	− 12.0°
Standard deviation	28.0°	28.1°	31.4°
Radial limits of agreement			
Exclusion zone 5%	− 56.4° to 42.2°	−65.1° to 46.6°	−70.2° to 50.8°

Data points representing percentage changes lower than 5% (exclusion zone 5%) or 10% (exclusion zone 10%) were not included in the analysis. n: number of observations

the four-quadrant or the polar plot analysis. The limits reported in our study to define acceptable concordance rate and trending ability were set on previous literature in human medicine that in turn uses limits to assess cardiac output monitors [13, 15]. Moreover the refinement of the exclusion zone by Receiver Operating Characteristic (ROC) curve analysis was recommended for cardiac output monitoring although literature is lacking in a suitable exclusion zone for trending ability of blood pressure monitor. The exclusion zone used in our study has been reported previously although an optimal value for NIBP monitor is not yet outlined [13, 15]. The trending ability in this study may also have been affected by a low agreement between measurement methods especially at high blood pressure. Minimal changes in IBP might be associated with opposite changes of high magnitude in NIBP. Those changes, included in the analysis, may have caused a dispersion of data in the four-quadrant and polar plot analysis affecting the concordance rate and the trending ability. Moreover hypotensive episodes in some rabbits responded poorly to a decrease in end-tidal isoflurane and as no other treatments were performed, the assessment of trending ability in our study might be difficult to quantify.

Rabbits are particularly sensitive to the vasodilatatory effects of volatile anaesthetics despite an ongoing surgical procedure or the application of a supramaximal electrical stimulation [4, 16]. Harvey et al. arbitrarily defined hypotension in anaesthetized rabbits as invasive SAP or MAP lower than 60 mmHg and/or 80 mmHg respectively [4], and based on these criterion most of the rabbits in the study were classified as hypotensive. Because mean bias between NIBP and IBP for MAP and SAP were almost 5 and 10 mmHg, it was decided to evaluate the performance of the device describing hypotension with a cutoff of 65

and 90 mmHg respectively. Using the cutoff of 65 mmHg for MAP the device showed a superior sensitivity in detecting mean IBP lower than 60 mmHg. The new analysis indeed showed an increase in sensitivity for MAP of almost 92% while the sensitivity to detect a systolic IBP lower than 80 mmHg remains lower regardless the cutoff considered, although it increases from 46 to 74%.

Our study presents some limitations: first the agreement between IBP and NIBP was evaluated only in the front limb, while hind limb may have resulted in a different outcome. Ypsilantis et al. demonstrated a good correlation between the oscillometric pressures measured on the front limb with that recorded on the abdominal aorta rather the one recorded on the hind limb [7]. For neutering procedure the positioning of the cuff on the hind limb was considered less suitable because it proves difficult to reach in case of dislodgment or detachment.

All the rabbits enrolled in this study were owned patients undergoing elective neutering. While the use of such cases may provide a good evaluation of the oscillometric device in a clinical setting, on the other hand this represents a limitation because these may have introduced confounding factors due to a different haemodynamic status based on the surgical stimulations.

Another limitation is that during the surgical procedure, the intensity of the cardiovascular stimulation may have varied rapidly on the base of the manoeuvre performed. The dynamic response test was performed at the beginning of each anaesthesia but it was not repeated during the surgical procedure. The fundamental frequency, represented by the pulse rate (170–200 beats/min), was almost 6 times the natural frequency measured. This contributed to reduce the underdamping of the fluid-filled pressure transducer system due to the low damping coefficient recorded in most of rabbits [10]. Underdamping of a system used to measure IBP tends to overestimate SAP while the opposite is observed in a system that demonstrates overdamping. It cannot be excluded that according to the increase in the haemodynamic status a change in the damping coefficient may have influenced the agreement particularly at high blood pressure values.

Conclusion

Agreement is poor between the systolic arterial blood pressure measured with the non-invasive device and that measured invasively at the level of ear artery. Invasive MAP is overestimated at high pressure values although bias decreases if only measurements lower than 60 mmHg obtained invasively were considered and match the requirement of good agreement based on ACVIM and AACI guidelines. Trending ability of the new device is

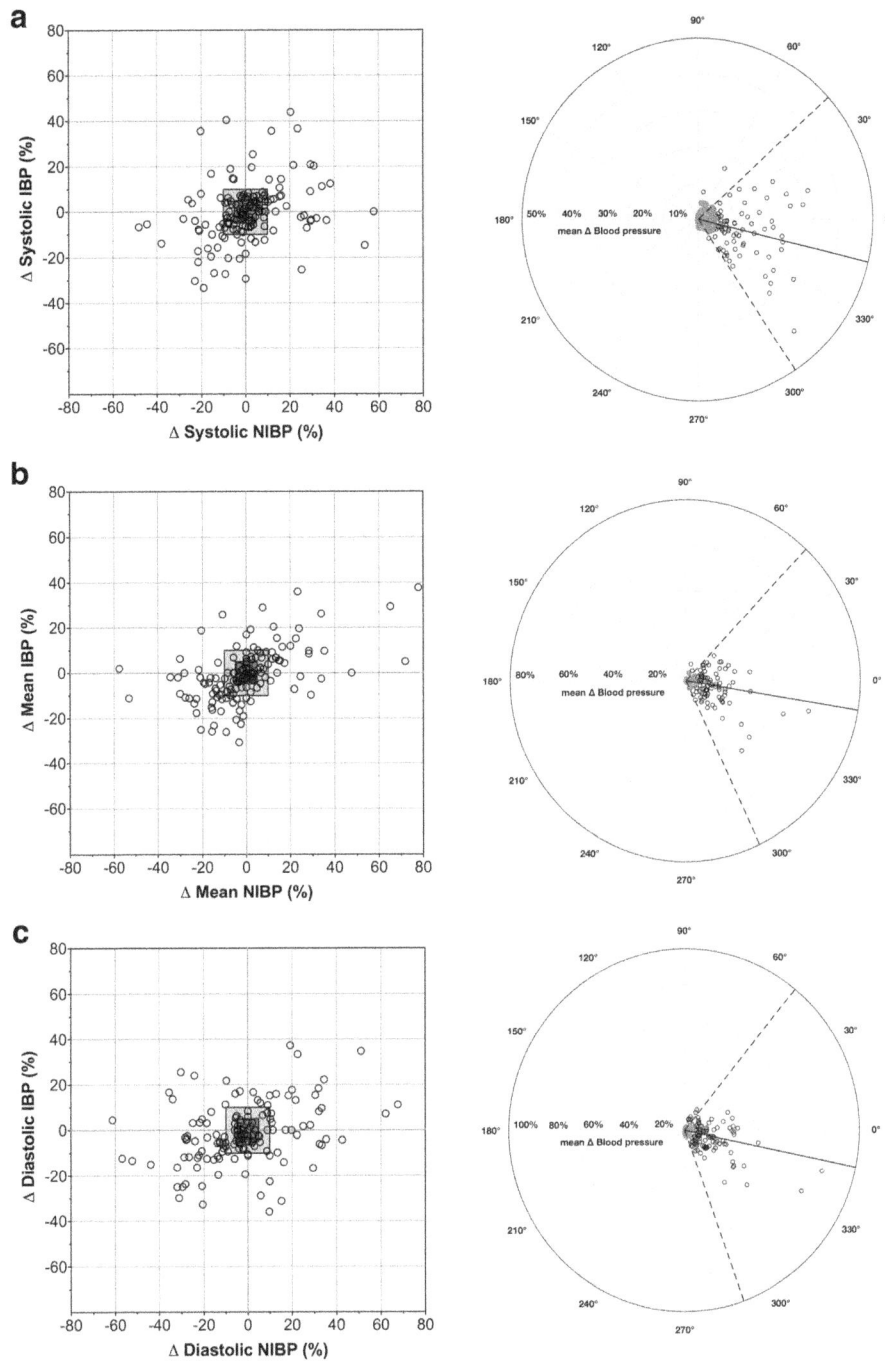

Fig. 2 Four-quadrant (left) and polar plot (right) for systolic (a), mean (b) and diastolic (c) arterial blood pressure measured in 18 pet rabbits undergoing elective neutering surgery. In the concordance plot, each point represents a percentage changes in arterial blood pressure measured with an oscillometric device (Δ NIBP) or invasively (Δ IBP). In the 4-quadrant plot the grey areas limit the 10% and 5% exclusion zone where percentage changes in arterial blood pressure are ≤10% and 5% respectively. Dots in the upper left or lower right quadrant represent inaccurate trending between methods. The positive half circle polar plots show the values for the mean changes of arterial blood pressure measurement obtained non-invasively and invasively. The distance of each point from the center represents the mean change in arterial blood pressure calculated as absolute value of Δ NIBP+Δ IBP/2; the angle with the horizontal axis shows the concordance of the methods. Solid line defines the mean angular bias and the dotted lines the upper and lower radial limit of agreement (bias ±1.96 × standard deviation) obtained for the data points in black. The grey points represent arterial blood pressure changes ≤5% (exclusion zone 5%) and were excluded from the analysis. Good agreement between the two methods is considered with a mean angular bias and a radial limit of agreement < 5° and < 30° respectively

Table 3 Ability of the oscillometric monitor in detecting systolic or mean invasive pressure lower than 80 or 60 mmHg

	Sensitivity	Specificity	Positive predictive value	Negative predictive value
Systolic arterial blood pressure				
Cutoff of 80 mmHg for NIBP	46.3% (37.3%–5.56%)	77.6% (63.4%–88.2%)	83.8% (72.9%–91.6%)	36.5% (27.3%–46.6%)
Cutoff of 90 mmHg for NIBP	74.0% (65.3%–81.5%)	57.1% (42.2%–71.2%)	81.3% (72.8%–88.0%)	46.7% (33.7%–60.0%)
Mean arterial blood pressure				
Cutoff 60 of mmHg for NIBP	73.8% (63.0%–82.8%)	78.4% (68.4%–86.5%)	76.5% (65.8%–85.3%)	75.8% (65.7%–84.2%)
Cutoff 65 of mmHg for NIBP	91.8% (83.6%–96.6%)	61.4% (50.4%–71.6%)	69.4% (59.9%–77.8%)	88.5% (77.8%–95.3%)

Specificity, sensitivity, positive and negative predictive value of the non-invasive oscillometric blood pressure (NIBP) device in detecting a systolic and a mean invasive blood pressure lower than 80 mmHg and 60 mmHg at different cutoff limits. Data are expressed as percentage (95% confidential interval)

poor although for MAP concordance rate is superior than SAP and DAP. The sensitivity of the device is higher in detecting invasive MAP lower than 60 mmHg if a cutoff value of 65 mmHg is considered and may be used to identify hypotension in anaesthetized rabbits although it has a poor ability to identify false positive.

Abbreviations
DAP: Diastolic arterial blood pressure; IBP: Invasive arterial blood pressure; IV: Intravenous; MAP: Mean arterial blood pressure; NIBP: Non-invasive arterial blood pressure; SAP: Systolic arterial blood pressure

Acknowledgments
None.

Funding
Not applicable.

Authors' contributions
LB, study design, data collection and interpretation and preparation of manuscript; IAV, data management and preparation of manuscript; MS, data collection and preparation of manuscript; MC, data collection and management and preparation of manuscript; AM, study design, data collection and interpretation and preparation of manuscript. All authors read and approved the final manuscript.

Consent for publication
Not applicable.

Competing interests
The authors declare that they have no competing interests.

Author details
[1]Veterinary Teaching Hospital, University of Padua, Viale dell'Università 16, 35020 Legnaro, PD, Italy. [2]Department of Animal Medicine, Production and Health, University of Padua, Viale dell'Università 16, 35020 Legnaro, PD, Italy.

References
1. Brodbelt DC, Blissitt KJ, Hammond RA, Neath PJ, Young LE, Pfeiffer DU, et al. The risk of death: the confidential enquiry into perioperative small animal fatalities. Vet Anaesth Analg. 2008;35:365–73.
2. Barter LS, Epstein SE. Comparison of Doppler, oscillometric, auricular and carotid arterial blood pressure measurements in isoflurane anesthetized New Zealand white rabbits. Vet Anaesth Analg. 2014;41:393–7.
3. Bellini L, Banzato T, Contiero B, Zotti A. Evaluation of sedation and clinical effects of midazolam with ketamine or dexmedetomidine in pet rabbits. Vet Rec. 2014;175(15):372.
4. Harvey L, Knowles T, Murison PJ. Comparison of direct and Doppler arterial blood pressure measurements in rabbits during isoflurane anaesthesia. Vet Anaesth Analg. 2012;39:174–84.
5. Love L, Harvey R. Arterial blood pressure measurement: physiology, tools, and techniques. Comp Contin Edu Pr Vet. 2006;28:450–61.
6. Allweiler SI. How to improve anesthesia and analgesia in small mammals. Vet Clin North Am Exot Anim Pract. 2016;19:361–77.
7. Ypsilantis P, Didilis VN, Politou M, Bougioukas I, Bougioukas G, Simopoulos C. A comparative study of invasive and oscillometric methods of arterial blood pressure measurement in the anesthetized rabbit. Res Vet Sci. 2005;78:269–75.
8. Lakhal K, Ehrmann S, Runge I, Legras A, Dequin PF, Mercier E, et al. Tracking hypotension and dynamic changes in arterial blood pressure with brachial cuff measurements. Anesth Analg. 2009;109:494–501.
9. Ehrmann S, Lakhal K, Boulain T. Pression artérielle non invasive : principes et indications aux urgences et en réanimation. Réanimation. 2009;18:267–73.
10. Cerejo SA, Teixeira-Neto FJ, Garofalo NA, Rodrigues JC, Celeita-Rodríguez N, Lagos-Carvajal AP. Comparison of two species-specific oscillometric blood pressure monitors with direct blood pressure measurement in anesthetized cats. J Vet Emerg Crit Care. 2017; https://doi.org/10.1111/vec.12623.
11. Brown S, Atkins C, Bagley R, Carr A, Cowgill L, Davidson M, et al. ACVIM consensus statement guidelines for the identification, evaluation, and management of systemic hypertension in dogs and cats; 2007. p. 542–58.
12. Bland JM, Altman DG. Agreement between methods of measurement with multiple observations per individual. J Biopharm Stat. 2007;17:571–82.
13. Smolle K, Schmid M, Prettenthaler H, Weger C. The accuracy of the CNAP® device compared with invasive radial artery measurements for providing continuous noninvasive arterial blood pressure readings at a medical intensive care unit: a method-comparison study. Anesth Analg. 2015;121:1508–16.
14. Critchley LA, Lee A, Ho AM. A critical review of the ability of continuous cardiac output monitors to measure trends in cardiac output. Anesth Analg. 2010;111:1180–92.
15. Lakhal K, Martin M, Faiz S, Ehrmann S, Blanloeil Y, Asehnoune K, et al. The CNAP™ finger cuff for noninvasive beat-to-beat monitoring of arterial blood pressure: an evaluation in intensive care unit patients and a comparison with 2 intermittent devices. Anesth Analg. 2016;123:1126–35.
16. Barter LS, Epstein SE. Cardiopulmonary effects of three concentrations of isoflurane with or without mechanical ventilation and supramaximal noxious stimulation in New Zealand white rabbits. Am J Vet Res. 2013;74:1274–80.

A comparison of microRNA expression profiles from splenic hemangiosarcoma, splenic nodular hyperplasia, and normal spleens of dogs

Janet A. Grimes[1,5*], Nripesh Prasad[2], Shawn Levy[2], Russell Cattley[3], Stephanie Lindley[1], Harry W. Boothe[1], Ralph A. Henderson[1] and Bruce F. Smith[4]

Abstract

Background: Splenic masses are common in older dogs; yet diagnosis preceding splenectomy and histopathology remains elusive. MicroRNAs (miRNAs) are short, non-coding RNAs that play a role in post-transcriptional regulation, and differential expression of miRNAs between normal and tumor tissue has been used to diagnose neoplastic diseases. The objective of this study was to determine differential expression of miRNAs by use of RNA-sequencing in canine spleens that were histologically confirmed as hemangiosarcoma, nodular hyperplasia, or normal.

Results: Twenty-two miRNAs were found to be differentially expressed in hemangiosarcoma samples (4 between hemangiosarcoma and both nodular hyperplasia and normal spleen and 18 between hemangiosarcoma and normal spleen only). In particular, mir-26a, mir-126, mir-139, mir-140, mir-150, mir-203, mir-424, mir-503, mir-505, mir-542, mir-30e, mir-33b, mir-365, mir-758, mir-22, and mir-452 are of interest in the pathogenesis of hemangiosarcoma.

Conclusions: Findings of this study confirm the hypothesis that miRNA expression profiles are different between canine splenic hemangiosarcoma, nodular hyperplasia, and normal spleens. A large portion of the differentially expressed miRNAs have roles in angiogenesis, with an additional group of miRNAs being dysregulated in vascular disease processes. Two other miRNAs have been implicated in cancer pathways such as PTEN and cell cycle checkpoints. The finding of multiple miRNAs with roles in angiogenesis and vascular disease is important, as hemangiosarcoma is a tumor of endothelial cells, which are driven by angiogenic stimuli. This study shows that miRNA dysregulation is a potential player in the pathogenesis of canine splenic hemangiosarcoma.

Keywords: Splenic mass, Hemangiosarcoma, Canine, MicroRNA, RNA-sequencing, Angiogenesis

Background

Splenic masses are common in older dogs and may be malignant, benign, or non-neoplastic; yet diagnosis preceding splenectomy and histopathology remains elusive. Several studies have reported approximately 70% of dogs with non-traumatic hemoperitoneum had hemangiosarcoma [1–3]. Hemoperitoneum is reported in 63–80% of dogs with hemangiosarcoma, compared with only 30% of dogs with benign splenic masses [4, 5]. This has led to the 'double 2/3 rule,' which is currently used to give owners a prediction of the odds of each of the possibilities [6]. According to this rule, approximately 2/3 of splenic masses are malignant, and of those that are malignant, 2/3 are hemangiosarcoma. Other malignant splenic masses include various sarcomas, lymphoma, and histiocytic sarcoma [1, 7]. Benign and non-malignant splenic conditions include hemangioma, nodular hyperplasia, formerly classified as a subset of fibrohistiocytic nodules, and hematoma [1, 8].

* Correspondence: jgrimes@uga.edu
[1]Department of Clinical Sciences, Auburn University College of Veterinary Medicine, Auburn University, Auburn, AL, USA
[5]Department of Small Animal Medicine and Surgery, College of Veterinary Medicine, University of Georgia, 2200 College Station Road, Athens, GA 30602, USA
Full list of author information is available at the end of the article

Many studies have attempted to identify repeatable measures or other techniques that might distinguish malignant from benign masses [5, 9–14]. For instance, mass-to-splenic volume ratio and splenic weight as a percentage of body weight have been used to differentiate malignant from benign splenic lesions, with hemangiosarcoma masses being smaller in both categories [5]. However, these values can only be calculated after splenectomy, and splenic size can change due to contraction or engorgement in response to medications or hemoperitoneum. Diagnostic imaging has been evaluated for its ability to differentiate malignant from benign lesions with contrast harmonic ultrasound, CT, and MRI showing promise [9–11]. Such modalities may differentiate malignant from benign lesions but do not diagnose a specific disease process. Prognosis and survival times between various malignancies can be quite varied and availability of these treatment modalities is limited and may be cost prohibitive [1, 12, 15]. While splenic aspirates may be beneficial for certain neoplasms such as lymphosarcoma, they usually fail to aid in the diagnosis of many splenic tumors due to blood contamination and poor exfoliation. Also, some clinicians recommend not aspirating the spleen in suspected cases of hemangiosarcoma due to risk of tumor rupture and seeding of the tumor into the abdomen [5, 6]. Testing of blood with multi-parameter flow cytometry and measuring levels of vascular endothelial growth factor and thymidine kinase have been evaluated, but have not been found to be definitive diagnostic tools [12–14]. It is clear that additional work needs to be done to develop a minimally invasive pre-surgical diagnostic test to differentiate hemangiosarcoma from other splenic masses.

Hemangiosarcoma, a tumor of vascular endothelial origin, is the most common splenic tumor, and the prognosis is poor: dogs that undergo surgery alone as a treatment for splenic hemangiosarcoma have a median survival time of three months; this extends to six months if chemotherapy is used in conjunction with surgery [6]. The decision to proceed with surgery can be difficult for owners because although there are rare long-term survivors, median survival times are typically short, and currently there is no ability to give a definitive diagnosis prior to surgery and histopathology.

MicroRNAs (miRNAs) are 18–25 nucleotide, single stranded, non-coding RNAs that play a role in post-transcriptional regulation [16–18]. MicroRNAs inhibit expression of target genes by binding to the 3' untranslated region of certain messenger RNAs (mRNAs) [16, 17]. MicroRNAs have a role in cell growth, cell differentiation, apoptosis, and oncogenesis [17]. Expression profiles give information on the identities and quantities of particular miRNAs within a given tissue; such profiles are consistent between like-tissue samples [19].

MicroRNAs in tumor samples have been used to diagnose tumors, provide prognostic information, and aid in targeted treatments in human medicine [18–22]. Many tumor types have been evaluated for differential miRNA expression, including ovarian carcinomas, breast cancer, cervical cancer, non-small cell lung cancer, leukemias, colorectal tumors, squamous cell carcinoma, and hepatocellular carcinoma [21–28]. Use of miRNAs in support of other diagnostic methods is currently in its infancy, with miRNA signatures having been developed in people to distinguish melanoma and metastatic breast cancer from healthy controls and higher risk groups in breast cancer and prostate cancer [29–32]. There are few reports of miRNA involvement in cancer of veterinary patients, but interest in this area will likely increase with the rapid growth of this topic in human medicine [33–35].

MicroRNAs have excellent stability in serum, and miRNAs representative of cancer tissue have been identified in the circulation of patients with cancer [20]. Such identification allows for the potential to develop a noninvasive diagnostic test to diagnose cancers, without having to obtain a tissue sample of the tumor of interest. The objective of this study was to identify and compare expression profiles of miRNAs from canine splenic hemangiosarcoma, splenic nodular hyperplasia, and normal splenic tissues using RNA-sequencing. We hypothesized that there would be differences in miRNA expression among the three groups. This work is the first step in determining altered miRNA expression in canine splenic masses. Once altered miRNA expression has been identified in the tissues, future studies can be performed to evaluate these same altered miRNAs in the serum of patients with splenic masses. The end goal of this research is to develop a blood-based diagnostic test to determine the nature of canine splenic masses. Ultimately, this work may also provide insight into pathways that are dysregulated in hemangiosarcoma, allowing a better understanding of both tumorigenesis and potential therapies.

Methods
Sample collection
Splenic mass samples: Samples were collected from spleens removed from client-owned animals undergoing splenectomy for a splenic mass. After removal of the spleen, the mass was trimmed to obtain two samples: one for the study and an adjacent piece of tissue for histopathologic evaluation to confirm a diagnosis and ensure that representative tissue was present in the sample. Samples to be used for the study were flash frozen with liquid nitrogen within 30 min of splenectomy and stored in a −80 °C freezer until further use. Only masses confirmed to contain tissue from hemangiosarcoma or

nodular hyperplasia were used for the study. Five samples in each category (hemangiosarcoma and nodular hyperplasia) were collected.

Normal spleen samples: Archived fresh frozen tissue samples were utilized to analyze normal splenic tissue. Samples were collected within 30 min of splenectomy, flash frozen in liquid nitrogen, and stored in a −80 °C freezer. Histopathology of adjacent tissue performed at the time of sample collection confirmed these five spleens to be normal.

Histopathology

Tissues (splenic masses and normal spleens) were trimmed and fixed in 10% neutral-buffered formalin for 24–72 h prior to processing by paraffin impregnation. Sections approximately 4–5 microns thick were prepared by microtomy, mounted on glass slides, deparaffinized, and stained with hematoxylin and eosin prior to applying glass coverslips. Each slide was evaluated by light microscopy for diagnosis by a board-certified (ACVP) pathologist. Cases of hemangiosarcoma were confirmed by demonstration of CD31 by immunohistochemistry (Dako, Denmark). Sections were mounted onto slides, deparaffinized, heat-treated for antigen retrieval, and labeled with CD31 using FLEX monoclonal mouse anti-human CD31 clone JC70A visualized by peroxidase-mediated oxidation of diaminobenzidine (EnVision FLEX + Mouse High pH Link system, Dako, Denmark). Slides were coverslipped, counterstained with hematoxylin, and examined by light microscopy.

RNA isolation

The Qiagen miRNeasy kit (Qiagen Inc., Valencia, CA, USA) was utilized to extract RNA from the frozen tissue sections. Extraction was performed according to manufacturer protocol using the Bullet Blender (Next Advance Inc., Averill Park, NY, USA) for homogenization, and one modification to the protocol, where the Buffer RWT step was repeated for a second time. The NanoDrop (ThermoScientific, Wilmington, DE, USA) was used to confirm an appropriate 260/280 and 260/230 ratio for the sample (>1.8 in each case).

RNA Sequencing and smRNA library prep protocol

RNA samples were sent to the Genomic Services Laboratory at the HudsonAlpha Institute for Biotechnology for miRNA-sequencing analysis. NEBNext® Small RNA Library Prep Set for Illumina® (New England Bio-Labs Inc., Ipswich, MA, USA) was utilized. Three prime adapters were ligated to total input RNA followed by hybridization of multiplex SR RT primers and ligation of multiplex 5` SR adapters. Reverse Transcription (RT) was done using SuperScript III RT (Life Technologies, Grand Island, NY, USA) for 1 h at 50 °C. Immediately

after RT reaction, indexed primers were added to uniquely barcode each sample and PCR amplification was done for 12 cycles using LongAmp Taq 2X master mix. Post PCR material was then purified using QIAquick PCR purification kit (Qiagen Inc., Valencia, CA, USA). Post PCR yield and concentration of the prepared libraries was assessed using Qubit® 2.0 Fluorometer and DNA 1000 chip on Agilent 2100 Bioanalyzer.

Size selection of small RNA libraries with a target size range of 140 base pairs was done on a 3% agarose gel using Pipin prep instrument (Sage Science, Boston, MA, USA). Accurate quantification for sequencing applications was performed using the qPCR-based KAPA Biosystems Library Quantification kit. Each library was diluted to a final concentration of 12.5 nM and pooled equimolar prior to clustering. Cluster generation was carried out on a cBot v1.4.36.0 using Illumina's Truseq Single Read (SR) Cluster Kit v3.0. Single End (SE) sequencing was performed on an Illumina HiSeq2000, running HiSeq Control Software (HCS) v1.5.15.1, using a 50 cycle TruSeq SBS HS v3 reagent kit. The clustered flowcells were sequenced for 56 cycles, consisting of a 50 cycle read, followed by a 6 cycle index read. Image analysis and base calling was performed using the standard Illumina Pipeline consisting of Real Time Analysis (RTA) version v1.13 and demultiplexed using bcl2fastq converter with default settings.

Analysis

Post-processing of the sequencing reads from miRNA-sequencing experiments from each sample was performed as per unique in-house pipelines. Briefly, quality control checks on raw sequence data from each sample was performed using FastQC (Babraham Bioinformatics, London, UK). Raw reads were imported on a commercial data analysis platform CLCbio (Qiagen Inc., Valencia, CA, USA). Adapter trimming (GTGACTGGAGTTCAGACGTGTG CTCTTCCGATCT) was done to remove ligated adapters from the 3' end of the sequenced reads with only one mismatch allowed; poorly aligned 3' ends were also trimmed. Sequences shorter than 15 nucleotides length were excluded from further analysis. Trimmed reads with low qualities (base quality score less than 30, alignment score less than 95, mapping quality less than 40) were removed. Filtered reads were used to extract and count the small RNA that were annotated with miRNAs from the miRBase release 20 database [36, 37].

The quantification operation carried out measurement at both the gene level and at the active region level. Active region quantification considered only reads whose 5' end matched the 5' end of the mature miRNA annotation. Samples were grouped as patient and control identifiers, and differential expression of miRNA was calculated on the basis of their fold change observed between individual patients and averaged control samples. The p-value of differentially expressed miRNAs was estimated by implementing t-tests with Benjamini Hochberg false discovery rate corrections of 0.05 [38].

Results

Principal component analysis was performed compiling the miRNA data from all five samples within each group. This revealed hemangiosarcoma samples grouped independently from nodular hyperplasia and normal spleen, indicating hemangiosarcoma samples were distinctly different than the other two categories (Fig. 1). When hemangiosarcoma samples were removed from the analysis, nodular hyperplasia and normal spleen samples also showed differential expression, indicating that it may be possible to distinguish between these two conditions with further analyses (Fig. 2). Volcano plots were created of the comparison groups highlighting miRNAs that were significantly over or underexpressed between the groups. Significant over and underexpression of various miRNAs was found for each of the three groups: hemangiosarcoma compared to normal spleen (Fig. 3), hemangiosarcoma compared to nodular hyperplasia (Fig. 4), and nodular hyperplasia compared to normal spleen (Fig. 5).

Individual microRNA results were evaluated, significance was set at $p < 0.05$, and data were limited to microRNAs with a fold change $\geq \pm 2$. With these criteria, 51 unique miRNAs were found to be differentially expressed across the three groups (Fig. 6), with 4 miRNAs being potential candidates specific to hemangiosarcoma (Table 1) and 18 being differentially expressed between hemangiosarcoma and normal spleen only (Table 2). No miRNAs were significantly differentially expressed between all of the three possible pairings.

Hemangiosarcoma compared to both normal spleen and nodular hyperplasia

Four miRNAs were significantly different between hemangiosarcoma samples and both normal spleens and spleens with nodular hyperplasia, indicating these miRNAs may be markers specific for hemangiosarcoma (Table 1). Of these miRNAs, two were significantly overexpressed (mir-126, mir-452) and two significantly underexpressed (mir-150, mir-203) in hemangiosarcoma samples compared to both normal spleens and spleens with nodular hyperplasia.

Hemangiosarcoma compared to normal spleen

Eighteen miRNAs were differentially expressed between hemangiosarcoma and normal spleen only (without also

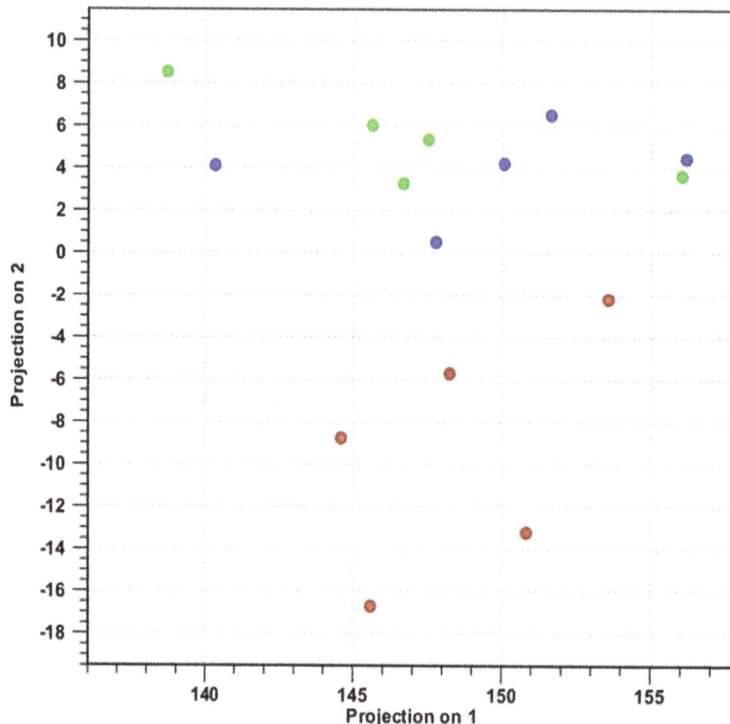

Fig. 1 Principal component analysis of hemangiosarcoma, nodular hyperplasia, and normal spleen samples. The hemangiosarcoma samples (*red*) showed differential expression from both nodular hyperplasia (*blue*) and normal spleen (*green*) samples. The axes correspond to principal component 1 (x-axis) and principal component 2 (y-axis)

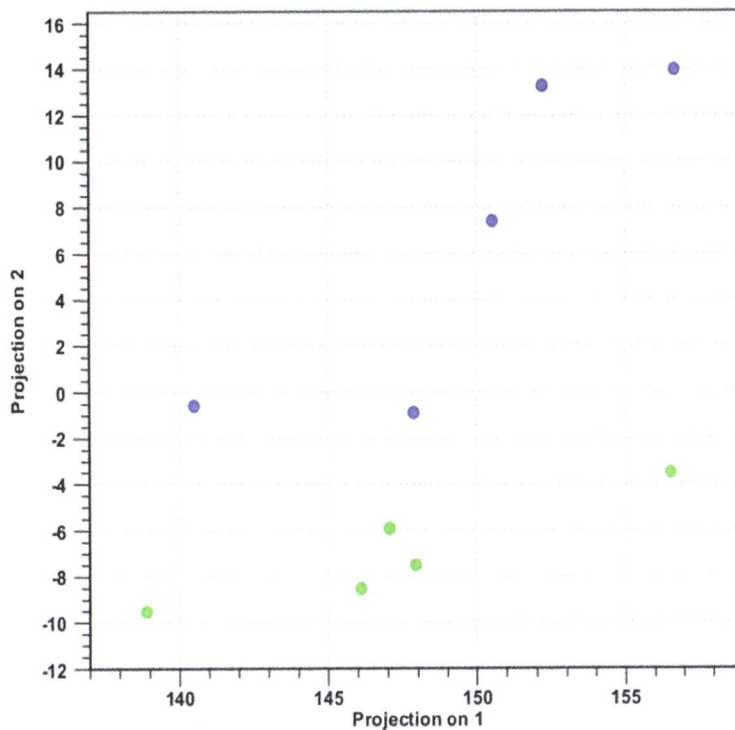

Fig. 2 Principal component analysis of nodular hyperplasia and normal spleen samples. The nodular hyperplasia samples (*blue*) showed differential expression from normal spleen samples (*green*). The axes correspond to principal component 1 (x-axis) and principal component 2 (y-axis)

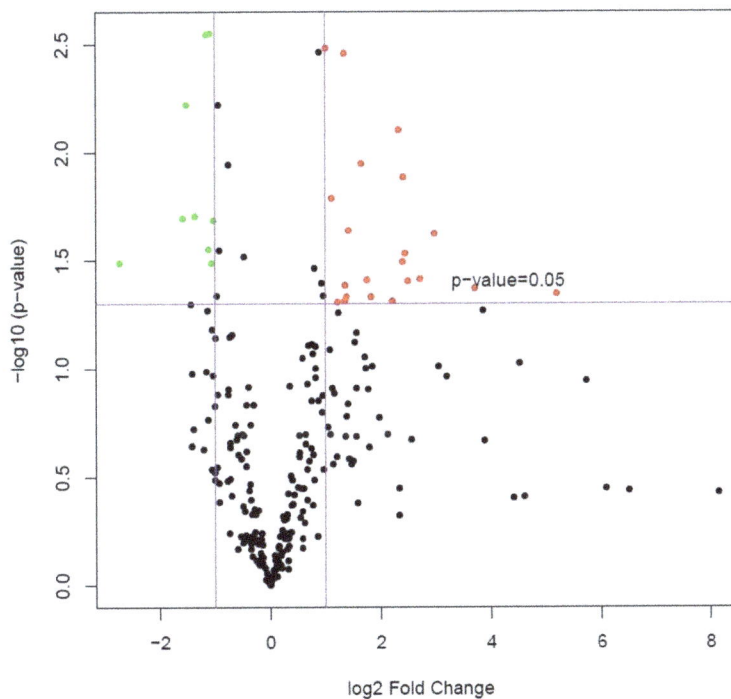

Fig. 3 Volcano plot showing significantly overexpressed (*red*) and significantly underexpressed (*green*) miRNAs between hemangiosarcoma and normal spleen. The axes correspond to $\log_2$ (fold change) (x-axis) and $-\log_{10}$ (*p*-value) (y-axis)

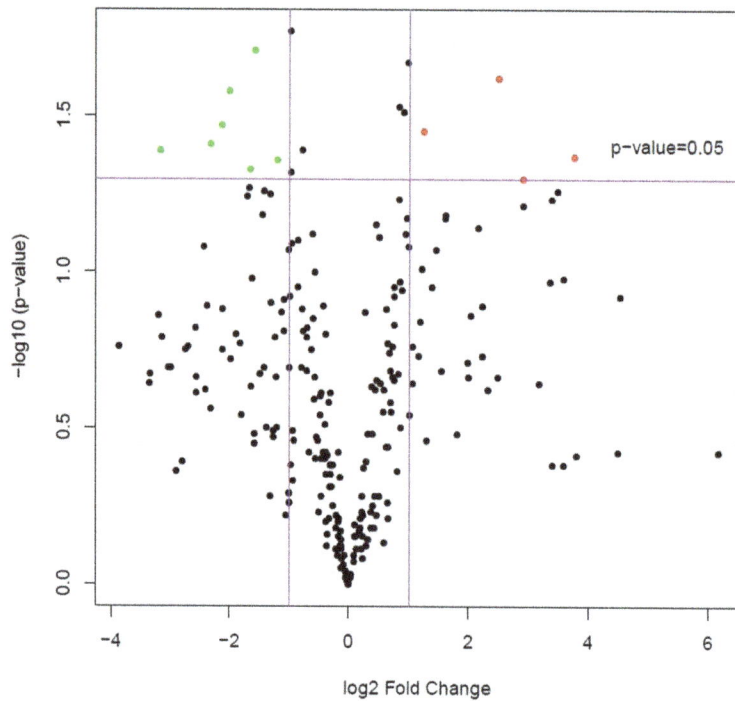

Fig. 4 Volcano plot showing significantly overexpressed (*red*) and significantly underexpressed (*green*) miRNAs between hemangiosarcoma and nodular hyperplasia. The axes correspond to $\log_2$ (fold change) (x-axis) and $-\log_{10}$ (*p*-value) (y-axis)

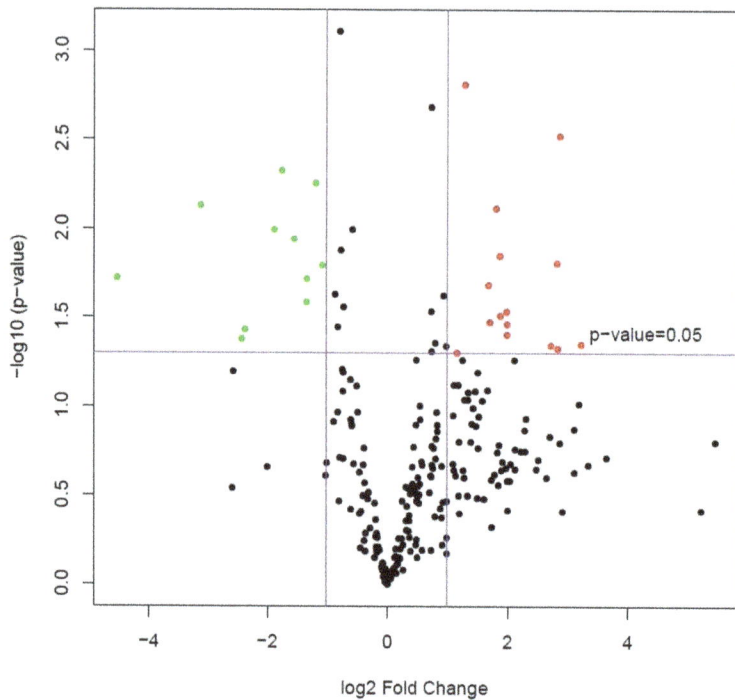

Fig. 5 Volcano plot showing significantly overexpressed (*red*) and significantly underexpressed (*green*) miRNAs between nodular hyperplasia and normal spleen. The axes correspond to $\log_2$ (fold change) (x-axis) and $-\log_{10}$ (*p*-value) (y-axis)

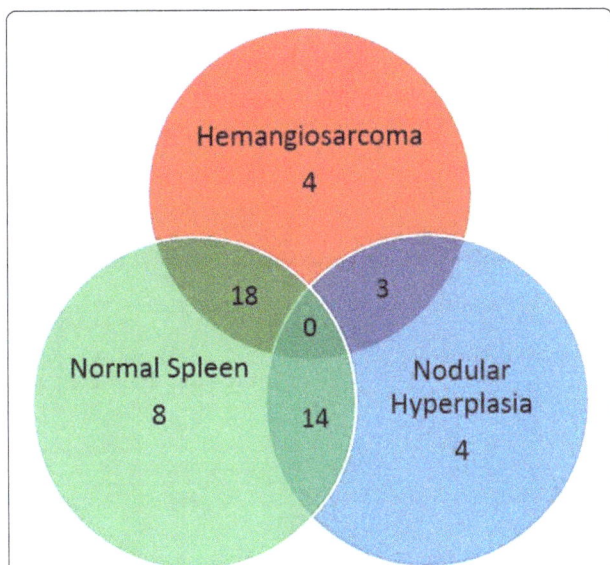

Fig. 6 Venn diagram demonstrating miRNAs differentially expressed between hemangiosarcoma, nodular hyperplasia, and normal spleen (fold change ≥ ± 2, significance set a $p < 0.05$). Eighteen miRNAs were differentially expressed solely between hemangiosarcoma and normal spleen samples. Fourteen miRNAs were differentially expressed solely between nodular hyperplasia and normal spleen samples. Three miRNAs were differentially expressed solely between hemangiosarcoma and nodular hyperplasia samples. Four miRNAs were determined to be potential markers of hemangiosarcoma as they were differentially expressed between hemangiosarcoma and nodular hyperplasia samples and also hemangiosarcoma and normal spleen samples. Four miRNAs were determined to be potential markers of nodular hyperplasia as they were differentially expressed between hemangiosarcoma and nodular hyperplasia samples and also nodular hyperplasia and normal spleen samples. Eight miRNAs were determined to be potential markers of normal splenic tissue as they were differentially expressed between hemangiosarcoma and normal spleen samples and also nodular hyperplasia and normal spleen samples

canines with splenic hemangiosarcoma, splenic nodular hyperplasia, and normal spleens.

Four miRNAs were identified as potential markers of hemangiosarcoma, as they were differentially expressed in hemangiosarcoma samples compared to both normal spleen and nodular hyperplasia samples: mir-126, mir-150, mir-203, and mir-452. Mir-126 and mir-452 were significantly overexpressed in hemangiosarcoma samples, while mir-150 and mir-203 were significantly underexpressed in hemangiosarcoma samples compared to normal spleen and nodular hyperplasia samples. Three of these miRNAs, mir-126, mir-150, and mir-203 have previously been found to have roles in angiogenesis [39–47]. Previous reviews have confirmed that mir-126 is expressed in higher numbers in vascular tissues such as heart, liver, and lung and also in endothelial cell lineage cells [39, 43, 48]. Additional work has shown that mir-126 levels are increased in endothelial precursor cells, which are the cells of origin of hemangiosarcoma, explaining their upregulation in this particular tumor type [12, 40–43]. Mir-126 can behave in both pro- and anti-angiogenic ways, but is pro-angiogenic in endothelial precursor cells and actively proliferating and migrating endothelial cells [41]. Mir-126 enhances angiogenesis by increasing VEGF expression through its targeting of the PI3K regulatory subunit 2 (p85β) [39, 40, 43, 49]. Dogs with hemangiosarcoma have higher plasma VEGF levels than healthy controls, which correlates with the findings of increased mir-126 expression in hemangiosarcoma samples [13]. The PI3K pathway has been previously implicated in canine hemangiosarcoma as well, with mutations in PTEN leading to increased phosphorylated Akt [50]. Mir-126 may be acting in concert with other mediators to influence this pathway, leading to increased VEGF production and a pro-survival state. Mir-126 also targets regulator of G-protein signaling (RGS16) which inhibits CXCR4, an important protein in angiogenesis [41, 51]. When CXCR4 is activated, both circulating hematopoietic stem cells and prostate cancer cells have increased endothelial cell adhesion and transendothelial migration, indicating this pathway may direct metastasis [52, 53]. Mir-150 also plays a role in regulation of CXCR4, with decreased

playing a role in nodular hyperplasia samples), with 15 being significantly overexpressed in hemangiosarcoma samples and three being underexpressed (Table 2).

Discussion

The results of this study confirm the hypothesis that miRNAs are differentially expressed in the tissues of

Table 1 MiRNAs significantly differentially expressed between hemangiosarcoma and both nodular hyperplasia and normal spleen[a]

MicroRNA	Fold Change (HSA vs. NS)	p-value (HSA vs. NS)	Fold Change (HSA vs. NH)	p-value (HSA vs. NH)	HSA (Means)	NH (Means)	NS (Means)
mir-126	3.382336	0.038943	5.614515	0.023733	40134.8	7148.4	11866
mir-150	−2.84562	0.006069	−9.05708	0.040751	3097.6	28055.2	8814.6
mir-203	−2.56436	0.01982	−2.29043	0.043515	60.6	138.8	155.4
mir-452	13.06709	0.042741	13.54305	0.042579	818	60.4	62.6

[a] fold change ≥ ± 2 and significance set a $p < 0.05$
HSA hemangiosarcoma, *NS* normal spleen, *NH* nodular hyperplasia

Table 2 MiRNAs significantly differentially expressed between hemangiosarcoma and normal spleen only[a]

MicroRNA	Fold Change	p-value	Hemangiosarcoma (Means)	Normal Spleen (Means)
mir-139	3.554455	0.046672	71.8	20.2
mir-140	−2.21531	0.002865	12837.4	28438.8
mir-188	2.539683	0.003478	192	75.6
mir-193a	5.277433	0.013137	509.8	96.6
mir-22	2.010375	0.003289	65029.2	32346.8
mir-26a-2//mir-26a-1	−2.03635	0.020626	118478.2	241263.2
mir-301b	2.34	0.049404	46.8	20
mir-30e	−2.1239	0.002838	2931.4	6226
mir-33b	2.569892	0.041145	47.8	18.6
mir-365-2//mir-365-1	4.615929	0.048929	1043.2	226
mir-424	4.978495	0.007939	92.6	18.6
mir-450a	7.765751	0.023887	3673.2	473
mir-450b	2.68626	0.023021	3519	1310
mir-503	5.391026	0.029408	168.2	31.2
mir-505	2.169014	0.016269	30.8	14.2
mir-542	5.563845	0.039428	2326.8	418.2
mir-758	3.142857	0.011275	4.4	1.4
mir-876	6.5	0.038656	2.6	0.4

[a] fold change $\geq \pm 2$ and significance set a $p < 0.05$

expression of mir-150 (as was seen in the hemangiosarcoma samples) leading to increased expression of CXCR4 protein [45, 46]. VEGF has also been confirmed to be a direct target of mir-150, and downregulation of mir-150 led to increased VEGF expression in brain microvascular endothelial cells, leading to increased proliferation and migration of these cells [44]. Mir-203, which was downregulated in the hemangiosarcoma samples, has been shown to be a tumor suppressor that targets VEGFA, with increased expression of mir-203 leading to suppression of VEGFA in cervical cancer [47]. Although mir-452 has not been previously associated with angiogenic-specific pathways, it has been shown to target cyclin-dependent kinase inhibitor 1B, an inhibitor of the cell cycle checkpoint from G1 to S [54]. Hepatocellular carcinoma cells significantly overexpress mir-452, leading to increased cell invasion and migration and inhibition of apoptosis [54]. This miRNA was overexpressed by 13-fold in hemangiosarcoma samples compared to both nodular hyperplasia and normal spleen samples, indicating dysregulation of the cell cycle checkpoints may be a key player in the transition to hemangiosarcoma.

The 18 miRNAs significantly different between hemangiosarcoma and normal spleen only were further investigated for potential downstream targets. Seven of these, mir-139, mir-140, mir-26a, mir-424, mir-503, mir-505, and mir-542 have been shown to be involved in angiogenesis [55–63]. Although mir-139 has been reported to act as a tumor suppressor in most studies, its role in angiogenesis is becoming clearer [55, 56, 64, 65]. Mir-139 was found to increase cancer endothelial cell migration and promote vessel formation in pancreatic cancer [55]. Mir-139 was also found to negatively regulate CXCR4, playing a role in tightly regulating angiogenesis to prevent over-activation of endothelial cells [56]. It is possible that mir-139 is upregulated in response to the increased CXCR4 levels associated with mir-126 and mir-150 overexpression. Both mir-140 and mir-26a directly target VEGFA to repress its expression [57, 58]. These 2 miRNAs were underexpressed in the hemangiosarcoma samples compared to normal spleen, which fits with previous findings of increased VEGF expression in patients with hemangiosarcoma [13]. Mir-424 was found to be increased in tissues undergoing vascular remodeling after hypoxia, resulting in increased cell migration, and blockade of mir-424 led to decreased proliferation and vascular tube formation [59]. Another group found a contradictory function, in that mir-424 regulated VEGF and bFGF signaling by reducing expression of receptors for those cytokines and increased expression of mir-424 led to reduced proliferation and migration of endothelial cells [60]. This group also found that VEGF and bFGF had stimulatory effects on mir-424 expression, indicating that increased levels of VEGF, as seen in hemangiosarcoma, may have led to the finding of mir-424 being overexpressed, participating in a negative feedback loop [14, 60]. While it remains clear that mir-424 plays a role in angiogenesis, further studies are warranted to evaluate its specific role in canine hemangiosarcoma. Mir-503 is transcribed with mir-424 due to their close proximity, and mir-503 has also been shown to be anti-angiogenic by targeting VEGFA [61–63]. Mir-505, which was increased in the hemangiosarcoma samples, has been shown to decrease endothelial cell migration and vascular tube formation [66]. One study found that mir-542-3p targeted angiopoietin-2 and acted as an anti-angiogenic signal [67]. Angiogenesis requires a delicate balance of its mediators, and mir-424, mir-503, mir-505, and mir-542 may be overexpressed in these samples due to the effects of the multitude of other miRNAs acting in a pro-angiogenic manner. Vessel formation in hemangiosarcoma should not be strictly compared to normal angiogenesis, as tumor vessels are tortuous and leaky [68]. It is feasible that mixed angiogenic signaling leads to the abnormal vessel formation found in canine hemangiosarcoma. Mir-503 has also been shown to target the PI3K pathway by inhibiting the regulatory subunit, PI3K p85, acting as a tumor suppressor [69]. Again, this finding may be a regulatory negative feedback loop in response to mir-126 overexpression. Further work should be done to evaluate the interrelated roles of these miRNAs.

Mir-22, which was overexpressed in the hemangiosarcoma samples, has been shown to downregulate PTEN, which parallels the previous finding of PTEN inactivation in canine hemangiosarcoma [50, 70–72]. Mir-30e has been shown to be an endogenous miRNA in human microvascular endothelial cells and plays a role in human atherosclerosis by altering differentiation pathways [73–75]. Mir-33b and mir-758, which were overexpressed in the hemangiosarcoma samples, have also been shown to regulate gene expression in human atherosclerotic plaques [76]. Another miRNA, mir-365, which was overexpressed in these samples, has been shown to decrease vascular smooth muscle production in vascular injury repair [77]. It is clear that mir-30e, mir-33b, mir-365, and mir-758 are involved in the vasculature, but their specific role in canine hemangiosarcoma is unclear.

The remaining 6 miRNAs have been previously implicated in neoplasia, but more specific information relating specifically to hemangiosarcoma and/or angiogenesis could not be found [78–83].

Another group has evaluated miRNA expression in canine hemangiosarcoma, specifically looking at mir-214 [84]. This miRNA was found to act as a tumor suppressor by promoting apoptosis, and was downregulated in their samples [84]. Later work by the same group found overexpression of mir-214 in the media of canine hemangiosarcoma and human angiosarcoma cell lines, which contradicted their previous findings of

underexpression within the cells themselves [85]. They also found increased expression of mir-214 in the plasma of canine patients with hemangiosarcoma, which decreased after tumor removal [85]. The explanation for the contradictory findings in these studies was that intracellular and extracellular concentrations of miRNAs can be different and because miRNAs can have a multitude of downstream targets, they may act differently depending on their location and the disease state. Mir-214 was not significantly different in expression in the samples reported here. One reason for this may have been the methods used to evaluate for differential expression of miRNA. In the study reported here, RNA-sequencing was used to determine differentially expressed miRNAs, compared to the previously reported studies which used qRT-PCR to evaluate for miRNAs [84, 85]. Both the study reported here and the previously published works had relatively small sample numbers, and evaluation of a larger sample size may help to clarify these confounding results [84, 85]. Despite the lack of agreement in the findings of mir-214, the results reported here agree with the findings of mir-126 reported by the previous group, in which they found overexpression of mir-126 in plasma samples of canine patients with hemangiosarcoma [85]. These previous studies only evaluated mir-214 and mir-126 expression and did not evaluate for other miRNAs, but the finding of mir-126 overexpression, similar to the findings of the current study, is noteworthy. It is important to note that disease stage was not evaluated in the study reported here nor in the previously reported studies evaluating miRNA in canine hemangiosarcoma. This may also help to explain the contradictory findings regarding mir-214, as patients with different disease stages may have different miRNA expression levels. The long-term goal of the study presented here is to identify these dysregulated miRNAs in the circulation of patients with hemangiosarcoma. Mir-126 was overexpressed in these tissue samples, and work by others has shown it to be overexpressed in the serum of canine patients with splenic hemangiosarcoma. The hope is that with additional investigation, other miRNAs that were identified in the current study will be found in the circulation, allowing use of a minimally invasive diagnostic test for canine splenic hemangiosarcoma.

Conclusions

Results of the current study confirm the hypothesis that miRNAs are significantly differentially expressed between canine splenic hemangiosarcoma, nodular hyperplasia, and normal spleen samples. Ten of the 22 miRNAs dysregulated in hemangiosarcoma samples have been shown to have roles in angiogenesis (mir-26a, mir-126, mir-139, mir-140, mir-150, mir-203, mir-424, mir-503, mir-505, and mir-542). This is of particular importance for this tumor specifically, as it is a tumor of endothelial cells. An additional 4 miRNAs (mir-30e, mir-33b, mir-758, and mir-365) have been shown to be dysregulated in vascular disease processes. Two additional miRNAs (mir-22 and mir-452) have been implicated in cancer pathways, with mir-22 downregulating PTEN, a tumor suppressor that plays a role in hemangiosarcoma, and mir-452 altering cell cycle checkpoints to increase cell replication [54, 70–72]. Although the sample numbers in this study were small, the results point to clear roles of miRNAs in the pathogenesis of hemangiosarcoma via alteration of angiogenic signaling and cancer pathways. Further work needs to be done to evaluate these miRNA in a larger sample size and to elucidate the specific roles these miRNAs play in the angiogenic alterations leading to development of hemangiosarcoma, as the majority of these miRNAs have not been previously implicated in hemangiosarcoma. Further exploration is indicated to identify these miRNA in circulation to allow delineation of a specific miRNA panel that may become useful as a minimally invasive, pre-surgical diagnostic test to differentiate canine splenic hemangiosarcoma from other masses of the spleen.

Acknowledgements
None.

Funding
This research was funding through an American Kennel Club Canine Health Foundation ACORN grant. The funding body had no role in study design, data collection, analysis, interpretation, or writing of the manuscript.

Authors' contributions
JAG: made substantial contributions to conception and design, or acquisition of data, or analysis and interpretation of data, involved in drafting the manuscript, gave final approval of the version to be published, agreed to be accountable for all aspects of the work in ensuring that questions related to the accuracy or integrity of any part of the work are appropriately investigated and resolved. NP: made substantial contributions to conception and design, or acquisition of data, or analysis and interpretation of data, involved in revising the manuscript critically for important intellectual content, gave final approval of the version to be published, agreed to be accountable for all aspects of the work in ensuring that questions related to the accuracy or integrity of any part of the work are appropriately investigated and resolved. SL: made substantial contributions to conception and design, or acquisition of data, or analysis and interpretation of data, involved in revising the manuscript critically for important intellectual content, gave final approval of the version to be published, agreed to be accountable for all aspects of the work in ensuring that questions related to the accuracy or integrity of any part of the work are appropriately investigated and resolved. RC: made substantial contributions to conception and design, or acquisition of data, or analysis and interpretation of data, involved in revising the manuscript critically for important intellectual content, gave final approval of the version to be published, agreed to be accountable for all aspects of the work in ensuring that questions related to the accuracy or integrity of any part of the work are appropriately investigated and resolved. SL: made substantial contributions to conception and design, involved in revising the manuscript critically for important intellectual content, gave final approval of the version to be published, agreed

to be accountable for all aspects of the work in ensuring that questions related to the accuracy or integrity of any part of the work are appropriately investigated and resolved. HWB: made substantial contributions to conception and design, involved in revising the manuscript critically for important intellectual content, gave final approval of the version to be published, agreed to be accountable for all aspects of the work in ensuring that questions related to the accuracy or integrity of any part of the work are appropriately investigated and resolved. RAH: made substantial contributions to conception and design, involved in revising the manuscript critically for important intellectual content, gave final approval of the version to be published, agreed to be accountable for all aspects of the work in ensuring that questions related to the accuracy or integrity of any part of the work are appropriately investigated and resolved. BFS: made substantial contributions to conception and design, or acquisition of data, or analysis and interpretation of data, involved in revising the manuscript critically for important intellectual content, gave final approval of the version to be published, agreed to be accountable for all aspects of the work in ensuring that questions related to the accuracy or integrity of any part of the work are appropriately investigated and resolved.

Authors' information
None.

Competing interests
The authors declare that they have no competing interests.

Consent for publication
Not applicable – canine study, no human subjects.

Author details
[1]Department of Clinical Sciences, Auburn University College of Veterinary Medicine, Auburn University, Auburn, AL, USA. [2]Genomics Services Laboratory, HudsonAlpha Institute for Biotechnology, Huntsville, AL, USA. [3]Department of Pathobiology, Auburn University College of Veterinary Medicine, Auburn University, Auburn, AL, USA. [4]Scott Ritchey Research Center, Auburn University College of Veterinary Medicine, Auburn University, Auburn, AL, USA. [5]Department of Small Animal Medicine and Surgery, College of Veterinary Medicine, University of Georgia, 2200 College Station Road, Athens, GA 30602, USA.

References
1. Hammond TN, Pesillo-Crosby SA. Prevalence of hemangiosarcoma in anemic dogs with a splenic mass and hemoperitoneum requiring a transfusion: 71 cases (2003–2005). J Am Vet Med Assoc. 2008;232(4):553–8.
2. Pintar J, Breitschwerdt EB, Hardie EM, Spaulding KA. Acute nontraumatic hemoabdomen in the dog: a retrospective analysis of 39 cases (1987–2001). J Am Anim Hosp Assoc. 2003;39(6):518–22.
3. Aronsohn MG, Dubiel B, Roberts B, Powers BE. Prognosis for acute nontraumatic hemoperitoneum in the dog: a retrospective analysis of 60 cases (2003–2006). J Am Anim Hosp Assoc. 2009;45(2):72–7.
4. Prymak C, McKee LJ, Goldschmidt MH, Glickman LT. Epidemiologic, clinical, pathologic, and prognostic characteristics of splenic hemangiosarcoma and splenic hematoma in dogs: 217 cases (1985). J Am Vet Med Assoc. 1988;193(6):706–12.
5. Mallinckrodt MJ, Gottfried SD. Mass-to-splenic volume ratio and splenic weight as a percentage of body weight in dogs with malignant and benign splenic masses: 65 cases (2007–2008). J Am Vet Med Assoc. 2011;239(10):1325–7.
6. Thamm DH. Miscellaneous Tumors. In: Withrow S, Vail D, editors. Small Animal Clinical Oncology. 5th ed. St. Louis: Elsevier; 2013. p. 679–88.
7. Eberle N, von Babo V, Nolte I, Baumgartner W, Betz D. Splenic masses in dogs. Part 1: Epidemiologic, clinical characteristics as well as histopathologic diagnosis in 249 cases (2000–2011). Tierarztl Prax Ausg K Kleintiere Heimtiere. 2012;40(4):250–60.

8. Moore AS, Frimberger AE, Sullivan N, Moore PF. Histologic and immunohistochemical review of splenic fibrohistiocytic nodules in dogs. J Vet Intern Med. 2012;26(5):1164–8.

9. O'Brien RT, Iani M, Matheson J, Delaney F, Young K. Contrast harmonic ultrasound of spontaneous liver nodules in 32 dogs. Vet Radiol Ultrasound. 2004;45(6):547–53.

10. Fife WD, Samii VF, Drost WT, Mattoon JS, Hoshaw-Woodard S. Comparison between malignant and nonmalignant splenic masses in dogs using contrast-enhanced computed tomography. Vet Radiol Ultrasound. 2004; 45(4):289–97.

11. Clifford CA, Pretorius ES, Weisse C, Sorenmo KU, Drobatz KJ, Siegelman ES, Solomon JA. Magnetic resonance imaging of focal splenic and hepatic lesions in the dog. J Vet Intern Med. 2004;18(3):330–8.

12. Lamerato-Kozicki A, Helm K, Modiano J. Early detection of hemangiosarcoma. In: American College of Veterinary Internal Medicine: 2005; Baltimore, MD; 2005.

13. Clifford CA, Hughes D, Beal MW, Mackin AJ, Henry CJ, Shofer FS, Sorenmo KU. Plasma vascular endothelial growth factor concentrations in healthy dogs and dogs with hemangiosarcoma. J Vet Intern Med. 2001;15(2):131–5.

14. Thamm DH, Kamstock DA, Sharp CR, Johnson SI, Mazzaferro E, Herold LV, Barnes SM, Winkler K, Selting KA. Elevated serum thymidine kinase activity in canine splenic hemangiosarcoma*. Vet Comp Oncol. 2012;10(4):292–302.

15. Stefanello D, Valenti P, Zini E, Comazzi S, Gelain ME, Roccabianca P, Avallone G, Caniatti M, Marconato L. Splenic marginal zone lymphoma in 5 dogs (2001–2008). J Vet Intern Med. 2011;25(1):90–3.

16. Fazi F, Nervi C. MicroRNA: basic mechanisms and transcriptional regulatory networks for cell fate determination. Cardiovasc Res. 2008;79(4):553–61.

17. Esquela-Kerscher A, Slack FJ. Oncomirs - microRNAs with a role in cancer. Nat Rev Cancer. 2006;6(4):259–69.

18. He L, Thomson JM, Hemann MT, Hernando-Monge E, Mu D, Goodson S, Powers S, Cordon-Cardo C, Lowe SW, Hannon GJ, et al. A microRNA polycistron as a potential human oncogene. Nature. 2005;435(7043):828–33.

19. Wijnhoven BP, Michael MZ, Watson DI. MicroRNAs and cancer. Br J Surg. 2007;94(1):23–30.

20. Chen X, Ba Y, Ma L, Cai X, Yin Y, Wang K, Guo J, Zhang Y, Chen J, Guo X, et al. Characterization of microRNAs in serum: a novel class of biomarkers for diagnosis of cancer and other diseases. Cell Res. 2008;18(10):997–1006.

21. Wang Y, Li L, Qu Z, Li R, Bi T, Jiang J, Zhao H. The expression of miR-30a* and miR-30e* is associated with a dualistic model for grading ovarian papillary serious carcinoma. Int J Oncol. 2014;44(6):1904–14.

22. Gasparini P, Cascione L, Fassan M, Lovat F, Guler G, Balci S, Irkkan C, Morrison C, Croce CM, Shapiro CL, et al. microRNA expression profiling identifies a four microRNA signature as a novel diagnostic and prognostic biomarker in triple negative breast cancers. Oncotarget. 2014;5(5):1174–84.

23. Yu Q, Liu S, Wang H, Shi G, Yang P, Chen X. miR-126 suppresses the proliferation of cervical cancer cells and alters cell sensitivity to the chemotherapeutic drug bleomycin. Asian Pac J Cancer Prev. 2013;14(11): 6569–72.

24. Yuan Y, Shen Y, Xue L, Fan H. miR-140 suppresses tumor growth and metastasis of non-small cell lung cancer by targeting insulin-like growth factor 1 receptor. PLoS One. 2013;8(9), e73604.

25. Palacios F, Abreu C, Prieto D, Morande P, Ruiz S, Fernandez-Calero T, Naya H, Libisch G, Robello C, Landoni AI, et al. Activation of the PI3K/AKT pathway by microRNA-22 results in CLL B-cell proliferation. Leukemia. 2015; 29(1):115–25.

26. Chen X, Guo X, Zhang H, Xiang Y, Chen J, Yin Y, Cai X, Wang K, Wang G, Ba Y, et al. Role of miR-143 targeting KRAS in colorectal tumorigenesis. Oncogene. 2009;28(10):1385–92.

27. Yu ZW, Zhong LP, Ji T, Zhang P, Chen WT, Zhang CP. MicroRNAs contribute to the chemoresistance of cisplatin in tongue squamous cell carcinoma lines. Oral Oncol. 2010;46(4):317–22.

28. Weng Z, Wang D, Zhao W, Song M, You F, Yang L, Chen L. microRNA-450a targets DNA methyltransferase 3a in hepatocellular carcinoma. Exp Ther Med. 2011;2(5):951–5.

29. Greenberg E, Besser MJ, Ben-Ami E, Shapira-Frommer R, Itzhaki O, Zikich D, Levy D, Kubi A, Eyal E, Onn A, et al. A comparative analysis of total serum miRNA profiles identifies novel signature that is highly indicative of metastatic melanoma: a pilot study. Biomarkers. 2013; 18(6):502–8.

30. van Schooneveld E, Wouters MC, Van der Auwera I, Peeters DJ, Wildiers H, Van Dam PA, Vergote I, Vermeulen PB, Dirix LY, Van Laere SJ. Expression profiling of cancerous and normal breast tissues identifies microRNAs that are differentially expressed in serum from patients with (metastatic) breast cancer and healthy volunteers. Breast Cancer Res. 2012;14(1):R34.

31. MacKenzie TA, Schwartz GN, Calderone HM, Graveel CR, Winn ME, Hostetter G, Wells WA, Sempere LF. Stromal expression of miR-21 identifies high-risk group in triple-negative breast cancer. Am J Pathol. 2014;184(12):3217–25.

32. Nguyen HC, Xie W, Yang M, Hsieh CL, Drouin S, Lee GS, Kantoff PW. Expression differences of circulating microRNAs in metastatic castration resistant prostate cancer and low-risk, localized prostate cancer. Prostate. 2013;73(4):346–54.

33. Boggs RM, Wright ZM, Stickney MJ, Porter WW, Murphy KE. MicroRNA expression in canine mammary cancer. Mamm Genome. 2008;19(7–8):561–9.

34. Gioia G, Mortarino M, Gelain ME, Albonico F, Ciusani E, Forno I, Marconato L, Martini V, Comazzi S. Immunophenotype-related microRNA expression in canine chronic lymphocytic leukemia. Vet Immunol Immunopathol. 2011; 142(3–4):228–35.

35. Noguchi S, Mori T, Hoshino Y, Yamada N, Maruo K, Akao Y. MicroRNAs as tumour suppressors in canine and human melanoma cells and as a prognostic factor in canine melanomas. Vet Comp Oncol. 2013;11(2):113–23.

36. Griffiths-Jones S, Saini HK, van Dongen S, Enright AJ. miRBase: tools for microRNA genomics. Nucleic Acids Res. 2008;36(Database issue):D154–158.

37. Kozomara A, Griffiths-Jones S. miRBase: integrating microRNA annotation and deep-sequencing data. Nucleic Acids Res. 2011;39(Database issue): D152–157.

38. Benjamini Y, Hochberg Y. Controlling the false discovery rate: a practical and powerful approach to multiple testing. J R Statist Soc. 1995;57(1):289–300.

39. Ebrahimi F, Gopalan V, Smith RA, Lam AK. miR-126 in human cancers: clinical roles and current perspectives. Exp Mol Pathol. 2014;96(1):98–107.

40. Fish JE, Santoro MM, Morton SU, Yu S, Yeh RF, Wythe JD, Ivey KN, Bruneau BG, Stainier DY, Srivastava D. miR-126 regulates angiogenic signaling and vascular integrity. Dev Cell. 2008;15(2):272–84.

41. Chistiakov DA, Orekhov AN, Bobryshev YV. The role of miR-126 in embryonic angiogenesis, adult vascular homeostasis, and vascular repair and its alterations in atherosclerotic disease. J Mol Cell Cardiol. 2016;97: 47–55.

42. Song L, Li D, Gu Y, Wen ZM, Jie J, Zhao D, Peng LP. MicroRNA-126 Targeting PIK3R2 Inhibits NSCLC A549 Cell Proliferation, Migration, and Invasion by Regulation of PTEN/PI3K/AKT Pathway. Clin Lung Cancer. 2016.

43. Wang S, Aurora AB, Johnson BA, Qi X, McAnally J, Hill JA, Richardson JA, Bassel-Duby R, Olson EN. The endothelial-specific microRNA miR-126 governs vascular integrity and angiogenesis. Dev Cell. 2008;15(2):261–71.

44. He QW, Li Q, Jin HJ, Zhi F, Suraj B, Zhu YY, Xia YP, Mao L, Chen XL, Hu B. MiR-150 Regulates Poststroke Cerebral Angiogenesis via Vascular Endothelial Growth Factor in Rats. CNS Neurosci Ther. 2016;22(6):507–17.

45. Tano N, Kim HW, Ashraf M. microRNA-150 regulates mobilization and migration of bone marrow-derived mononuclear cells by targeting Cxcr4. PLoS One. 2011;6(10), e23114.

46. Rolland-Turner M, Goretti E, Bousquenaud M, Leonard F, Nicolas C, Zhang L, Maskali F, Marie PY, Devaux Y, Wagner D. Adenosine stimulates the migration of human endothelial progenitor cells. Role of CXCR4 and microRNA-150. PLoS One. 2013;8(1):e54135.

47. Zhu X, Er K, Mao C, Yan Q, Xu H, Zhang Y, Zhu J, Cui F, Zhao W, Shi H. miR-203 suppresses tumor growth and angiogenesis by targeting VEGFA in cervical cancer. Cell Physiol Biochem. 2013;32(1):64–73.

48. Meister J, Schmidt MH. miR-126 and miR-126*: new players in cancer. ScientificWorldJournal. 2010;10:2090–100.

49. Sessa R, Seano G, di Blasio L, Gagliardi PA, Isella C, Medico E, Cotelli F, Bussolino F, Primo L. The miR-126 regulates angiopoietin-1 signaling and vessel maturation by targeting p85beta. Biochim Biophys Acta. 2012; 1823(10):1925–35.

50. Dickerson EB, Thomas R, Fosmire SP, Lamerato-Kozicki AR, Bianco SR, Wojcieszyn JW, Breen M, Helfand SC, Modiano JF. Mutations of phosphatase and tensin homolog deleted from chromosome 10 in canine hemangiosarcoma. Vet Pathol. 2005;42(5):618–32.

51. Mondadori dos Santos A, Metzinger L, Haddad O, M'Baya-Moutoula E, Taibi F, Charnaux N, Massy ZA, Hlawaty H, Metzinger-Le Meuth V. miR-126 Is Involved in Vascular Remodeling under Laminar Shear Stress. Biomed Res Int. 2015;2015:497280.

52. Kucia M, Reca R, Miekus K, Wanzeck J, Wojakowski W, Janowska-Wieczorek A, Ratajczak J, Ratajczak MZ. Trafficking of normal stem cells and metastasis

of cancer stem cells involve similar mechanisms: pivotal role of the SDF-1-CXCR4 axis. Stem Cells. 2005;23(7):879–94.

53. Kukreja P, Abdel-Mageed AB, Mondal D, Liu K, Agrawal KC. Up-regulation of CXCR4 expression in PC-3 cells by stromal-derived factor-1alpha (CXCL12) increases endothelial adhesion and transendothelial migration: role of MEK/ERK signaling pathway-dependent NF-kappaB activation. Cancer Res. 2005; 65(21):9891–8.

54. Zheng Q, Sheng Q, Jiang C, Shu J, Chen J, Nie Z, Lv Z, Zhang Y. MicroRNA-452 promotes tumorigenesis in hepatocellular carcinoma by targeting cyclin-dependent kinase inhibitor 1B. Mol Cell Biochem. 2014;389(1–2): 187–95.

55. Li L, Li B, Chen D, Liu L, Huang C, Lu Z, Lun L, Wan X. miR-139 and miR-200c regulate pancreatic cancer endothelial cell migration and angiogenesis. Oncol Rep. 2015;34(1):51–8.

56. Papangeli I, Kim J, Maier I, Park S, Lee A, Kang Y, Tanaka K, Khan OF, Ju H, Kojima Y, et al. MicroRNA 139-5p coordinates APLNR-CXCR4 crosstalk during vascular maturation. Nat Commun. 2016;7:11268.

57. Sun J, Tao S, Liu L, Guo D, Xia Z, Huang M. miR1405p regulates angiogenesis following ischemic stroke by targeting VEGFA. Mol Med Rep. 2016;13(5):4499–505.

58. Chai ZT, Kong J, Zhu XD, Zhang YY, Lu L, Zhou JM, Wang LR, Zhang KZ, Zhang QB, Ao JY, et al. MicroRNA-26a inhibits angiogenesis by down-regulating VEGFA through the PIK3C2alpha/Akt/HIF-1alpha pathway in hepatocellular carcinoma. PLoS One. 2013;8(10), e77957.

59. Ghosh G, Subramanian IV, Adhikari N, Zhang X, Joshi HP, Basi D, Chandrashekhar YS, Hall JL, Roy S, Zeng Y, et al. Hypoxia-induced microRNA-424 expression in human endothelial cells regulates HIF-alpha isoforms and promotes angiogenesis. J Clin Invest. 2010;120(11):4141–54.

60. Chamorro-Jorganes A, Araldi E, Penalva LO, Sandhu D, Fernandez-Hernando C, Suarez Y. MicroRNA-16 and microRNA-424 regulate cell-autonomous angiogenic functions in endothelial cells via targeting vascular endothelial growth factor receptor-2 and fibroblast growth factor receptor-1. Arterioscler Thromb Vasc Biol. 2011;31(11):2595–606.

61. Caporali A, Emanueli C. MicroRNA-503 and the extended microRNA-16 family in angiogenesis. Trends Cardiovasc Med. 2011;21(6):162–6.

62. Caporali A, Meloni M, Vollenkle C, Bonci D, Sala-Newby GB, Addis R, Spinetti G, Losa S, Masson R, Baker AH, et al. Deregulation of microRNA-503 contributes to diabetes mellitus-induced impairment of endothelial function and reparative angiogenesis after limb ischemia. Circulation. 2011;123(3):282–91.

63. Zhou B, Ma R, Si W, Li S, Xu Y, Tu X, Wang Q. MicroRNA-503 targets FGF2 and VEGFA and inhibits tumor angiogenesis and growth. Cancer Lett. 2013; 333(2):159–69.

64. Watanabe K, Amano Y, Ishikawa R, Sunohara M, Kage H, Ichinose J, Sano A, Nakajima J, Fukayama M, Yatomi Y, et al. Histone methylation-mediated silencing of miR-139 enhances invasion of non-small-cell lung cancer. Cancer Med. 2015;4(10):1573–82.

65. Zhang HD, Jiang LH, Sun DW, Li J, Tang JH. MiR-139-5p: promising biomarker for cancer. Tumour Biol. 2015;36(3):1355–65.

66. Yang Q, Jia C, Wang P, Xiong M, Cui J, Li L, Wang W, Wu Q, Chen Y, Zhang T. MicroRNA-505 identified from patients with essential hypertension impairs endothelial cell migration and tube formation. Int J Cardiol. 2014;177(3):925–34.

67. He T, Qi F, Jia L, Wang S, Song N, Guo L, Fu Y, Luo Y. MicroRNA-542-3p inhibits tumour angiogenesis by targeting angiopoietin-2. J Pathol. 2014; 232(5):499–508.

68. Gamlem H, Nordstoga K. Canine vascular neoplasia–histologic classification and inmunohistochemical analysis of 221 tumours and tumour-like lesions. APMIS Suppl. 2008;125:19–40.

69. Yang Y, Liu L, Zhang Y, Guan H, Wu J, Zhu X, Yuan J, Li M. MiR-503 targets PI3K p85 and IKK-beta and suppresses progression of non-small cell lung cancer. Int J Cancer. 2014;135(7):1531–42.

70. Bar N, Dikstein R. miR-22 forms a regulatory loop in PTEN/AKT pathway and modulates signaling kinetics. PLoS One. 2010;5(5), e10859.

71. Tan G, Shi Y, Wu ZH. MicroRNA-22 promotes cell survival upon UV radiation by repressing PTEN. Biochem Biophys Res Commun. 2012;417(1):546–51.

72. Xu XD, Song XW, Li Q, Wang GK, Jing Q, Qin YW. Attenuation of microRNA-22 derepressed PTEN to effectively protect rat cardiomyocytes from hypertrophy. J Cell Physiol. 2012;227(4):1391–8.

73. Kriegel AJ, Baker MA, Liu Y, Liu P, Cowley Jr AW, Liang M. Endogenous microRNAs in human microvascular endothelial cells regulate mRNAs encoded by hypertension-related genes. Hypertension. 2015;66(4):793–9.

74. Ding W, Li J, Singh J, Alif R, Vazquez-Padron RI, Gomes SA, Hare JM, Shehadeh LA. miR-30e targets IGF2-regulated osteogenesis in bone marrow-derived mesenchymal stem cells, aortic smooth muscle cells, and ApoE–/– mice. Cardiovasc Res. 2015;106(1):131–42.

75. Han H, Wang YH, Qu GJ, Sun TT, Li FQ, Jiang W, Luo SS. Differentiated miRNA expression and validation of signaling pathways in apoE gene knockout mice by cross-verification microarray platform. Exp Mol Med. 2013;45, e13.

76. Mandolini C, Santovito D, Marcantonio P, Buttitta F, Bucci M, Ucchino S, Mezzetti A, Cipollone F. Identification of microRNAs 758 and 33b as potential modulators of ABCA1 expression in human atherosclerotic plaques. Nutr Metab Cardiovasc Dis. 2015;25(2):202–9.

77. Zhang P, Zheng C, Ye H, Teng Y, Zheng B, Yang X, Zhang J. MicroRNA-365 inhibits vascular smooth muscle cell proliferation through targeting cyclin D1. Int J Med Sci. 2014;11(8):765–70.

78. Zhang H, Qi S, Zhang T, Wang A, Liu R, Guo J, Wang Y, Xu Y. miR-188-5p inhibits tumour growth and metastasis in prostate cancer by repressing LAPTM4B expression. Oncotarget. 2015;6(8):6092–104.

79. Pu Y, Zhao F, Cai W, Meng X, Li Y, Cai S. MiR-193a-3p and miR-193a-5p suppress the metastasis of human osteosarcoma cells by down-regulating Rab27B and SRR, respectively. Clin Exp Metastasis. 2016;33(4):359–72.

80. Funamizu N, Lacy CR, Parpart ST, Takai A, Hiyoshi Y, Yanaga K. MicroRNA-301b promotes cell invasiveness through targeting TP63 in pancreatic carcinoma cells. Int J Oncol. 2014;44(3):725–34.

81. Castilla MA, Moreno-Bueno G, Romero-Perez L, Van De Vijver K, Biscuola M, Lopez-Garcia MA, Prat J, Matias-Guiu X, Cano A, Oliva E, et al. Micro-RNA signature of the epithelial-mesenchymal transition in endometrial carcinosarcoma. J Pathol. 2011;223(1):72–80.

82. Zhao Z, Li R, Sha S, Wang Q, Mao W, Liu T. Targeting HER3 with miR-450b-3p suppresses breast cancer cells proliferation. Cancer Biol Ther. 2014;15(10): 1404–12.

83. Bienertova-Vasku J, Mazanek P, Hezova R, Curdova A, Nekvindova J, Kren L, Sterba J, Slaby O. Extension of microRNA expression pattern associated with high-risk neuroblastoma. Tumour Biol. 2013;34(4):2315–9.

84. Heishima K, Mori T, Sakai H, Sugito N, Murakami M, Yamada N, Akao Y, Maruo K. MicroRNA-214 Promotes Apoptosis in Canine Hemangiosarcoma by Targeting the COP1-p53 Axis. PLoS One. 2015;10(9), e0137361.

85. Heishima K, Mori T, Ichikawa Y, Sakai H, Kuranaga Y, Nakagawa T, Tanaka Y, Okamura Y, Masuzawa M, Sugito N, et al. MicroRNA-214 and MicroRNA-126 Are Potential Biomarkers for Malignant Endothelial Proliferative Diseases. Int J Mol Sci. 2015;16(10):25377–91.

Surgical treatment of traumatic eventration with polyester button and polypropylene mesh to strengthen the suture technique in equine

Carla Faria Orlandini, Denis Steiner, André Giarola Boscarato, Gabriel Coelho Gimenes and Luiz Romulo Alberton[*]

Abstract

Background: Defects in the abdominal wall of horses have high relapse rate. This is mainly in lateral eventrations and hernias caused by trauma from kicks of other horses or installation structures. The eventration region normally becomes swollen and there may be complications due to intestinal loop incarceration. The surgical treatment, consisting of reconstruction of the abdominal wall, frequently require biological or synthetic materials for the reinforcement of the suture line and tension support. Therefore, several studies have reported new materials for the repair of the abdominal wall, with the aim of improving the integration among adjacent tissues and reducing risks and complications such as rejection and infection. This report describes for the first time the use of a regular polypropylene mesh reinforced with polyester buttons for the herniorrhaphy.

Case presentation: A male, three-year-old, Appaloosa with 500 Kg presented to our hospital with a 10 days history of an increased volume on the left ventro-lateral region of the abdomen. During the physical examination, a deventration following traumatic rupture of the abdominal wall was diagnosed via ultrasonography. Then, the equine was anesthetized and moved to surgery for correction of the eventration which was performed according to conventional technique described in literature. Two days later, an eventration relapse was observed and confirmed via ultrasonography. After that, a second surgical intervention was performed using polyester buttons and polypropylene mesh. After the second surgical procedure, no complications related to eventration were observed either intra or postoperatively. After that, a recheck was performed thirty days later where satisfactory wound healing and total recovery were observed.

Conclusion: The use of polypropylene mesh reinforced with polyester buttons is an effective technique for the repair of traumatic eventration in horses. This technique provides effective reinforcement against the abdominal tension and was a good option for reconstruction of lacerated muscles in cases of equine post-traumatic eventration, including relapsing cases.

Keywords: Abdominal laceration, Equine, Eventration, Hernia, Hernioplasty, Surgery

* Correspondence: romulo@unipar.br
Department of Veterinary Medicine and Graduate Program in Animal Science, Universidade Paranaense, Praça Mascarenhas de Moraes 4282, Zona III, 87502-210 Umuarama, Paraná, Brazil

Background

The traumatic rupture of the abdominal wall, extending to one or more muscles, predispose to the escape of viscera that, when retained by the subcutaneous tissue and skin, form the so-called eventration, or lateral abdominal hernia [1, 2]. In horses, these are usually the result of trauma, associated with facility problems where the animal is maintained and trauma caused by kicks from other animals [2]. Eventrations are classified as partially or completely reducible and usually have slow or blunt onset. The opening region normally becomes swollen and some problems may occur due to retention or definitive incarceration of abdominal viscera [1]. Surgical treatment is effective for the reduction of the eventration content and reconstruction of the abdominal wall. This can be complex, mainly when there are alterations in the anatomic composition, adherences of structures and thin friable tissue. Moreover, the weight of the abdominal viscera on the peritoneal wall is an aggravating factor, predisposing the occurrence of relapse of the eventration, requiring the reinforcement of the suture line and, many times, the use of materials to enhance tension support [2].

Several synthetic or biological materials have been applied for the reconstitution of the abdominal wall, serving as reinforcement to tension or even to stimulate scarring and the tissue regeneration processes [3, 4]. However, these materials have been associated with severe adverse reactions such as infections and rejection [5]. Synthetic prosthesis have been commonly used since 1950, being divided into non absorbable, such as nylon, polytetrafluorethylene, silicone, polyester, polypropylene, polyvinyl sponge, and carbon fibers; and absorbable, such as polygalactin 910 and polyglycolic acid [5, 6]. More recently, biological materials have been used for the same purpose. Among these, swine small bowel submucosa [7, 8], swine urinary bladder submucosa [9], bovine peritoneum [10], microbial cellulose membrane [11], and bovine pericardium [4, 12] stand out. Collagen-based animal tissue has been more frequently used, associated to several conservation techniques to preserve its viability and reduce antigenicity [13].

New materials used for abdominal wall repair have been investigated and are associated with acceptable integration with adjacent tissues, improving performance in all interfaces and preventing complications. In this context, the aim of the present paper was to report a herniorraphy using polyester buttons to enforce a polypropylene mesh in a horse with eventration secondary to traumatic rupture of the abdominal muscles.

Case presentation

A male three-year-old, Appaloosa was admitted to the Universidade Paranaense, Veterinary Hospital presenting with a 10 days history of an increased volume of the left ventral-lateral region of the abdomen (Fig. 1).

Anamnesis showed injury due to trauma at the farm fence. The animal had already been treated with procaine benzylpenicillin (10.000 UI/Kg, IM, q24h), dexamethasone (1 mg/kg, IV, q24h) during four days and antitetanus serum. During physical examination, an increased volume with firm consistency, reducible and painful to touch was observed. Through ultrasonography, the presence of intestinal loops in the lesion area (Fig. 2) and peritoneal fluid and fibrin were observed, which confirmed the diagnostic of eventration. The animal was conducted to surgery on the day after admission.

Pre surgical preparation comprised of 8-h fasting of water and 12-h fasting for solids. Anesthesia was performed with xylazine 10 % (1 mg/kg, IV), ketamine (2 mg/kg, IV), and guaiacolglyceryl ether (50 g), diluted in 0.9 % saline solution (500 ml), all administered IV as pre anesthetic medication and also for induction of general anesthesia. After oro-tracheal intubation anesthesia

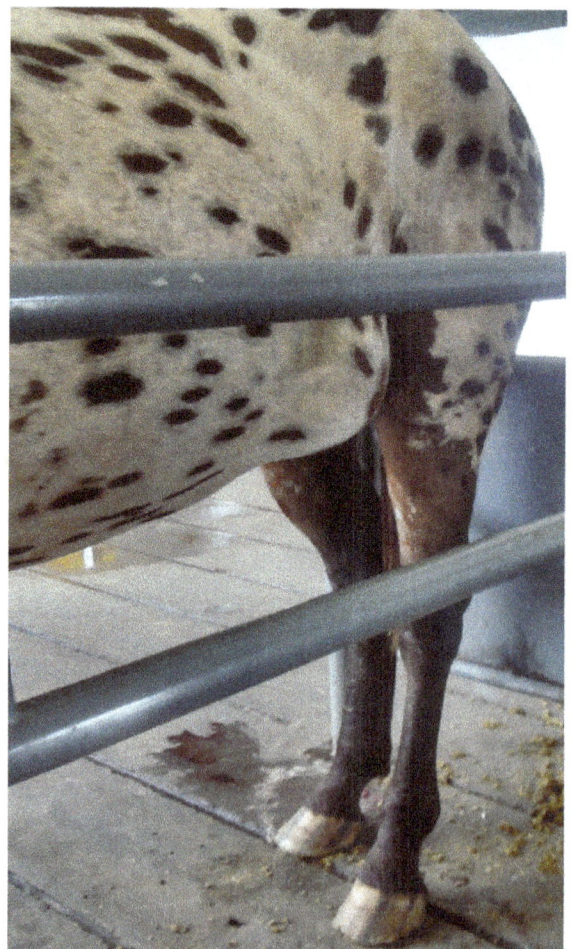

Fig. 1 Photograph demonstrating the equine presenting increased volume on the left ventral-lateral region due to trauma

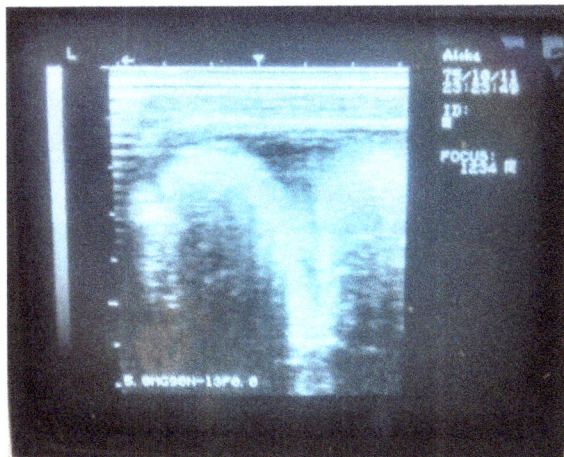

Fig. 2 Photograph illustrating an ultrassonography demonstrating the presence of intestinal loops in the subcutaneous region in the left ventral-lateral region of the abdomen of a horse with traumatic eventration

was maintained with isoflurane vaporized in oxygen and animal was positioned in dorsal recumbency for the surgical procedure. Then, hair clipping and preoperative antisepsis on the ventral and left ventral-lateral regions of the abdomen were performed. An incision of approximately 15-cm was performed, comprising skin and subcutaneous tissue, on the eventration region, through which it was possible to observe lacerations of the obliquusabdominis and transverses abdominus muscles, allowing the passage of intestinal loops to the subcutaneous space. To reduce the eventrated content, another incision, of approximately 20-cm was performed in the retro-umbilical region, comprising skin, subcutaneous, línea alba of the rectus abdominis and peritoneum (Fig. 3). As the lesion was located on the left ventrolateral region, the lateral position did not favor its manipulation and correction, hindering access and technique execution. In addition, the laceration of the abdominal muscles and the way the intestinal loops were eventrated impaired their anatomical replacement, with the need for a second access to aid this technique. It is noteworthy that due to the degree of muscle laceration and the time elapsed since trauma to the moment the animal was treated, the muscles abdominal oblique and transverse were extremely friable, hindering the approach of its edges, and hence difficulty to the suture of these tissues to close the laceration. Thus, the option of increasing the incision in such musculature to facilitate the repositioning of the bowel was ruled out, since this technique would make muscle reconstitution even more difficult.

After the repositioning of the intestinal loops, the peritoneum was closed in both openings of the abdominal region, using chromed catgut-4 suture line in a simple

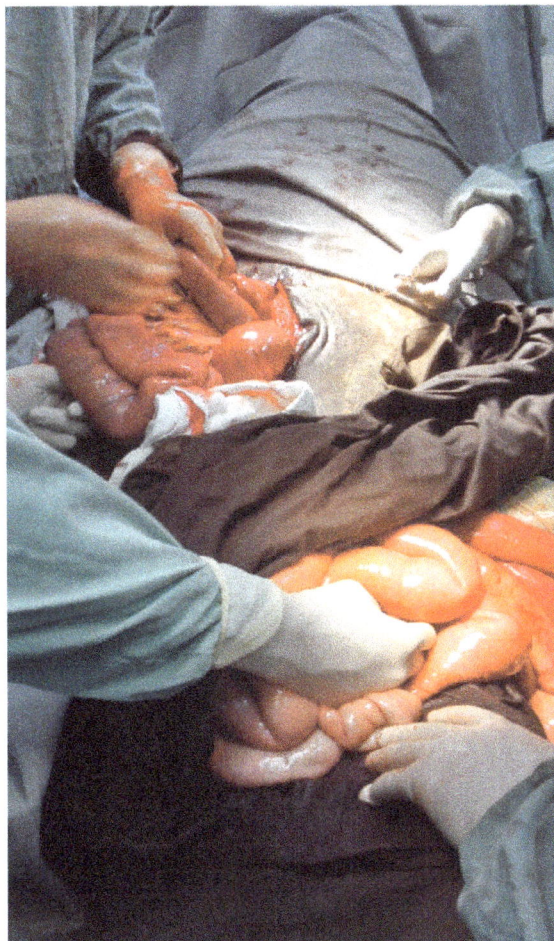

Fig. 3 Photograph illustrating a horse undergoing surgery for treatment of traumatic eventration, showing the passage of intestinal loops through lacerations of the abdominal muscles on the left ventral-abdominal region, and incision through the retro-umbilical region for traction and repositioning of eventrated tissues

continuous pattern. Subsequently, the lacerated muscles were repaired using nylon-4 and an anchored simple continuous pattern (Reverdin suture). For the suture of the rectus abdominis muscle, nylon-4 suture material was used in a Sultan suture pattern. The subcutaneous tissue was closed with vycril-1 in a simple continuous suture patern. Skin incisions were sutured with nylon-3 in a simple interrupted pattern.

Post-surgical treatment was performed by applying cold water on the suture regions and prepuce, cleaning of the surgical wounds with iodine povidone (PVPI), PVPI solution and anointment, and administration of flunixin meglumine (1.1 mg/kg, IV, q24h) and trimethoprim-sulfamethoxazole (15 mg/kg, IV, q12h). Two days after the procedure, eventration relapse was observed and confirmed by ultrasonography. Sodium heparin (30 UI/kg, SC, q24h) was administered for two days, associated to other postoperative medication to prevent possible adherence of eventrated intestinal loops. Four days after the first surgery, a second surgical intervention was performed. The preoperative procedures, anesthesia, as well as surgical access were performed as previously described. Rupture of sutures of lacerated muscles and peritoneum was observed, the latter was closed using the same procedure as in the first surgery. For the synthesis of the obliquus and transverse abdominis, ten 12.7 mm polyester buttons and a 15 x 15 cm polypropylene mesh were used, associated to simple continuous suture stitches with nylon-4 (Fig. 4).

The closure of the subcutaneous space and skin were performed using the same procedure as in the first surgery. Postoperative treatment was made with flunixin meglumine (1.1 mg/kg, IV, q24h), for three days, ceftiofur (2.2 mg/kg, IV, q24h) and gentamicin (6.6 mg/kg, IV, q24h) during 15 days. Three days after the second surgical procedure, another dehiscence of the

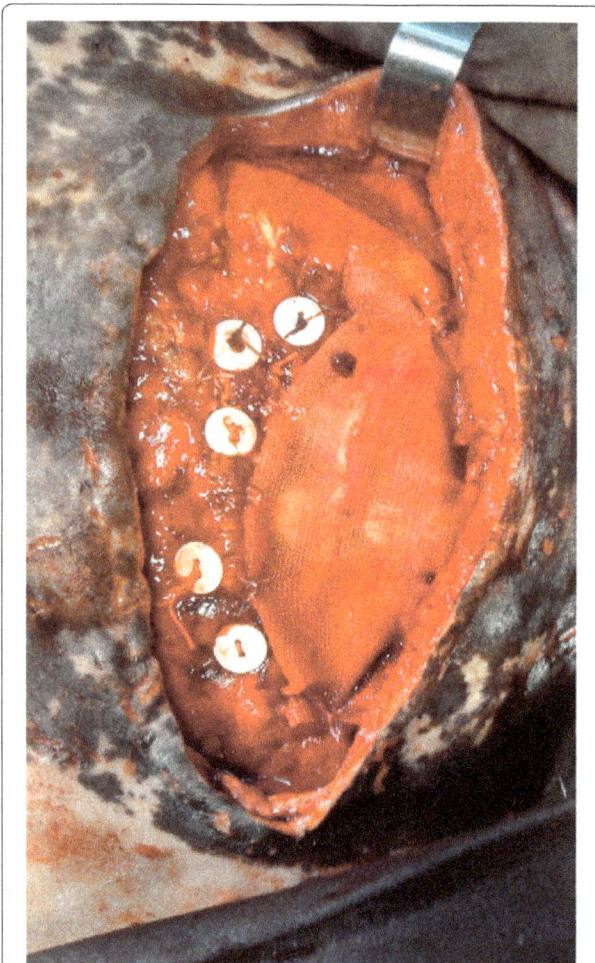

Fig. 4 Photograph illustrating a horse undergoing surgery for treatment of traumatic eventration demonstrating the synthetic materials, polyester buttons and polypropylen mesh used for reconstruction of the obliquus and transverse abdominis

cutaneous suture was observed. However, with daily cleanings of the wound as previously described, application of frozen total plasma, obtained from the animal, and compressive abdominal bandages, satisfactory wound healing and total recovery were observed within 30 days.

The first surgical intervention was performed 11 days after animal had suffered the trauma and thus presenting with eventration. During this period, probably there was not enough time for strong collagen formation to support the suture performed [14], which may have contributed to the lesion recurrence, with suture rupture of lacerated muscles and peritoneum. Nevertheless, surgical procedure was performed as soon as the animal was admitted, since the presence of peritoneal fluid and fibrin, visualized through ultrasonography, indicated possible adhesion formation and hence incarceration of eventrated bowel loops, which may have contribute to the onset of acute abdomen and possible further complications. Some authors have reported surgical techniques suitable for ventral hernia repair in horses including the attempt of primary defect closure, without the use of implants [15]. In this case, primary defect closure failure due to the size of the laceration and the animal's size [15]. The materials used to reinforce the abdominal suture were easy to apply, had good interaction with the suture and excellent resistance to traction, even when inserted in heavily lacerated muscle due to trauma and to surgical procedures. Moreover, materials were easy to acquire and had low cost. Similar results were described by using bovine pericardium preserved in 98 % glycerine for reinforcement of the peritoneal suture in horses with traumatic eventration [4]. According to authors, glycerin has low cost and is easily acquired and stored. Nevertheless, the conservation of biological membranes used as implants may be more demanding than simple sterilization used for the antisepsis of synthetic materials.

In a study comparing the use of bovine pericardium and polyester mesh for the repair of abdominal wall in rats, the authors concluded that the synthetic material used offered greater structural resistance and fibroblastic response; however, it showed higher adherence of abdominal viscera, when compared to bovine pericardium [16]. The implant of synthetic prothesis significantly stimulates the inflammatory response [16, 17]. The results confirm the hypothesis that biomaterials induce less inflammatory response [18]. The authors used hemicellulose membrane for reconstitution of defects in the abdominal wall induced in rats and found satisfactory results. Once the biomaterial establish a certain balance with adjacent tissues, minimal inflammatory response and few intestinal adherences are observed. These responses are desirable characteristics in any kind of implant. Comparing the use of synthetic material and biomaterial for the reconstruction of abdominal defects in rats, there is no histological difference between materials in relation to inflammatory process, classified as granulomatous regardless of material used [19]. Defects in the abdominal wall in equines, corrected only by suture, present great chance of relapse and, in such cases, polypropylene meshes are a good option for reconstruction and resistance of the abdominal wall [17]. However, despite the risk of complications and relapses, most hernia or eventration lesions in large animals are corrected with the use of sutures, various techniques and wires. In cattle, some authors have reported no significant difference between synthetic nonabsorbable sutures (nylon) and organic nonabsorbable sutures (cotton) for the suturing of muscles in animals with umbilical hernia [20]. However, the authors also reported that suture with cotton wire, provides higher recovery rate when compared to nylon, arguing that the texture of organic wire is not able to fray abdominal fascia, although suture has exerted pressure on tissues. However, it should be taken into consideration that due to its physical and chemical characteristics, this type of wire may trigger greater number of complications and predispose to possible contamination. According to some authors, the failure of abdominal suture techniques in cases of hernia and the high recurrence rate are due to the individual response of animals, postoperative failure and suture patterns [21]. The suture patterns chosen for the synthesis of lacerated muscle, in the case described here were based on the fact that a tension relaxation suture cannot be used due to the difficulty in anchoring the suture with the muscle fiber. The anchored continuous suture (Reverdin suture) allowed greater sealing of the laceration site, since the infiltration of peritoneal fluid could predispose to contamination and, consequently, point dehiscence. The Sultan suture technique provided stability to the incision line, since it is supported by four points, and lower chance of muscle laceration. The occurrence of hernia recurrence after the first surgery is probably related to the weakness presented by the lacerated muscles, with high friability and inflammation.

In the present case report, buttons were used to provide resistance to laceration. However, a polypropylene mesh in combination with buttons was chosen to reinforce the suture line. The tearing and rupture of muscles were associated with higher predisposition of further abdominal defect; this required greater approximation in the wound. According to the same authors, the technique used ensures good healing for abdominal reconstruction and good recovery of patients, which can return to normal activities, requiring approximately 60 days of movement restriction. However, in the case reported here, the animal returned to its normal routine 30 days after the procedure.

Conclusion

The use polyester buttons and polypropylene mesh, provided effective reinforcement to the abdominal tension and was deemed an effective option for reconstruction of lacerated muscles after post-traumatic eventration in a horse.

Consent

The surgical procedure was performed after the agreement of the horse owner.

Competing interests
The authors declare that they have no competing interests.

Authors' contributions
LRA was the mentor and principal advisor and proposed the concept of the study. CFO, DS, AGB and LRA were responsible for the surgical procedure. CFO, DS, AGB, GCG and LRA were involved in the drafting and writing of the manuscript. All authors have read, commented and approved the final article.

Acknowledgements
We would like to thank the Veterinary Hospital of the Universidade Paranaense and Graduate Program in Animal Science of the Universidade Paranaense, Brazil. Also we would like to thank the Coordenação de Aperfeiçoamento de Pessoal de Ensino Superior (CAPES) for funding the Programa de Suporte à Pós-Graduação de Instituições de Ensino Superior Particulares (PROSUP).
We would like to thank Dr. Anderson da Cunha from the Louisiana State University, School of Veterinary Medicine, Department of Veterinary Clinical Sciences for his help with the manuscript translation.

References
1. Knottenbelt DC, Pascoe RR. Afecções e distúrbios do cavalo. São Paulo: EditoraManole; 1998.
2. Auer JA, Stick JA. Equine surgery. 4th ed. St Louis: Elsevier Saunders; 2012.
3. Vulcani VAS, Macoris DG, Plepis AMG. Biomateriais para reparação cirúrgica da parede abdominal emanimais domésticos revisão. Arq Ciênc Vet Zool. 2009;12:141–7. UNIPAR, Umuarama.
4. Stelmann UJP, Silva AA, Souza BG,Hess TM, Aguiar GC, Santos AE. Utilização de pericárdio bovino como reforço da ráfia do peritônio no tratamento cirúrgico de eventração em equino: relato de caso. Rev. Cient. Elet. Med. Vet.2010. http://faef.revista.inf.br/imagens_arquivos/arquivos_destaque/deUhbGJWXS4U9Ib_2013-6-25-15-5-8.pdf. Accessed 23 Sept 2014.
5. Bellón JM. Propuesta de una nuevaclasificación de prótesis destinadas a La reparación de defectosherniarios em lapared abdominal. CirEspan. 2005;78:148–51.
6. BaergJ KG, TonitaJ PP, Reid D. Gastroschisis: a sixteen-year review. JPediatrSurg. 2003;38:771–4.
7. BadylakS KK, Tullius B, Simmons-ByrdA MR. Morphologic study of small intestinal submucosa as a body wall repair device. JSurg Res. 2002;103:190–202.
8. Greca FH, Souza Filho ZAS, Rocha SL, Borsato KS, Fernandes HAD, Niiside MA. Submucosa de intestino delgado no reparo de defeito em parede abdominal de ratos. ActaCirBras. 2004;19:471–7.
9. Soiderer EE, Lantz GC, Kazacos EA, Hodde JP, Wiegand RE. Morphologic study of three collagen materials for body wall repair. JSurg Res. 2004;118:161–75.
10. Bastos ELS, Fagundes DJ, Taha MO, Novo NF, Silvado RAB. Peritônio bovino conservado na correção de hérnia ventral em ratos: uma alternativa para tela cirúrgica biológica. Rev Col Bras Cir. 2005;32:256–60.
11. Falcão SC, Coelho ARB, EvêncioNeto J. Biomechanical evaluation of microbial cellulose (Zoogloeasp.) and expanded polytetrafluoroethylenemembranesas implants in repair of produced abdominal wall defectsin rats. Acta CirBras. 2008;23:184–91.

12. Yamatogi RS, RahalSC GJM, TagaR CTM, Lima AFM. Histologia da associação de membranas biológicas de origembovina implantadas no tecido subcutâneo de ratos. Cienc Rural. 2005;5:837–42.

13. VulcaniVAS MDG, Plepis AMG, Martins VCA, Franzo VS, RabeloRE S'a FJF. Implantação de biomembrana de colágeno tratada em solução alcalina ou conservada em glicerina a 98 % na parede abdominal de equinos. Cienc Rural. 2013;43:1422–8.

14. Smeak DD. Management and prevention of surgical complications associated with small animal abdominal herniorraphy. Probl Vet Med. 1989;1:254–67.

15. Haupt J, García-Lopez JM, Chope K. Use of a novel silk mesh for ventral midline hernioplasty in a mare. BMC Vet Res. 2015;11:58.

16. Quitzan JG, Rahal DC, RochaNS CAJ. Comparação entre pericárdio bovino preservado em glicerina e malha de poliéster no reparo de falhas da parede abdominal em ratos. Acta Cir Bras. 2003;18:297–301.

17. Ober C, Muste A, Mates N, Oana L, Beteg F, Vancea C. Techniques of implant of prosthetic meshes of polypropylene in repair of the abdominal wall defects in horses. Bull UnivAgric Sci Vet Med Cluj Napoca. 2007;64:509–13.

18. Andrade FAG, Cavalcanti CEO, Mota PKV, Plech R, Ferreira LM. Hemicelulose em reconstrução da parede abdominal em ratos. Rev Bras CirPlást. 2011;26:104–15.

19. Paulo NML, Lima FG, Siqueira Júnior JT, FleuryLFF S'a FJF, Borges AC, Telles TC. Membrana de látex da seringueira (*Hevea brasiliensis*), com e sem polilisina a 0,1 % e tela de marlex na reconstrução de defeitos iatrogênicos da parede abdominal de ratos. Acta CirBras. 2005;20:305–10.

20. Silva LAF, Eurides D, Souza LA, Oliveira BJA, Helou JB, Fonseca AM, Cardoso LL, Freitas SLR. Tratamento de hérnia umbilical em bovinos. Rev Ceres. 2012;59:39–47.

21. Silva LAF, Neto JBP, Chiquetto CE, Fioravanti MCS, Eurides D, Borges GV, Atayde IB, Rabelo RE. Herniorrafia umbilical em bovinos e avaliação do pós-operatório. Ciênc Anim Bras. 2000;1:126.

Faecal transplantation for the treatment of *Clostridium difficile* infection in a marmoset

Yumiko Yamazaki[1,2]* (iD), Shinpei Kawarai[3], Hidetoshi Morita[4], Takefumi Kikusui[5] and Atsushi Iriki[2,6]

Abstract

Background: The common marmoset has been used as an experimental animal for various purposes. Because its average weight ranges from 250 to 500 g, weight loss quickly becomes critical for sick animals. Therefore, effective and non-stressful treatment for chronic diseases, including diarrhoea, is essential.

Case presentation: We report a case in which faecal microbiota transplantation (FMT) led to immediate recovery from chronic and recurrent diarrhoea caused by *Clostridium difficile* infection. A male common marmoset experienced chronic diarrhoea after antibiotic treatments. The animal experienced severe weight loss, and a faecal sample was confirmed to be *C. difficile*-positive but was negative for protozoa. Metronidazole was partially effective at the first administration but not after the recurrence of the clinical signs. Then, oral FMT was administered to the subject by feeding fresh faeces from healthy individuals mixed with the marmoset's usual food. We monitored the faeces by categorization into four groups: normal, loose, diarrhoea, and watery. After the first day of FMT treatment, the marmoset underwent a remarkable recovery from diarrhoea, and after the fourth day of treatment, a test for *C. difficile* was negative. The clinical signs did not recur. The marmoset recovered from sinusitis and bilateral dacryocystitis, which also did not recur, as a by-product of the improvement in its general health caused by the cessation of diarrhoea after the FMT.

Conclusion: This is the first reported case of successful treatment of a marmoset using oral FMT. As seen in human patients, FMT was effective for the treatment of recurrent *C. difficile* infection in a captive marmoset.

Keywords: *Clostridium difficile*, Common marmoset, Diarrhoea, Faecal microbiota transplantation, Metronidazole

Background

Clostridium difficile is a major cause of severe diarrhoea, especially in hospitalized patients receiving antibiotic therapy [1]. Metronidazole is the first choice for *C. difficile* infections [1] in humans and small animals [2]. However, some patients suffer from recurrent infections after repeated treatments [1, 3].

Faecal microbiota transplantation (FMT) is an emergent treatment for diarrhoea caused by various pathogens [4]. Although the success rate of the therapy is variable and the techniques applied in the studies vary widely [5], a few studies have reported immediate recovery after several recurrent *C. difficile* infections (e.g., within 24 h after FMT) [6].

Here, we present a report of successful recovery from severe chronic diarrhoea after FMT in a male common marmoset (*Callithrix jacchus*). This species of small New World monkey has been used as an experimental animal for various purposes, including medical [7], neuroscientific [8], and cognitive studies [9], and the recent establishment of genetically modified animals [10] has enhanced the use of this species in additional research areas. Because their average weight ranges from 250 to 500 g, weight loss quickly becomes critical for sick animals. Therefore, effective and non-stressful treatment for chronic diseases, such as diarrhoea, is necessary. Thus, we administered oral FMT to an animal with chronic diarrhoea caused by *C. difficile*; this is a novel method for the treatment of gut microbiota disturbances in this species.

Case presentation

A male colony-bred common marmoset weighing 420 g that was 2 y and 2 m of age experienced chronic

---

* Correspondence: yumyam@a5.keio.jp
[1]Advanced Research Centres, Keio University, 35 Shinanomachi, Shinjuku-ku, Tokyo 160-8582, Japan
[2]Laboratory for Symbolic Cognitive Development, RIKEN BSI, 2-1 Hirosawa, Wako-shi, Saitama 351-0198, Japan
Full list of author information is available at the end of the article

diarrhoea after a 6-day treatment with ampicillin (Viccillin S-100, Meiji Seika Pharma, Tokyo, Japan, 25 mg/h, i.m., every 24 h) to prevent infection after craniotomy for neural recording; this study was a component of the neurocognitive study projects approved by the Animal Experiment Committees at the RIKEN Brain Science Institute and was conducted in accordance with the Guidelines for Conducting Animal Experiments of the RIKEN Brain Science Institute (H27–2-303). This animal had been housed singly for a few months in preparation for the surgery. The breeding room was maintained at 26–28 °C with 50–60% humidity. Due to the chronic diarrhoea, the animal experienced severe weight loss (BW 360 g; approximately 60 g lost compared to the pre-surgery weight) and was given an oral nutritional supplement (ELENTAL P, EA Pharma, Tokyo, Japan, 2 g per day) and a *Lactobacillus* preparation (Bioymbuster, Kyoritsu Seiyaku, Tokyo, Japan, 50mg/h, p.o., per day) in addition to the standard food regimen. The subject recovered from diarrhoea 1 month after termination of the antibiotic. This antibiotic has also been shown to cause *C. difficile*-associated disease in human patients [11]. A faecal sample collected 3 weeks after surgery was confirmed to be *C. difficile*-positive by anaerobic culture. The sample was negative for protozoa by zinc sulphate flotation performed at a commercial veterinary diagnostic laboratory (Monoris Inc., Tokyo, Japan). Diarrhoea was intermittent (occurrence on 11.3% of days, no watery appearance) for one and a half months after treatment. However, after that period, diarrhoea recurred on 65% of 20 days and was often watery and muddy

(dark brown appearance with little solid content). At this point, we tested the faecal sample (Techlab C Diff Quick Chek Complete, Alere, Chiba, Japan) and confirmed that it was positive for *C. difficile* antigen and toxin. Figure 1 shows the time course of the disease. We categorized the faeces into four groups as follows: normal (solid, with little liquid), loose (blobby with liquid but still formed), diarrhoea (mostly blobby, large amount of liquid, partially muddy), and watery (almost liquid, with small pieces of solids), as photographically represented next to the y-axis in Fig. 1. When there were no faeces, no score was assigned. We scored each day by the worst stool of the day; for instance, if both normal faeces and diarrhoea occurred during a day, then we recorded "diarrhoea" for that day.

The marmoset received metronidazole (Flagyl 250 mg, Shionogi, Osaka, Japan, 25 mg/h, every 24 h) [12] for 10 days (2 5-day periods separated by 2 weekend days). The diarrhoea decreased slightly during and after the medication, as illustrated by "After Metronidazole I (AMI) -10" in Fig. 2, although the *C. difficile* test was still positive for antigen and toxin. However, the diarrhoea quickly worsened within 10 days after termination of the medication. We re-administered the metronidazole 23 days after the end of the first medication cycle for 10 days as described above, with little evidence of recovery (Figs. 1 and 2).

Because the metronidazole was no longer effective, we decided to perform a FMT. Faeces from healthy individuals were administered orally by mixing with the pellet food (CMS-1M, CLEA Japan, Tokyo, Japan). Specifically,

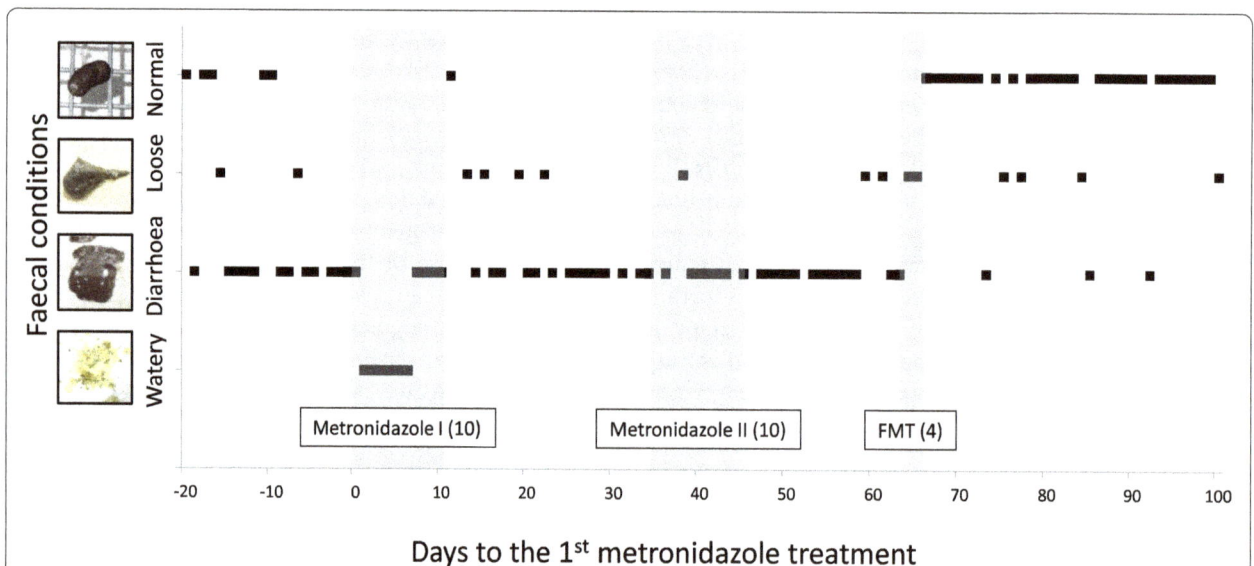

Fig. 1 Time course of diarrhoea before, during, and after the treatments. The "0" on the *horizontal axis* indicates the first day of the first metronidazole treatment. The faeces were divided into four categories (normal, loose, diarrhoea, and watery) as represented in the pictures next to the *vertical axis*. *Shaded vertical lines* show the two periods of metronidazole treatment and the faecal microbiota transplantation. The *numbers* next to the names of the treatments indicate the period in days

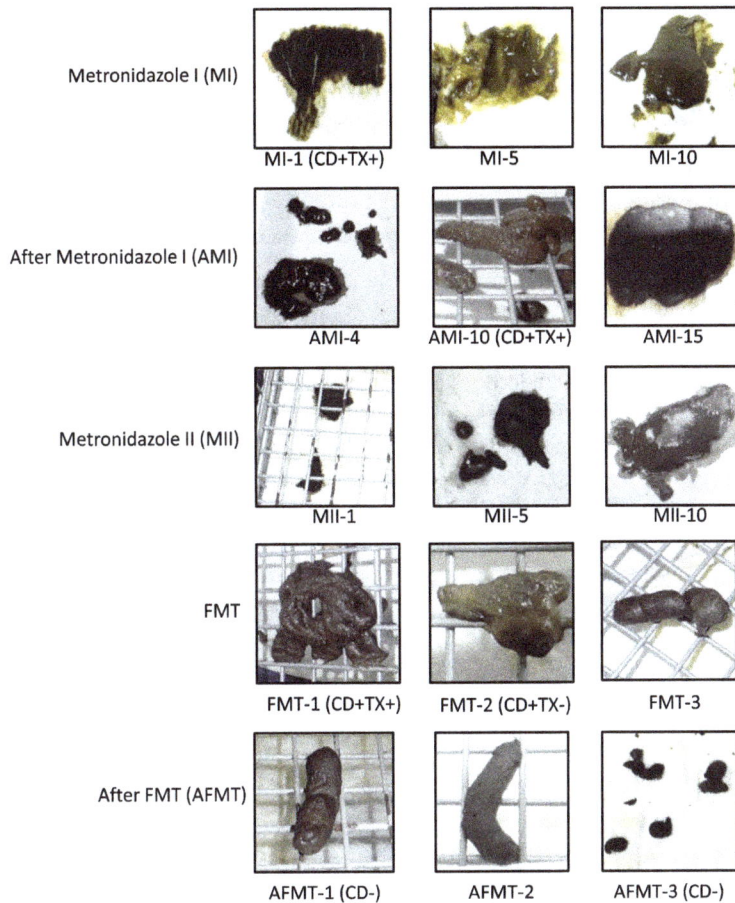

Fig. 2 Representative faecal samples during and after the treatments. Under each picture, the *numbers* next to the abbreviated names of the treatments (e.g., MI) show the day within a given treatment or phase. The results of the tests for *Clostridium difficile* antigen and toxin are shown in *parentheses* next to the legend. CD: *C. difficile* antigen; TX: *C. difficile* toxin

3 g of faeces from marmosets, 4 g of powdered marmoset food, 2 g of honey, and 8 ml of lukewarm water were mixed to make a wet mash. The donors were seven healthy marmosets with no history of medication for at least 3 months. Multiple donors were selected to increase the diversity of the microbiota in the faeces, which is thought to be key for effective FMT [4]. Faecal samples from the marmosets were collected within 30 min after defecation. The FMT treatment continued for four consecutive days, and at least two donors were selected per day. This method was chosen because the faecal samples were not consistently available.

The consistency of the subject's faeces changed quickly (Fig. 1). The faeces became more solid the day after the first FMT treatment (FMT-1 in Fig. 2), although the tests were still positive for *C. difficile* antigen and toxin. After the second treatment, the tests were *C. difficile*-positive but toxin-negative. The faeces were almost normal after the third treatment (FMT-3 in Fig. 2). Finally, the test results were negative for both *C. difficile* antigen and toxin after the

fourth day of FMT treatment (After FMT (AFMT)-1 in Fig. 2). Thereafter, the marmoset completely recovered from chronic diarrhoea and remained healthy for the subsequent 10 months, as shown in Fig. 1. No adverse effects were observed during or after the FMT treatment. *C. difficile* infection has not been observed in other animals in that breeding room.

In addition to the cessation of diarrhoea after the FMT treatment, the marmoset recovered from sinusitis and bilateral dacryocystitis, which had developed after the surgery for unknown reasons. The presence of sinusitis, epiphora, and mild conjunctivitis and the location of the swelling at the inner corners of eyes (especially the areas around the lacrimal punctum) indicated a tentative diagnosis of dacryocystitis. A bacteriological examination (Monoris Inc., Tokyo, Japan) of the discharge from the nose 1 month after the surgery confirmed the presence of a Gram-negative bacillus that showed sensitivity to enrofloxacin. Therefore, enrofloxacin (Baytril 15 mg, Bayer, Tokyo, Japan, 2.5 mg/kg, p.o., every 24 h) was administered

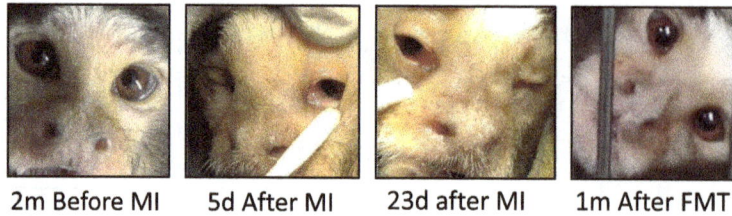

| 2m Before MI | 5d After MI | 23d after MI | 1m After FMT |

Fig. 3 Nasal and ocular signs before and after the treatments. *Swelling* between the eyes and nose was prominent after the first administration of metronidazole; FMT: faecal microbiota transplantation; m: month; d: day

for 10 days. Three months after this treatment, which was concurrent with the recovery from diarrhoea, the clinical signs became worse, and the swelling around the eyes and nose was significantly worse than the signs observed 2 months prior to the treatment (Fig. 3). The swelling did not improve after the first or second metronidazole treatment. On the first day of FMT, a large amount of nasal mucus was evident. However, the marmoset rapidly recovered, with no nasal mucus or lacrimation by the third day of FMT. Finally, these clinical signs resolved 1 month after treatment (Fig. 3), with no recurrence during the 10 months after FMT.

Discussion and Conclusions

Chronic and severe diarrhoea caused by *C. difficile* infection was terminated after 4 days of oral intake of faecal microbiota collected from healthy individuals. The subject readily accepted the treatment because the faeces were mixed with the usual marmoset food. This treatment showed marked benefits without the stress of drug administration by intragastric tube or a probe. Additionally, the FMT food was more palatable than metronidazole (which is extremely bitter); thus, a full dose could be administered every day (we determined that the food was palatable because the subject continued to eat the FMT food; if the food was not palatable, like metronidazole, the subject stopped eating, started salivating excessively, and wiped the food on the cage wires or perches). This immediate recovery was similar to the recovery observed in some human subjects [4, 6], with improvement starting within 24 h after the first treatment. These improvements in the clinical signs were correlated with the recovery from sinusitis and dacryocystitis. However, because no direct causal relationship existed between these clinical signs and the FMT, the general improvement in the animal's health condition after the cessation of diarrhoea most likely contributed to its recovery from these signs.

Of course, many questions remain unanswered. For example, we do not know the origin of the *C. difficile* infection. To this end, an analysis of the microbiota

of the infected and healthy animals is needed. A comparison of the microbiota of the donors with the microbiota of the patient after recovery could reveal the most desirable distribution of microbiota for FMT. Information on the Bifidobacteria in the common marmoset microbiome has been accumulating [13–16]. Bifidobacteria are widely used as probiotic organisms and may confer a health benefit to the host when an effective amount is administered to balance the host microbiome. This information would support a more detailed analysis of the healthy microbiome of this animal.

In conclusion, FMT appeared to be effective for the treatment of recurrent *C. difficile* infection in a captive marmoset, as seen in human patients. This small primate could be a valid model for the study of *C. difficile* infections and effective treatments, including FMT, in human patients.

Abbreviations
FMT: Faecal microbiota transplantation; *C. difficile*: *Clostridium difficile*

Acknowledgements
The authors thank Masakado Saiki, Masayuki Inada, Taku Koike, and Reiko Nakatomi for the data collection.

Funding
This work was supported by Brain Mapping by Integrated Neurotechnologies for Disease Studies (Brain/MINDS) at RIKEN, Japan, and the Science Research Promotion Fund for Private University at Azabu University, Japan, from the Ministry of Education, Culture, Sports, Science, and Technology of Japan (MEXT).

Authors' contributions
YY designed and executed the experiments; YY and SK wrote the main manuscript text and prepared the figures; and HM, TK, and AI coordinated the manuscript writing. All authors reviewed the manuscript. All authors read and approved the final manuscript.

Competing interests
A.I. is the President and CEO and Y.Y. is a director of RIKÆNALYSIS Corporation (RIKEN Venture Company). The other authors declare no competing financial interests.

Consent for publication
Not applicable.

Author details
[1]Advanced Research Centres, Keio University, 35 Shinanomachi, Shinjuku-ku, Tokyo 160-8582, Japan. [2]Laboratory for Symbolic Cognitive Development, RIKEN BSI, 2-1 Hirosawa, Wako-shi, Saitama 351-0198, Japan. [3]Laboratory of Small Animal Clinics, Veterinary Teaching Hospital, Azabu University, 1-17-71 Fuchinobe, Chuo-ku, Sagamihara-shi, Kanagawa 252-5201, Japan. [4]Graduate School of Environmental and Life Science, Okayama University, 1-1-1 Tsushimanaka, Kita-ku, Okayama-shi, Okayama 700-8530, Japan. [5]Companion Animal Research, School of Veterinary Medicine, Azabu University, 1-17-71 Fuchinobe, Chuo-ku, Sagamihara-shi, Kanagawa 252-5201, Japan. [6]RIKEN-NTU Research Centre for Human Biology, Nanyang Technological University, Singapore 639798, Singapore.

References
1. Aslam S, Hamill RJ, Musher DM. Treatment of Clostridium Difficile-associated disease: old therapies and new strategies. Lancet Infect Dis. 2005;5:549–57. doi:10.1016/S1473-3099(05)70215-2.
2. Willard MD. Disorders of the intestinal tract. In: Nelson R, Couto CG, editors. Small animal internal medicine. 5th ed. St. Louis: Elsevier; 2013. p. 455–91.
3. Musher DM, Aslam S, Logan N, Nallacheru S, Bhaila I, Borchert F, et al. Relatively poor outcome after treatment of Clostridium Difficile colitis with metronidazole. Clin Infect Dis. 2005;40:1586–90. doi:10.1086/430311.
4. van Nood E, Vrieze A, Nieuwdorp M, Fuentes S, Zoetendal EG, de Vos WM, et al. Duodenal infusion of donor feces for recurrent Clostridium Difficile. N Engl J Med. 2013;368:407–15. doi:10.1056/NEJMoa1205037.
5. Cammarota G, Ianiro G, Bibbò S, Gasbarrini A. Fecal microbiota transplantation: a new old kid on the block for the management of gut microbiota-related disease. J Clin Gastroenterol. 2014;48:S80–4. doi:10.1097/MCG.0000000000000244.
6. Kahn SA, Young S, Rubin DT. Colonoscopic fecal microbiota transplant for recurrent Clostridium Difficile infection in a child. Am J Gastroenterol. 2012;107:1930–1. doi:10.1038/ajg.2012.351.
7. Fernández-Oliva A, Finzi A, Haim H, Menéndez-Arias L, Sodroski J, Pacheco B. HIV-1 adapts to replicate in cells expressing common marmoset APOBEC3G and BST2. J Virol. 2015;90:725–40. doi:10.1128/JVI.02431-15.
8. Mitchell JF, Leopold DA. The marmoset monkey as a model for visual neuroscience. Neurosci Res. 2015;93:20–46. doi:10.1016/j.neures.2015.01.008.
9. Yamazaki Y, Saiki M, Inada M, Iriki A, Watanabe S. Transposition and its generalization in common marmosets. J Exp Psychol Anim Learn Cogn. 2014;40:317–26. doi:10.1037/xan0000027.
10. Sasaki E, Suemizu H, Shimada A, Hanazawa K, Oiwa R, Kamioka M, et al. Generation of transgenic non-human primates with germline transmission. Nature. 2009;459:523–7. doi:10.1038/nature08090.
11. McFarland LV, Surawicz CM, Stamm WE. Risk factors for Clostridium Difficile carriage and C. Difficile-associated diarrhea in a cohort of hospitalized patients. J Infect Dis. 1990;162:678–84. doi:10.1093/infdis/162.3.678.
12. Johnson-Delaney CA. Primates. Vet Clin North Am Small Anim Pract. 1994;24:121–56. doi:10.1016/S0195-5616(94)50007-X.
13. Endo A, Futagawa-Endo Y, Schumann P, Pukall R, Dicks LM. Bifidobacterium reuteri sp. nov., Bifidobacterium callitrichos sp. nov., Bifidobacterium saguini sp. nov., Bifidobacterium stellenboschense sp. nov. and Bifidobacterium biavatii sp. nov. isolated from faeces of common marmoset (Callithrix Jacchus) and red-handed tamarin (Saguinus Midas). Syst Appl Microbiol. 2012;35:92–7.
14. Modesto M, Michelini S, Stefanini I, Ferrara A, Tacconi S, Biavati B, et al. Bifidobacterium aesculapii sp. nov., from the faeces of the baby common marmoset (Callithrix Jacchus). Int J Syst Evol Microbiol. 2014;64:2819–27. doi:10.1099/ijs.0.056937-0.
15. Michelini S, Modesto M, Oki K, Stenico V, Stefanini I, Biavati B, et al. Isolation and identification of cultivable Bifidobacterium spp. from the faeces of 5 baby common marmosets (Callithrix Jacchus). Anaerobe. 2015;33:101–4. doi:10.1016/j.anaerobe.2015.03.001.
16. Toh H, Yamazaki Y, Tashiro K, Kawarai S, Oshima K, Nakano A, et al. Draft genome sequence of bifidobacterium aesculapii DSM 26737T, isolated from feces of baby common marmoset. Genome Announc. 2015;3 doi:10.1128/genomeA.01463-15.

Efficacy of oral meloxicam suspension for prevention of pain and inflammation following band and surgical castration in calves

M. E. Olson[1*], Brenda Ralston[2], Les Burwash[2], Heather Matheson-Bird[3] and Nick D. Allan[4]

Abstract

Background: Castration is one of the most common procedures performed on beef and dairy cattle. The objective of the study was to determine the efficacy of meloxicam oral suspension in reducing pain and inflammation in calves following band or surgical castration.

Methods: Two identical trials with the exception of the method of castration (Band Castration Study 1 and Surgical Castration Study 2) were conducted. Sixty (60) healthy Holstein calves 4 to 5 months of age (138–202 Kg) were used. Animals received either Meloxicam Oral Suspension at a dose of 1 mg/kg BW ($n = 15$ Study 1 and 15 Study 2) or Saline ($n = 15$ Study 1 and 15 Study 2) 2 h before castration. Physiological (Heart Rate, Plasma Cortisol and Plasma Substance P) and Behavioral (Visual Analog Scale (VAS), Accelerometers and tail Pedometers) evaluations were conducted before (day -1) and after Castration (Day 0, 1, 2, 3). Inflammation was evaluated daily by providing an individual animal score (Study1) or with a measurement of scrotal thickness (Study 2).

Results: Heart rates were significantly greater in control animals following band and surgical castration. Plasma cortisol and substance P were significantly reduced in animals receiving Meloxicam Oral Suspension. Control animals had significantly greater VAS scores. Accelerometers showed that meloxicam treated animals had a significantly greater motion index and number of steps as well as less % time lying and number of lying bouts. The scrotal inflammation (based on scrotal swelling) was significantly decreased in the meloxicam treated animals compared to the control animals on day 1, day 2 and 3.

Conclusion: Meloxicam Oral Suspension was able to significantly reduce the display of painful behaviors and physiological responses to pain in band castrated and surgical castrated calves for up to 72 h following a single oral treatment of 1 mg/kg body weight. Meloxicam Oral Suspension was able to significantly reduce scrotal inflammation in band castrated and surgical castrated calves.

Keywords: Oral meloxicam, Castration, Behavior, Pain, Calves

* Correspondence: merle@avetlabs.com
[1]Alberta Veterinary Laboratories, 411 19th Street SE, Calgary, Alberta T2E 6J7, Canada
Full list of author information is available at the end of the article

Background

Castration is one of the most common procedures performed on male beef and dairy cattle. The benefits of castration are well established and include population control, reduced aggressive and mounting behaviors and improved carcass quality. Regardless of the method, castration has been shown to produce physiological, behavioral and neuroendocrine alteration associated with pain and distress [1–5]. Currently, approved North American local and general anesthetics available to veterinarians and producers to control pain and stress associated with castration effects are only short term [3]. Recently, oral meloxicam has been demonstrated to provide effective pain relief in calves following dehorning and castration [6, 7] with efficacy duration of up to 3 days and a plasma half-life of 27 h [8]. Meloxicam is a nonsteroidal anti-inflammatory drug (NSAID) of the oxicam class which acts by inhibition of prostaglandin synthesis, thereby exerting anti-inflammatory, analgesic and anti-pyretic properties [8, 9]. Meloxicam preferentially inhibits the COX-2 isoenzyme and has been shown to be safer than non-selective NSAIDs like aspirin, flunixin and ketoprofen [10]. Meloxicam Oral Suspension is a new product that has been developed and recently registered in Canada. Meloxicam Oral Suspension has advantages over injectable formulations: 1) The onset of therapeutic activity is similar between injectable and oral formulations but the oral formulation has a significantly longer duration of activity (8), 2) Injection site reactions and needle stick injuries can be avoided with the use of an oral formulation, 3) Meloxicam Oral Suspension is highly palatable and is readily taken by oral gavage and it can be top dressed onto feed as a delivery method. 4) Meloxicam Oral Suspension is suitable for use in a number of domestic and wildlife mammalian species where restraint required for injection is not possible. The objective of the study was to determine the efficacy of meloxicam oral suspension in reducing pain and inflammation in calves following band or surgical castration. This study contributed to the registration of Meloxicam Oral Suspension in Canada for "alleviation of pain and inflammation following surgical and band castration in cattle".

Methods

The study was conducted in compliance with the guidelines of the Canadian Council on Animal Care after the appropriate review by the Institutional Animal Care and Use Committee. In evaluation of the study consideration was given that no local anesthetic was provided to animals and although not advocated it is standard of practice in North America. The early behavioral and physiological effects (first 3 h) of meloxicam oral suspension could not be evaluated if local anesthesia was employed. A pre-study power calculation was performed to determine the number of animals required to generate meaningful results. Procedures were designed to avoid or minimize discomfort, distress and pain to the animals.

Two identical trials, with the exception of the method of castration, were conducted during the month of August, 2014. The trails were run at separate times and there was no overlap of trials. Animals received Meloxicam Oral Suspension at an oral dose of 1 mg/kg BW ($n = 15$ Study 1 and $n = 15$ Study 2) or oral Saline 1 mL per 15 kg ($n = 15$ Study 1 and $n = 15$ Study 2) approximately 2 h before castration. The person in charge of the preparation of dosing syringes, treating the animals and randomization was not blinded. The persons caring for animals, collecting blood, downloading heart rate and accelerometer data, behavior scoring the animals, evaluating inflammation and analyzing the plasma were blinded.

Holstein calves were 4 to 5 months of age 138–186 Kg (Study 1, $n = 15$ for treatment, $n = 15$ for control); 142–202 Kg (Study 2, $n = 15$ for treatment, $n = 15$ for control). For each study animals were weighed, ranked by weight and allocated to treatment or control using random numbers. The animal was the experimental unit. All calves were brought to the facility from multiple sources in Southern Alberta, Canada at less than 4 weeks of age, fed a milk diet for 2–4 weeks and placed on solid feed. The feed at the time of study was a mixed barley grain and alfalfa hay ration (77.4 % dry matter, 12 % crude protein) with a mineral/vitamin supplement. Before and during the study, animals were comingled in a rectangular pen (24 m x 30 m) with 10 m of concrete feed bunk, automatic waterer and shelter (5 m x 10 m). Calves had free choice feed and were provided fresh feed twice daily. One animal was removed from the Meloxicam surgical castrated group due to a surgical complication which resulted in excess bleeding and the need for further care.

Castration procedure

In North America it is not standard practice to provide local or general anesthesia at the time of castration. All castrations were performed at time 0 (approximately two hours after receiving the treatment with Meloxicam Oral Suspension (Alberta Veterinary Laboratories, Calgary, AB) or saline (Baxter, Mississauga, ON, Canada). Band castrations were performed, without local anesthesia, by placing a latex band (UFA Coop, Calgary, Alberta) around the neck of the scrotum, employing a banding tool (UFA Coop, Calgary, Alberta)). Surgical castrations were performed without local anesthetics. The scrotum was disinfected with a chlorhexidine surgical scrub (Hibitane Skin Cleanser, Zoetis, Kirkland, Quebec, Canada). Longitudinal incisions were made on the lateral sides of the scrotum. The testes and spermatic cord were exteriorized by blunt dissection and the cremastor was broken using manual traction. Each testis was extracted with a slow steady pull.

Heart rate

The hair over the ventral girth was clipped. Girth heart rate recorders and Heart Rate Data loggers (WM Smartsync Heart Rate Logger, Oregon Scientific, PO box 1190, Cannon Beach Oregon) were placed around the girth of each animal on day 0 at the time of treatment (approximately -2 h). They were held in place with adhesive tape (3" Adhesive Ultra Elastic Tape, Covidien Canada, Saint Laurent, Quebec) wrapped loosely around the chest. Data loggers and straps were removed and data was downloaded on day 1, approximately 24 h after placement. Heart rates were continually collected with each data point representing the heart rate over a 10 s period. Heart Rates were downloading using a laptop computer and software supplied by the manufacturer (WM Smartsync Heart Rate Logger, Oregon Scientific, PO box 1190, Cannon Beach Oregon).

Blood collection and cortisol and substance P analysis

Blood (10 mL) was collected by jugular or tail vein venipuncture on day -1, t = 5 h, t = 24 h, t = 48 h and t = 72 h. Ten (10) mL of blood was collected for Cortisol and Substance P (SP) analysis. Blood was collected in heparinized tubes and aprotonin (0.1 mL) was immediately added. Blood samples were centrifuged at 1600 x g for 15 min in a refrigerated centrifuge. The plasma was separated and placed in microfuge tubes in a -80C freezer for analysis. Cortisol and Substance P were analyzed using validated assay kits (Assay Designs™ Cortisol enzyme immunoassay (EIA) kit, Assay Designs, Inc. Ann Arbor, MI, USA;

Parameter, Substance P Assay, R&D Systems, Inc.614 McKinley Place NE, Minneapolis, MN USA).

Accelerometer recording

Accelerometers (IceTags, www.icerobotics.com) were used to objectively measure movements of the animals. IceTags are a specialized activity monitoring system developed by IceRobotics Ltd, Edinburgh, Scotland, UK to support research into livestock behaviour, health and welfare. They have been validated for cattle, sheep and goats (www.icer obotics.com, [11]). The system consists of an IceTag Sensor which is a 3 axis accelerometer that is strapped to the hind leg of an animal and a download station. Data was collected continually over the study period. The sensor outputs include: 1) Standing/Lying: determined by the sensor passing a specific threshold between horizontal/vertical, 2) Lying bouts: exact start and end time of each lying bout, plus duration, 3) Motion index: indicates the overall activity of the animal calculated using the acceleration on each of the 3 axes. This is a manufacturer proprietary measure and is recommended over the step count as a measure of activity and 4) Step count: the number of times the calf lifts their tagged leg, based on the amount of force the animal uses.

ICE Tag recorders were placed on the left hind hock of each animal on day -1. The ICE tags were secured with tape (3" Adhesive Ultra Elastic Tape, Covidien Canada, Saint Laurent, Quebec). The time clock on the recorders was synchronized and set to the current date and time of the download station. ICE tags remained in place until day 3 (approximately 96 h after the treatment with meloxicam or saline placebo). The information was downloaded for analysis. Downloading was performed in the laboratory after using a reader, laptop computer and software supplied by the manufacturer IceRobotics (IceRobotics Ltd, Edinburgh, Scotland, UK).

After the data was downloaded the following data was excluded for analysis: 1.) The data from time of activating the ICE Tag until the device was placed on the animal's leg and the animal returned to the home pen. 2.) The data during the period of time animals were being processed (Blood collection, castration, tail pedometer placement and removal, heart rate monitor placement and removal, movement of animals to and from handling area) and 3.) The data from the time of ICE tag removal until downloading of the data. The sum of each activity (standing time, lying time, lying bouts, motion index and step counts) were tabulated for each study period.

Visual behavioral monitoring of pain

Behavioral data were obtained as described below. All samples were taken at the times relative to when (day and hour) a particular group was castrated. To assess treatment effects, behavioral observations were made by three experienced observers that were blind to the treatments. Observers were experienced animal scientists with training from an ethologist (Dr. Schwartzkopf -Gerswin) well recognized in recording painful behaviors. Observers used a Visual Analog Scale (VAS) to document behavioral responses indicative of pain and discomfort: Day 0: One (1) hour after castration for approximately 3 h (there were more painful behaviors so recording took more time); Day 1: Two hours of observation; Day 2: Two hours of observation; Day 3: Two hours of observation. The scoring was based upon the presence or absence of the following behaviors :belly kicking, stretching, changing of position, arching of the back, standing alone in pen, looking or attempting to lick the scrotum, frequent tail flicking, not alert and lack of interest in feed or water. The VAS was a 100 mm horizontal line with the far left indicating no pain response and the far right representing an extreme pain response. The observers placed a mark along this continuum that represented the amount of pain response an animal was exhibiting. The distance from the end point to the mark was measured to the nearest 0.1 cm and was recorded as the animal's response to the castration (VAS score).

Tail movement (tail pedometers)

Pedometers (Waterproof Step Movement Calorie Counter Multi-Function Digital Pedometer M2, China) were used to determine tail movements. Pedometers were secured to the tail of each animal (10 cm from the tail base) on day -1 with adhesive tape (2" Adhesive Ultra Elastic Tape, Covidien Canada, Saint Laurent, Quebec). Pedometer values were recorded and reset at approximate times t = 0, t = 24 h, t = 48 h and t = 72 h. The pedometers were manually read and the "steps" recorded. After recording, the pedometers were reset and placed on the tail for the data collection for the next day. Pedometers were removed on day 3.

Inflammation evaluation

In band castrated animals the scrotal tissue swelling above the band was scored post castration on day 0 (immediately after castration), day 1, day 2 and day 3 at the time of blood collection (when animal was restrained in head gate). These scores were recorded as: 0 = No swelling, 1 = slight swelling, 2 = moderate swelling and 3 = severe swelling. The diameter of the mid scrotum tissue was measured post castration in surgically castrated animals on day 0 (immediately after castration), day 1, day 2 and day 3 at the time of blood collection (when animal was restrained in head gate). This was performed using digital calipers.

Data analysis

A two-tailed Student's t test was used to compare treatment and control heart rates, cortisol concentrations, substance P concentrations, accelerometer data, pedometer data and scrotal thickness measurements. Nonparametric analysis (Mann–Whitney test) was used to compare scrotal thickness scores and visual analog scale values. Significance was established at a 95 % confidence interval and data is expressed as mean, standard error (SE) with P values.

Results

Heart rate

The mean heart rates were recorded between the following times: 1) 2 to 4 h after castration, 2) 6 to 8 h after castration and 3) 8 to 10 h after castration. The mean heart rate was calculated using the software provided by the Data Logger provider (WM Smartsync Heart Rate Logger, Oregon Scientific, PO box 1190, Cannon Beach Oregon). During these times animals were not being processed and the recordings were free of interference. In many of the animals signals could not be obtained after 10 h of recording so data was not analyzed past this time. The data is summarized in Table 1. The heart rates were significantly elevated in the control animals compared to the treated animals ($P < 0.05$) for both the band castrated and surgical castrated animals for all observation times.

Plasma cortisol and substance P

Animals were acclimated to be handled and minimal to no restraint was required to collect blood from the tail vein of calves. Therefore the act of blood collection had minimal effects on plasma cortisol and substance P. Plasma cortisol and substance P values in band and surgically castrated animals are provided in Table 2 and Fig. 1 The plasma cortisol values were significantly elevated in the control animals compared to the treated animals ($P < 0.05$) on day 0 and 1 for band castrated animals and day 0 for surgical castrated animals. The plasma substance P concentrations were significantly elevated in the control animals compared to the treated animals ($P < 0.05$) on day 0 and day 1 for both the band castrated animals and surgical castrated animals.

Accelerometer behavior data

Ice Tag data was downloaded from the accelerometers and only times that animals were in their home pen without any external disturbances were included for analysis. For Band Castrated calves (Study 1) analysis periods were: a) Day -1 (3:00 pm) to Day 0 (8:00 am), b) Day 0 (1:00 pm) to Day 1 (10:00 am), c) Day 1 (1:30 pm) to Day 2 (8:30 am); Day 2 (11:30 am) to Day 3 (9:00 am). For Surgical Castrated calves (Study 2) analysis periods were: a) Day -1 (1:30 pm) to Day 0 (8:00 am), b) Day 0 (2:15 pm) to Day 1 (9:00 am), c) Day 1 (10:30 am) to Day 2 (8:30 am); Day 2 (10:00 am) to Day 3 (9:00 am). The behavior data is provided in Table 3 and Fig. 2.

For band castrated calves, the motion index was significantly elevated in meloxicam treated animals compared to the control animals ($P < 0.05$) on day 0–1, day 1–2 and day 2–3. The percent of time lying was significantly lower in meloxicam treated animals compared to the control animals ($P < 0.05$) on day 0–1. The number of steps taken was significantly greater in meloxicam treated animals compared to the saline treated animals ($P < 0.05$) on day 0–1, day 1–2 and day 2–3. Band castration control animals had significantly more lying bouts than meloxicam treated animals ($P < 0.05$) on day 0–1, day 1–2 and day 2–3.

In surgically castrated animals the motion index was significantly elevated in meloxicam treated animals compared to the treated animals ($P < 0.05$) on day 0–1, day 1–2 and day 2–3. The percent of time lying was significantly greater in meloxicam treated animals compared to the saline treated animals ($P < 0.05$) on day 1–2 for surgically castrated animals. The number of steps taken was significantly elevated in meloxicam treated animals compared to the saline treated animals ($P < 0.05$) on day 0–1, day 1–2 and day 2–3. There was no difference in the number of lying bouts between control animals and meloxicam treated animals ($P > 0.05$).

Table 1 Heart Rates of Calves following Band or Surgical Castration

Time Post – Castration	Treatment	Band Castration			Surgical Castration		
		Mean (beats/min)	SE	P Value	Mean (beats/min)	SE	P Value
2–4 h	Meloxicam	119.3	2.2	0.0001	100.2	4.0	0.0019
	Control (Saline)	141.2	2.7		116.6	2.0	
6–8 h	Meloxicam	112.9	2.0	0.0005	98.4	5.1	0.0003
	Control (Saline)	131.3	3.4		122.9	3.0	
8–10 h	Meloxicam	113.3	3.9	0.0033	103.2	3.6	0.0026
	Control (Saline)	134.8	4.6		119.0	2.7	

Visual analog scale (VAS)

The mean total Visual Analog Scale (VAS) score the three experienced observers used to identify painful behaviors in cattle are provided in Table 4 and Fig. 3. The data is expressed as a percentage of the total line with 0 % assigned to animals with no observed pain associated behaviors and 100 % assigned to animals with severe pain behaviors (e.g. kicking, stretching, changing of position, arched back, standing alone in the pen). The VAS scores are higher in all band castrated animals compared to all surgical castrated animals. Band castrated animals receiving Meloxicam Oral Suspension demonstrated significantly less painful behaviors (P < 0.05) than saline treated controls on observation day 0, day 1 and day 2. Surgical castrated animals receiving Meloxicam Oral Suspension demonstrated significantly less painful behaviors (P < 0.05) than saline treated controls on observation for day 0, day 1 and day 2. The VAS was compared between band and surgical castrated calves. For both meloxicam and control castrated calves there was a significantly higher scores on days 0, 1 and 2 in Band castrated calves compared to surgical castration.

Tail pedometers

Tail pedometer data was collected on the belief that pain associated with castration in calves would result in more

tail swishes. Pedometers were easily attached to the tail base and tail swishes could be recorded. Animals rarely lost their pedometers and they were replaced the next day during processing. Data from animals that lost their pedometers was not used in the analysis. Pedometer data is provided in Table 5. There was no difference in the number of "steps" recorded on the tail pedometers between control animals and meloxicam treated animals (P > 0.05) following band and surgical castration. The "steps" on the pedometers represent the number of tail swishes.

Inflammation scoring and measurement

Generally, swelling in the band castrated calves was minimal proximal to the band in the inguinal area. The scrotal inflammation score was significantly less in the meloxicam treated animals compared to the control animals (P < 0.05) for band castrated animals on day 2 and 3 (Table 6). In surgical castrated animals the scrotal tissue swelling could be easily objectively evaluated using digital calipers (Table 6). The scrotal inflammation (based on scrotal swelling) was significantly less in the meloxicam treated animals compared to the control animals (P < 0.05) for surgical castrated animals on day 1, day 2 and 3. There was no evidence of infections in any animal in the study.

Table 2 Plasma Cortisol and Substance P values in Band and Surgically Castrated Animals

Day of Study	Treatment	Plasma Cortisol (ηmol/L)				Substance P (pg/L)			
		Band Castrated		Surgical Castrated		Band Castrated		Surgical Castrated	
		Mean (SE)	P value	Mean (SE)	P value	Mean (SE)	P value	Mean (SE)	P value
Day -1	Meloxicam	14.2 (1.6)	0.8519	16.4 (2.3)	0.6041	243.9 (16.4)	0.4679	249.8 (7.8)	0.4849
	Control (Saline)	13.2 (1.4)		18.7 (1.9)		268.2 (15.6)		244.5 (11.5)	
Day 0	Meloxicam	23.9 (1.2)	0.0032	39.6 (5.5)	0.0421	243.7 (13.9)	0.0012	267.9 (11.2)	0.0137
	Control (Saline)	36.1 (4.5)		58.0 (7.7)		340.5 (23.0)		314.7 (13.4)	
Day 1	Meloxicam	29.6 (5.3)	0.0340	14.1 (2.1)	0.8785	261.8 (15.5)	0.0181	260.6 (8.1)	0.0424
	Control (Saline)	38.4 (3.6)		18.2 (5.1)		335.5 (23.8)		304.4 (17.0)	
Day 2	Meloxicam	33.4 (5.4)	0.8846	9.3 (1.7)	0.0808	251.6 (14.9)	0.0680	273.2 (10.4)	0.3947
	Control (Saline)	33.6 (4.3)		13.7 (2.4)		295.2 (16.3)		301.1 (17.0)	
Day 3	Meloxicam	27.6 (6.7)	0.6783	14.9 (2.0)	0.4581	253.7 (12.7)	0.5338	333.7 (11.2)	0.8103
	Control (Saline)	28.7 (6.4)		19.6 (3.0)		264.9 (16.4)		334.8 (5.3)	

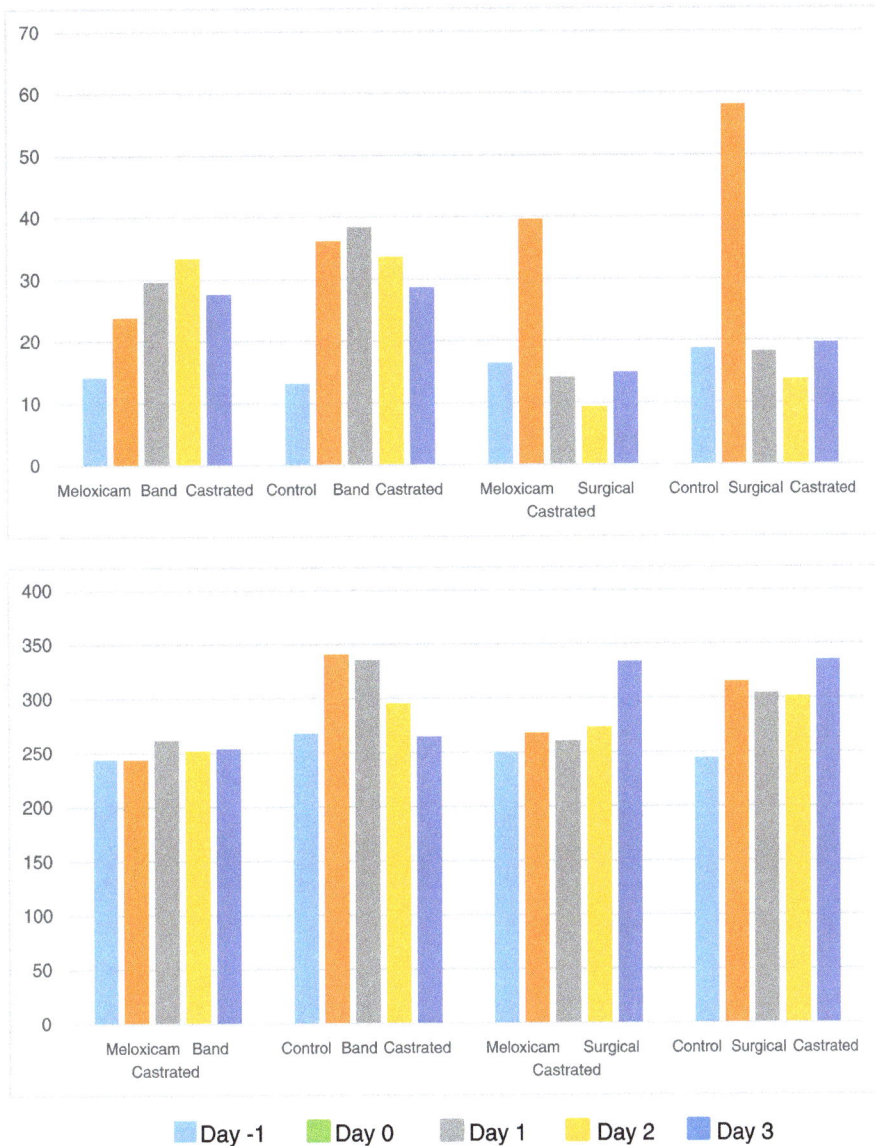

Fig. 1 Plasma Cortisol (Upper, ηmol/L) and Plasma Substance P (Lower, pg/L) in band and surgically castrated calves on day -1, 0, 1, 2 and 3

Discussion

Cattle are able to mask pain and stress as an important component to survival. The development of appropriate cattle pain model systems and robust markers are essential for the demonstration of pain and pharmacological relief of pain [3, 4]. The study protocol was designed to focus on robust indicators that have been established and validated previously [3, 4]. The investigators have also learned that the breed and age of animals also play a critical role in demonstration of pain and relief of pain. Beef breeds that are over 250 kg have difficulty in displaying demonstrations of pain [3, 4], but this does not mean that they do not feel pain. Well acclimated dairy calves which are 100 to 300 kg body weight appear to respond best to painful procedures such as castration and dehorning as well as interventions that reduce or eliminate the pain [3, 4]. For this reason we have selected dairy bull calves for this study. In this study the calves were brought to the study site at a young age and were handled daily and frequently by farm employees. These animals were ideal subjects as they were not stressed by handling and therefore the physiological and behavioral responses to the meloxicam could be readily measured [3, 4].

Compounded oral meloxicam preparations have been used previously in North America for control of pain and inflammation for dehorning and castration [3, 4]. Meloxicam Oral Suspension is the first commercial oral meloxicam available for cattle in North America. This formulation has proven to be stable, effective and safe for cattle as part of the regulatory submission. The long

Table 3 Accelerometer Behavioral Data in Band and Surgically Castrated Animals

Study Day	Variable	Treatment	Band Castrated			Surgical Castrated		
			Mean	SE	P Value	Mean	SE	P Value
Day -1 To Day 0 (pre-castration)	Motion Index	Meloxicam	6563	431.2	0.6783	5066	236.6	0.0771
		Control	6835	391.9		4510	200.2	
	% Time Lying	Meloxicam	62.2	1.1	0.6482	68.2	0.88	0.9131
		Control	61.4	1.6		67.9	0.95	
	Number of Steps	Meloxicam	1728	72.5	0.0537	1397	91.8	0.3051
		Control	2006	101.7		1197	54.3	
	Lying Bouts	Meloxicam	35	3.3	0.4303	23.21	1.5	0.5698
		Control	39	3.9		24.07	1.6	
Day 0 To Day 1	Motion Index	Meloxicam	6041	311.6	0.0144	5786	369.9	0.0001
		Control	4778	320.3		3836	218.8	
	% Time Lying	Meloxicam	62.5	1.1	0.0079	59.7	1.9	0.4450
		Control	68.1	1.5		60.4	1.2	
	Number of Steps	Meloxicam	1630	66.1	0.0340	1650	65.0	0.0028
		Control	1321	106.1		1293	68.4	
	Lying Bouts	Meloxicam	40.5	3.1	0.0095	24.0	1.6	0.1967
		Control	56.5	4.2		20.9	1.5	
Day 1 to Day 2	Motion Index	Meloxicam	4255	216.0	0.0003	6639	910.9	0.0011
		Control	3001	189.2		4114	212.6	
	% Time Lying	Meloxicam	62.4	1.4	0.4068	61.4	0.86	0.0154
		Control	64.5	1.4		58.9	0.66	
	Number of Steps	Meloxicam	1229	59.9	0.0055	1778	91.8	0.0424
		Control	953	75.5		1497	76.5	
	Lying Bouts	Meloxicam	29.7	3.2	0.0045	32.1	3.88	0.6940
		Control	51.7	5.3		33.07	2.53	
Day 2 To Day 3	Motion Index	Meloxicam	5030	379.2	0.0465	4985	382.9	0.0043
		Control	3769	314.4		3748	174.2	
	% Time Lying	Meloxicam	60.7	1.3	0.0815	61.34	1.0	0.6468
		Control	63.9	1.4		60.4	1.0	
	Number of Steps	Meloxicam	1639	71.9	0.0238	1666	81.6	0.0121
		Control	1351	83.0		1429	66.1	
	Lying Bouts	Meloxicam	45.1	8.9	0.0361	36.7	3.7	0.9652
		Control	72.9	12.6		36.3	2.7	

duration of activity (3 days) and versatility of oral delivery provides the veterinarian and producer a product that can address their animal welfare needs.

It has been demonstrated that heart rate increases over baseline levels by stressful events such as castration, dehorning, and branding [3, 12, 13]. The duration of the increased heart rate over baseline has been reported to last for several hours after the painful stimulation. Recently meloxicam was shown to significantly reduce heart rates in scoop dehorned cattle which was attributed to reduction in pain and stress associated with NSAID treatment [14]. In this study, there were no uncastrated control animals but the heart rate was significantly increased in control animals over meloxicam treated animals for 10 h after the castration procedure. This effect was observed in both band castrated and surgically castrated animals.

There are many studies that have shown an increase in plasma cortisol associated with castration in cattle [3, 15, 16]. The peak cortisol concentration is reported to occur within 30 min after castration [3]. Dairy calves also appear to be more responsive than beef bulls and it is believed that beef calves have a higher tolerance to pain [3]. Plasma

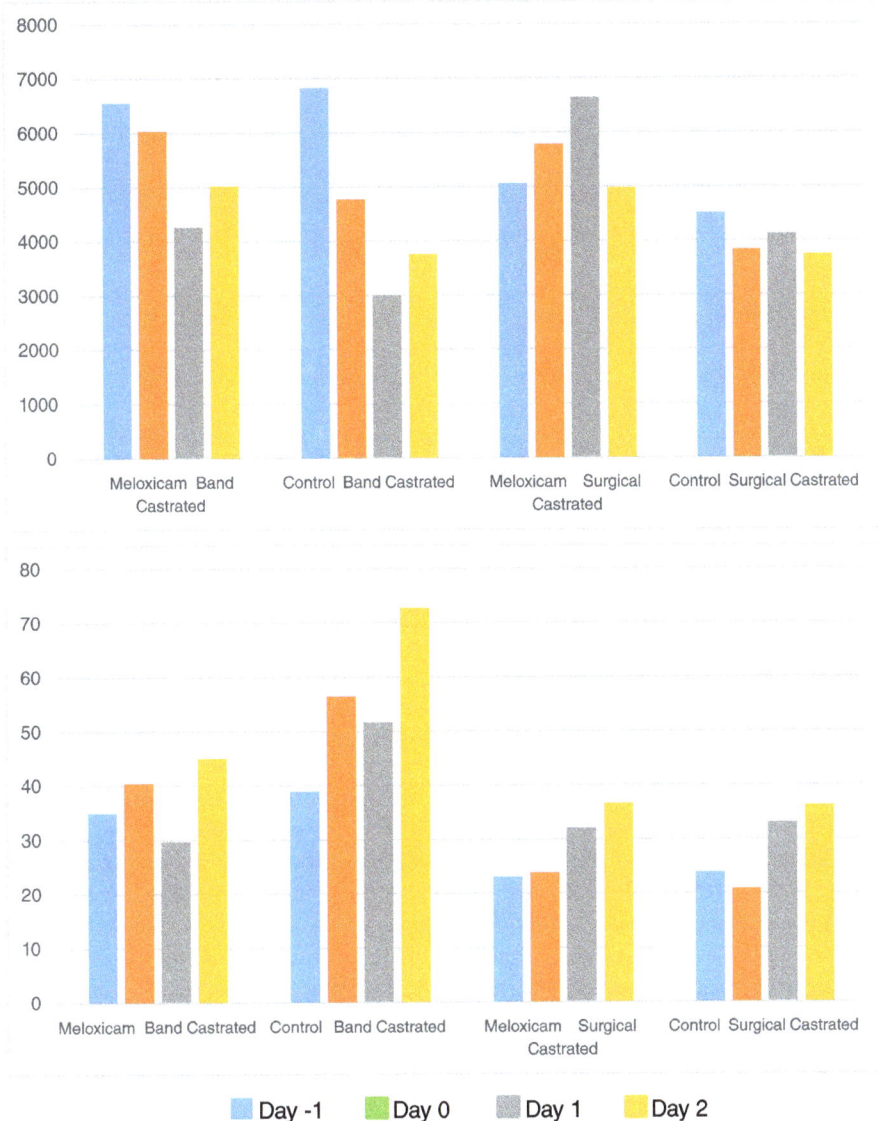

Fig. 2 Motion Index (Upper) and Number of Lying Bouts (Lower) in band and surgically castrated calves on day -1, 0, 1 and 2

cortisol has been shown to be significantly reduced in castrated calves receiving NSAIDs before castration [16]. In this study plasma cortisol was significantly reduced on day 0 and day 1 which indicates that animals receiving meloxicam are in less pain and are under less stress than control calves. As expected, the difference was most pronounced on day 0 (approximately 4 h after castration).

Substance P is an 11-amino acid neuropeptide that regulates the excitability of dorsal horn nociceptive neurons and is present in areas of neuroaxis involved in pain, stress and anxiety [3]. It has been shown to be elevated with soft tissue injury, castration and dehorning [3, 14, 17]. In this study, plasma substance P was elevated in control animals over meloxicam treated animals on day 0 (approximately 4 h after castration) and day 1

(approximately 20 h after castration). This is similar with that observed previously with dehorned dairy bulls [14].

There are several manufacturers of accelerometers that can be attached to the leg of cattle and provide long term, unbiased and validated behavioral data. The ICE tags used it this study have been validated and extensively used in cattle for behavioral assessment of pen designs and pharmaceutical intervention (www.icerobotics.com). The accelerometers allow objective monitoring of animal behavioral changes as animals in pain have certain behavioral characteristics: 1) they spend more time lying, 2) they stand up and lay down more frequently (uncomfortable), 3) they walk less (fewer steps). The ICE tag accelerometers are able to record these events as well as generate a movement index. The higher the movement index, the more

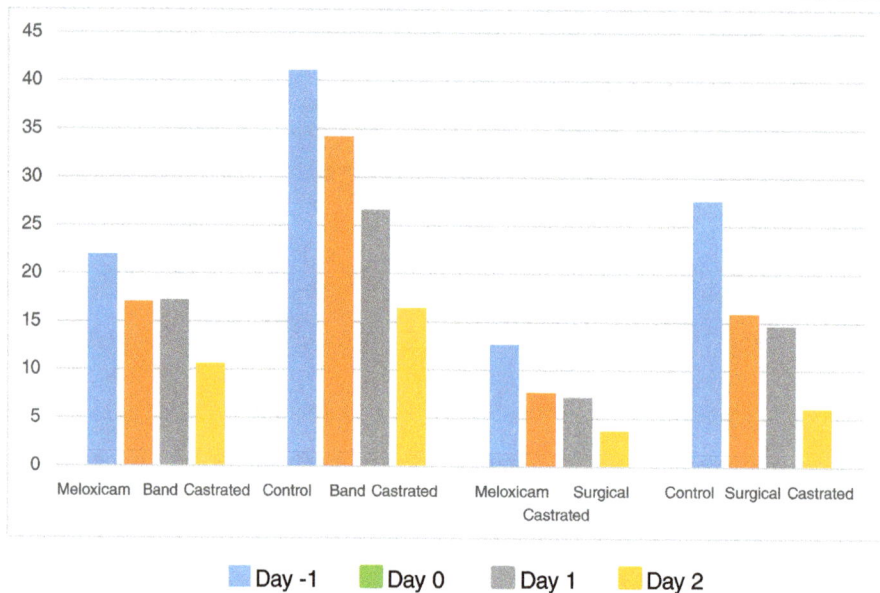

Fig. 3 Visual Analog Score (VAS) of in band and surgically castrated calves on day -1, 0, 1 and 2

the animal is moving throughout the pen. In this study meloxicam had a significant effect on several behavioral parameters: In both band and surgical castrated animals the motion index and the number of steps were significantly greater in meloxicam treated animals on day 0 (first 24 h after castration), day 1 (24 to 48 h after castration) and day 2 (48 to 72 h after castration). This suggests that animals receiving meloxicam were in less pain and there was less swelling allowing the animals to move more freely throughout the pen. There were a greater number of lying bouts in control animals over meloxicam treated animals in only the band castrated animal but this was observed on days 0, 1 and 2. This suggests that band castration makes it more uncomfortable for the animals to remain in

the lying position for extended periods of time. The percent of time lying was only significantly more in control animals on day 0 (band castrated) and day 1 (surgical castrated). These results are in agreement with observations previously published where meloxicam demonstrated evidence of changes in calf behavior associated with castration and dehorning [7, 18]. In these studies meloxicam treated animals spent more time walking and less time lying down. These studies concluded that lying behavior and movement are good indicators of animal well-being and pain.

Visual Analog Scale (VAS) score is a subjective method to rate the level of pain in animals. This method permits evaluation of the level of pain by observing

Table 4 Mean Visual Analog Scale scores Behavioral Data in Band and Surgically Castrated Animals

Study Day	Band vs Surgical Castration P value		Treatment	Band Castrated			Surgically Castrated		
				Mean (%)	Standard Error	P Value	Mean (%)	Standard Error	P Value
Day -1	Control	Meloxicam	Meloxicam	0	0	1.000	0	0	1.000
			Control (Saline)	0	0		0	0	
Day 0	0.0001	<0.0001	Meloxicam	21.97	3.10	0.0001	12.70	2.12	0.0001
			Control (Saline)	41.07	3.73		27.64	3.04	
Day 1	0.002	0.0002	Meloxicam	17.05	2.66	0.0001	7.67	1.53	0.002
			Control (Saline)	34.17	3.28		15.92	2.25	
Day 2	0.0136	0.0031	Meloxicam	17.25	2.88	0.0056	7.20	1.51	0.0136
			Control (Saline)	26.61	3.29		14.69	2.39	
Day 3	0.0515	0.1296	Meloxicam	10.61	1.78	0.0515	3.73	0.72	0.1296
			Control (Saline)	16.44	2.37		6.04	0.98	

Table 5 Mean Pedometer Recordings (Tail Swishes) in Band and Surgically Castrated Animals

Study Day	Treatment	Band Castration			Surgical Castration		
		Mean (swishes)	Standard Error	P Value	Mean (swishes)	Standard Error	P Value
Day −1 to 0	Meloxicam	5425	452	0.4068	16095	2567	0.0275
	Control (Saline)	7041	1094		9011	1297	
Day 0 to 1	Meloxicam	8575	1327	0.1161	19168	2414	0.058
	Control (Saline)	8135	1350		12934	1775	
Day 1 to 2	Meloxicam	7730	1402	0.6625	20674	3683	0.7107
	Control (Saline)	11961	2238		17559	2269	
Day 2 to 3	Meloxicam	12819	2172	0.1264	20394	4137	0.9085
	Control (Saline)	17865	2791		16945	2595	

behaviors that cannot be easily objectively recorded. These include, stretching, belly kicks, licking, foot stomping and ear position. The VAS scoring was significantly greater (more pain) in control calves over meloxicam treated animals on days 0, 1 and 2 for both band and surgical castrated animals. This supports the previous studies where behavioral evaluation demonstrated that meloxicam had a positive, ameliorative effect on behavioral changes in dehorned animals [7, 18].

Tail swishing is a response to a number of stimuli including 1) flies, 2) skin irritation and 3) local painful stimuli. Castrated animals generally swish their tails more frequently due to localized pain. It was hoped that tail pedometers would be able to identify positive behavioral effects of meloxicam by reducing tail swishing. In this study there was considerable variation among animals with respect the number of "steps" recorded on the tail pedometers. There was no difference between the number of steps in control and meloxicam treated animals. This method may not be sensitive enough to demonstrate a difference and/or the number of flies that stimulated tail swishing masked any swishing due to painful stimuli.

Meloxicam has been shown to be an effective anti-inflammatory agent in many veterinary species including cattle [19, 20]. This study permitted the subjective and objective evaluation of inflammation at the band and surgical wound site following castration. There was a pronounced effect of meloxicam in surgical castrated animals and the effect was less in band castrated animals. We have recently shown that oral meloxicam has a significant effect in reduction of swelling in castrated horses [21].

Conclusion

Meloxicam Oral Suspension was able to significantly reduce pain response behaviors and physiological responses to pain in band castrated and surgical castrated calves for up to 72 h following a single oral treatment of 1 mg/kg body weight. Meloxicam Oral Suspension was also able to significantly reduce inflammation in band castrated and surgical castrated calves. Now that oral meloxicam is available to Canadian Veterinarians and producers additional benefits to cattle and other food animal species may be recognized. The availability of this product should improve the welfare of cattle and other larger companion and food animal species.

Table 6 Mean Swelling Scores (Band Castrated Animals) and Mean Mid-Scrotal Diameter (Surgically Castrated Animals)

Study Day	Treatment	Band Castration			Surgical Castration		
		Mean Score	Standard Error	P Value	Mean (mm)	Standard Error	P Value
Day 0	Meloxicam	0	0	1.000	10.97	0.27	0.4845
	Control (Saline)	0	0		11.28	0.28	
Day 1	Meloxicam	0.067	0.067	0.1577	26.53	1.21	0.0001
	Control (Saline)	0.267	0.118		41.01	2.69	
Day 2	Meloxicam	0.200	0.107	0.0297	33.54	2.54	0.0154
	Control (Saline)	0.600	0.131		43.58	2.85	
Day 3	Meloxicam	0.467	0.165	0.0232	37.81	2.26	0.0246
	Control (Saline)	1.067	0.182		48.82	3.10	

Abbreviations
NSAID, nonsteroidal anti-inflammatory drug; VAS, visual analog score

Acknowledgements
The authors would like to acknowledge the assistance of Alberta Agriculture and Forestry, ALMA and Alberta Veterinary Laboratories in conducting this study. They also grateful for the assistance of the producer for allowing use of his animals and facilities.

Funding
The study was funded by Alberta Livestock and Meat Agency (ALMA), 2011R043R, and Alberta Veterinary Laboratories.

Authors' contributions
MO designed the studies and participated in the execution of the studies. He also analyzed the data. BR, LB and HM all participated in the animal phase of the study and assisted in data analysis. NA performed the analysis of plasma substance P and cortisol. MEO prepared the manuscript and all authors contributed to, read and approved the final manuscript.

Competing interests
BR, LB, HM and NA have no competing interests that could inappropriately have influenced or biased the content of the paper. MO is an employee of Alberta Veterinary Laboratories, the manufacturer of Meloxicam Oral Suspension.

Consent for publication
Not applicable.

Author details
[1]Alberta Veterinary Laboratories, 411 19th Street SE, Calgary, Alberta T2E 6J7, Canada. [2]Alberta Agriculture and Forestry, 97 East Lake Ramp NE, Airdrie, Alberta T4A 0C3, Canada. [3]Alberta Horse Industry Association, 97 East Lake Ramp NE, Airdrie, Alberta T4A 0C3, Canada. [4]Chinook Contract Research, 97 East Lake Ramp NE, Airdrie, Alberta T4A 0C3, Canada.

References
1. Fisher AD, Knight TW, Cosgrove GP. Effects of surgical or banding castration on stress responses and behavior of bulls. Aust Vet J. 2001;79:279–84.
2. González LA, Schwartzkopf-Genswein KS, Caulkett NA, Janzen E, McAllister TA, Fierheller E, Schaefer AL, Haley DB, Stookey JM, Hendrick S. Pain mitigation after band castration of beef calves and its effects on performance, behavior, Escherichia coli, and salivary cortisol. J Anim Sci. 2010;88:802–10.
3. Coetzee JF. A review of pain assessment techniques and pharmacological approaches to pain relief after bovine castration: Practical implications for cattle production within the United States. Appl Anim Behav Sci. 2011;135:192–213.
4. Coetzee JF. Assessment and management of pain associated with castration in cattle. Vet Clin Food Anim. 2013;29:75–101.
5. Stafford KJ Mellor DJ. The welfare significance of the castration of cattle: a review. NZ Vet J. 2005;53:271–8.
6. Heinrich A, Duffield TF, Lissemore KD, Millman ST. The effect of meloxicam on behavior and pain sensitivity of dairy calves following cautery dehorning with a local anesthetic. J Dairy Sci. 2010;93:2450–7.
7. Heinrich A, Duffield TF, Lissemore KD, Squires EJ, Millman ST. The impact of meloxicam on postsurgical stress associated with cautery dehorning. J Dairy Sci. 2009;92:540–7.
8. Coetzee JF, KuKanich B, Mosher R, Allen PS. Pharmacokinetics of Intravenous and Oral Meloxicam in Ruminant Calves. Vet Ther. 2009;10(4):E1–8.
9. Tegeder I, Pfeilschifter J, Geisslinger G. Cyclooxygenase-independent actions of cyclooxygenase inhibitors. FASEB J. 2001;15:2057–72.
10. Beretta C, Garavaglia G, Cavalli M. COX-1 and COX-2 inhibition in horse blood by phenylbutazone, flunixin, carprofen and meloxicam: An in vitro analysis. Pharmacol Res. 2005;52:302–6.
11. McGowan JE, Burke CR, Jago JG. Validation of technology of objectively measuring behavior in diary cows and its application for estrous detection. Proceedings New Zealand Soc Animal Production. 2007;67:136–42.
12. Schwartzkopf-Gerswin KS, Booth-McLean ME, McAllister TA, Mears GJ. Physiological and behavioral changes in Holstein calves during and after dehorning or castration. Can J Anim Sci. 2005;85:131–8.
13. Lay DC, Friend TH, Grissom KK, Jenkins OC. Behavioral and physiological effects of freeze or hot iron branding on crossbred cattle. J Anim Sci. 1992;70:330–6.
14. Coetzee JK, Mosher RA, KuKanich B, Gehring R, Robert B, Reinbold JB, White BJ. Pharmacokinetics and effect of intravenous meloxicam in weaned Holstein calves following scoop dehorning without local anesthesia. BMC Vet Res. 2012;8:153. http://www.biomedcentral.com/1746-6148/8/153.
15. Chase CC, Larsen RE, Randel RD, Hammond AC, Adams EL. Plasma cortisol and white blood cell responses in different breeds of bulls: a comparison of two methods of castration. J Anim Sci. 1995;73:975–80.
16. Stafford KJ, Mellor DJ, Todd SE, Bruce RA, Ward RN. Effects of local anesthesia or local anesthesia plus a NSAID on the acute cortisol response of calves to five different methods of castration. Res Vet Sci. 2002;73:61–70.
17. Coetzee JF, Lubbers BV, Toerber SE, Gehring R, Thomson DU, White BJ, Apley MD. Plasma concentrations of substance P and cortisol in beef calves after castration or simulated castration. Am J Vet Res. 2008;69:751–62.
18. Theurer ME, White BJ, Coetzee JF, Edwards LN, Mosher RA, Cull CA: Assessment of behavioral changes associated with oral meloxicam administration at time of dehorning in calves using remote triangulation device and accelerometers. BMC Vet Res. 2012;8:48. http://www.biomedcentral.com/1746-6148/8/48.
19. Laven R, Chambers P, Stafford K. Using non-steroidal anti-inflammatory drugs around calving: Maximizing comfort, productivity and fertility. Vet J. 2012;192:8–12.
20. Smith GW, Davis JL, Tell LA, Webb AI, Riviere JE. Extra label use of nonsteroidal anti-inflammatory drugs in cattle. J Am Vet Med Assoc. 2008;232:697–701.
21. Olson ME, Fierheller E, Burwash L, Ralston B, Schatz C, Matheson-Bird H. The efficacy of Meloxicam oral suspension for controlling pain and inflammation after castration in horses. J Equine Vet Sci. 2015;35:724–30.

Investigation of short-term surgical complications in a low-resource, high-volume dog sterilisation clinic in India

I. Airikkala-Otter[1], L. Gamble[1], S. Mazeri[2], I. G. Handel[2], B. M. de C. Bronsvoort[2], R. J. Mellanby[3] and N. V. Meunier[2*]

Abstract

Background: Surgical sterilisation is currently the method of choice for controlling free-roaming dog populations. However, there are significant logistical challenges to neutering large numbers of dogs in low-resource clinics. The aim of this study was to investigate the incidence of short-term surgical complications in a low-resource sterilisation clinic which did not routinely administer post-operative antibiotics.

The medical records of all sterilisation surgeries performed in 2015 at the Worldwide Veterinary Service International Training Centre in Tamil Nadu, India were reviewed (group A) to assess immediate surgical complications. All animals in this group were monitored for at least 24 h post-surgery but were not released until assessed by a veterinarian as having uncomplicated wound healing. In the second part of this study from August to December 2015, 200 free-roaming dogs undergoing sterilisation surgery, were monitored for a minimum of 4-days post-surgery to further assess postoperative complications (group B).

Results: Surgery related complications were seen in 5.4% (95%CI, 4.5–6.5%) of the 1998 group A dogs monitored for at least 24 h, and in 7.0% (3.9–11.5%) of the 200 group B dogs monitored for 4 days. Major complications were classed as those requiring an intervention and resulted in increased morbidity or mortality. Major complications were seen in 2.8% (2.1–3.6%) and 1.5% (3.1–4.3%) of group A and B, respectively. Minor complications requiring little or no intervention were recorded for 2.6% (1.9–3.4%) for group A and 5.5% (2.8–9.6%) for group B. There was no evidence for a difference in complication rates between the two groups in a multivariate regression model.

Conclusion: This study demonstrated that high volume, low-resource sterilisation of dogs can be performed with a low incidence of surgical complications and low mortality.

Keywords: Sterilisation surgery, Ovariohysterectomy, Castration, Surgical complications, Companion animal, Welfare

Background

Developing strategies to effectively control the size and impact of free-roaming dog populations is an important public health priority in many countries. Free-roaming dogs are susceptible to a number of welfare concerns such as malnutrition, disease, and traffic accidents [1]. In addition, large free-roaming dog populations can lead to conflicts with humans. These conflicts include zoonotic diseases such as rabies, nuisance through noise and pollution, aggressive behaviour towards people, especially children, and predation of livestock and wildlife [2, 3]. Implementing dog population control measures has been shown to reduce dog bites [4], lower the vaccination threshold required for effective rabies control [5], as well as increase body condition scores and decrease the prevalence of numerous diseases in the dog population [6].

A wide range of dog population control techniques have been reported. These include large-scale culling operations, which have now been shown to be ineffective because immigration and increased birth rates quickly compensate for the losses [7]. Additionally, culling dogs is not an effective approach to reduce the impact of zoonotic diseases such as rabies [7, 8]. Chemical castration has been used as an alternative

* Correspondence: natascha.meunier@ed.ac.uk
[2]The Epidemiology, Economics and Risk Assessment (EERA) Group, The Roslin Institute and the Royal (Dick) School of Veterinary Studies (R(D)SVS), Easter Bush, Midlothian EH25 9RG, UK
Full list of author information is available at the end of the article

to surgery [9] and immunocontraceptives are under development [10, 11]. Despite these advances, surgical sterilisation clinics are currently the main control method advocated to control free-roaming dog populations [12]. However, undertaking surgical sterilisation on a large scale is logistically challenging in many parts of the world, notably in low income settings where the need to control these populations is often the greatest. In addition, surgical sterilisation can be associated with major complications including haemorrhage, ovarian remnant syndrome, stump pyometra, adhesions, and wound dehiscence or infection, as well as anaesthetic complications and drug reactions [13, 14]. Moreover, there are few reports which describe the incidence of surgical complications in clinics which sterilise large numbers of dogs in low income settings.

The objective of this study was to investigate the incidence of surgical complications in dogs in a low-resource sterilisation clinic which did not administer routine postoperative antibiotics. This was done by assessing peri- and post-operative complications following sterilisation surgery, including deaths, iatrogenic surgical complications and wound breakdown in a cohort of 200 dogs over a period of 4 days. In addition, surgery records were assessed for all dogs in the same year for a minimum 24 h follow-up period.

Methods
Study site
The Worldwide Veterinary Service (WVS) International Training Centre (ITC) in India has been performing male and female dog sterilisation surgeries since 2010 to control the free-roaming dog population in the Nilgiris district of Tamil Nadu. The sterilisation programmes are conducted according to the Animal Birth Control (ABC) guidelines, as recommended by the Animal Welfare Board of India [15]. During 2010–2015, approximately 14,000 dogs were neutered in the training centre. The WVS ITC presented a regular two-week training course teaching high-standard sterilisation techniques to veterinarians and international veterinary student participants. All surgeries were conducted under the supervision of ITC veterinary instructors. Free-roaming dogs from the nearby towns and villages were caught and brought in to the clinic by the WVS ITC team of trained animal handlers. The average number of surgeries undertaken at the WVS ITC clinic was 20 surgeries per working day during the study period.

Ethics approval for this study was attained from the University of Edinburgh, Veterinary Ethics Research Committee (VERC 114.16). The neutering programme was approved by the Animal Welfare Board of India.

Study design
For the first part of this study, all surgical records at the WVS ITC from January to December 2015 were reviewed (group A). All dog sterilisation case record sheets were entered into a database using a purpose-designed form on a smartphone based application (The Rabies App, Mission Rabies; WVS Data Collection App, WVS; 2016). Records were excluded if details of surgical monitoring and recovery were missing.

In the second part of the study, 200 free-roaming dogs were monitored for complications after surgery for a minimum of 4 days between August and December 2015 (group B). Kennel space was a major limitation and dogs were enrolled as space became available. This resulted in batches of all dogs operated on certain days being included in the study as a kennel became free, with no dogs enrolled on other days even though surgery took place.

Surgical protocol
Premedication of xylazine (2 mg/kg IM) and butorphanol (0.1 mg/kg IM) was administered in the kennel based on an estimated weight. Once sedated, dogs were weighed for accurate medication dosages and an intravenous catheter was placed in all cases. Intravenous fluids (0.9% normal saline) were administered at 10 ml/kg/h throughout the surgery. Dogs were induced with propofol (1 mg/kg IV) and diazepam (0.25 mg/kg IV). After induction, all dogs received amoxicillin-cloxacillin (20 mg/kg IV), meloxicam (0.2 mg/kg IV), tramadol (4 mg/kg IV) and ivermectin (200μg/kg SC). Lignocaine was given as constant rate infusion for analgesia (1.2 mg/kg/h) and male dogs were injected subcutaneously with lignocaine as a prescrotal local block (20 mg SC). Maintenance of the anaesthesia was achieved with a propofol bolus (1 mg/kg IV) every 6–10 min to effect.

After induction dogs were prepared for surgery by manually shaving the surgical site and cleaning the surgical field with a chlorhexidine surgical scrub solution for 5 min. The preparation of the surgical field was completed with a final spray of isopropyl alcohol. Sterile drapes and surgical instruments were used for each patient. Surgical caps, masks and sterile gloves were worn by all surgeons. Standard aseptic technique was followed in all surgical procedures, including surgical scrubbing of hands with an iodine-based scrub solution and aseptic handling of instruments and consumables after autoclaving. Surgeons replaced their gloves if a break in aseptic technique occurred.

Animals were examined before surgery for pregnancy or cryptorchidism. Ovariohysterectomy was performed with a ventral midline incision according to standard techniques [16]. Bilateral orchidectomy was done with a midline prescrotal incision. Catgut was used for internal ligatures and absorbable suture material for closing the muscle, subcutaneous and intradermal layers in a continuous pattern. The majority of dogs were operated on by course participants (students or veterinary surgeons with limited experience) under the direct supervision of a surgically scrubbed veterinary instructor. A small number of animals were sterilised by experienced surgeons for demonstration purposes. The surgical protocol followed was the same for all dogs operated at the WVS ITC.

All ownerless dogs were kept overnight after surgery and received meloxicam (0.2 mg/kg SC) and a rabies vaccine on the following day. Meloxicam injections were repeated daily for dogs remaining on site. Post-operative antibiotics were not given unless clinically indicated such as in patients with visible signs of infection or systemic illness. All free-roaming dogs were monitored for at least 24 h post-surgery before being released.

Post-operative assessment

Dogs were monitored daily by WVS ITC veterinary instructors until release. Wound scores were recorded each morning on a scale 0–4 (Table 1, with 0 = perfect healing, and 4 = open wound) and any interventions or complications were recorded. Pain scores were additionally recorded dependant on the visual appearance of the dog and its reaction to gentle touch around the surgical wound, scored with a pain scale from '0' no pain, to '9' excruciating pain, based on the scale by Mathews, (2000) [17] (Table 2).

Free-roaming dogs were returned to their original location 1–5 days after surgery, depending on the healing of the wound as well as logistics and schedules of the release and catching vehicles. Dogs with a wound healing score of 0 or 1 would be marked for release. Dogs with a wound score of 2 or above, or any additional complications, were kept for monitoring or treatment as required. All dogs in group B were kept for a minimum of four days regardless of wound score.

Analysis

Complications were entered into the database as free text comments from the surgical monitoring and follow-

Table 1 Post-operative wound scoring scale used at the WVS ITC

Wound score	Wound description
0	Perfectly healing wound, edges in apposition
1	Mild redness on the skin around the wound
2	Swelling or discharge or exposed subcutis
3	Partial opening of the wound
4	Complete opening of the wound

Table 2 Post-operative pain scoring scale used at the WVS ITC

Pain score	Clinical signs often associated with degree of pain
0 No pain	Bright, eating, sleeping comfortably, grooming, affectionate
1 Mild discomfort	Eats, sleeps, resists surgical palpation, not depressed
2 Mild pain	Picks at food, guards surgical area, slightly depressed
3 Mild to moderate	Inappetant, guards/ looks/ licks/ chews surgical area, unrelaxed, whimpers
4 Moderate	Depressed, reluctant to move, aggressive, may vocalise, mydriasis
5 Increased moderate	As 4, but more pronounced
6 Moderate to severe	Very depressed, will not move even to urinate, vocalises often
7 Severe	Motionless, extremely depressed, vocalises
8 Increased severe	As 7, hyperalgesic wherever touched, trembling
9 Excruciating	Piercing screams, nearly comatose

up sheets. Any surgically related complication which developed during or after surgery in the follow-up period was categorised into a) major complications, requiring intervention or resulting in high morbidity or death; b) minor complications, requiring observation; and c) surgical site specific, relating to the incision wound. These categories were not mutually exclusive.

The excluded patient population, those with incomplete patient records, were compared to the study group with univariate analysis of factors with Pearson's Chi-square test, Fisher's exact test, or Students T-test, as appropriate. A logistic regression model was used to look at the association of study group, age, sex, weight, and surgery time (minutes), with an interaction term for sex and surgery time, on the three categories of complications versus uncomplicated surgery. Age was classified into three groups for the purpose of analysis: < 1 year, 1–2 years, > 3 years. All analysis was conducted in R Statistical Software [18].

Results

Total records

The records of 2395 surgically sterilised dogs were examined for 2015. Of these, 197 records were excluded due to incomplete information on wounds scores or surgical monitoring. There was no difference between those included or excluded with regard to: sex, age, surgery time, major, incidental or surgery site complications. Minor complications were lower in the excluded group ($p = 0.04$). Of those excluded from the study, 2 dogs were euthanised during surgery for pre-existing health conditions with poor prognosis.

Paper records were available for 2198 free-roaming dogs which were included in the study. Of these records, 1998 dogs were potentially monitored during and after surgery for at least 24 h until fit for release and 200 dogs were monitored for the minimum period of four days.

Group A 24-h monitoring

The short-term monitoring study comprised of 1998 surgical records of dogs sterilised at the WVS ITC clinic in 2015. There were 932 ovariohysterectomies and 1066 castrations, including 44 pregnant bitches and 12 cryptorchid dogs. The median age was 2 years (range 0.2–12.5). Mean surgical times were 95.7 min for ovariohysterectomy (SD 25.3) and 50.2 min for castration (SD 18.5). Based on assessment of the surgical wound on the first day following surgery, 70.2% of dogs were released, and subsequently, 91.2% of dogs had been released within two days of surgery.

In total, 108 dogs (5.4%; 95%CI 4.5–6.5%) had at least one surgery related complication in this group (Table 3). The major complications were seen in 56 dogs (2.8%; 2.1–3.6%). Two anaesthetic deaths were reported, and one dog died two days after surgery with haemorrhagic gastroenteritis. Dehiscence of the wound resulted in a scrotal ablation in one case. A further three scrotal ablations were performed at the time of the initial surgery, but the reasons for these were not clearly documented. Surgical intervention was required in three dogs intra-operatively with major haemorrhage, two specifically with torn ovarian ligaments, and one female dog re-operated immediately following ovariohysterectomy due to suspected internal bleeding; all recovered without further incident. Anaesthetic reasons for intervention included tremors or seizures requiring diazepam (n = 10). Further interventions including wound flushing (n = 17) and further antibiotic administration (n = 4). Where an alternative reason was not given for post-operative antimicrobial use, these were considered related to the surgical wound (n = 6). Pyometra was diagnosed at surgery and treated in 11 dogs. Minor complications were seen in 52 dogs (2.6%; 1.9–3.4%). These included mild wound swelling or discharge, notable blood loss during surgery, the development of diarrhoea, and postoperative hypothermia (Table 4). Complications specifically related to the surgical site were seen in 54 of 1996 dogs (2.7%; 2.0–3.5%).

This case number was supported by 92.8% of dogs having a wound healing score of '0–1' (good healing to mild redness) on the first day post-op, 7.1% with a score of '2' (swelling or discharge), and only one animal with a score of '3' (partial opening). The pain score was '0' (no pain) in 72.3% of dogs, '1' (mild discomfort) in 25.0%, and '2–3' (mild to moderate) in 2.7% of dogs.

Group B 4-day monitoring

The 4-day follow-up study evaluated the immediate surgical complications and short-term wound healing of 200 dogs with complete monitoring records (86 females and 114 males) operated on between August and December 2015. Two females were pregnant and one male was a cryptorchid. The median age was 2 years (range 0.3–12.0 years). The mean surgical times were 92.2 (SD 22.5) and 52.2 (SD 19.8) minutes for the ovariohysterectomy and castrations, respectively.

Fourteen of the 200 dogs (7.0%, 95%CI 3.9–11.5) had at least one surgery related complication (Table 3). Three major complications, 1.5% (3.1–4.3%), were seen in the prospective group. These included one scrotal ablation which was performed in a dog at the time of the initial surgery due to a scrotal incision made during shaving, and two further cases required flushing of the surgical wound. Minor complications were seen in 11 of 200 dogs (5.5%; 2.8–9.6%), including moderate scrotal swelling (n = 3), wound discharge (n = 3), diarrhoea (n = 3), one shaving inflicted wound, and postoperative hypothermia (n = 1). Nine cases were specifically related to the surgical site (4.5%, 2.1–8.4%). No wound breakdown or post-operative wound infection was observed. These results can be seen in Table 4.

Wounds scores were '0–1' in 89.5% of dogs on the first day post-op, and '2' in 10.5% of dogs. By day two, the number of dogs with a score of '2' had decreased to 7.1%. The pain score was '1' in 20.5% of dogs, and '2' in 0.5% on the day following surgery. No dogs showed a pain score of '2' or more by the second day post-op, and 8.1% showed a score of '1' (mild discomfort). The results are summarised over the four days in Fig. 1, indicating

Table 3 Complication frequency of dogs undergoing sterilisation surgery in 2015

Complications	Group A – 24 h monitoring			Group B – 4 day monitoring		
	n (N = 1998)	Percent	95% CI	n (N = 200)	Percent	95% CI
Surgical (Any)	108	5.4	4.5–6.5	14	7.0	3.9–11.5
Major surgical (required intervention)	56	2.8	2.1–3.6	3	1.5	3.1–4.3
Minor surgical (observation only)	52	2.6	1.9–3.4	11	5.5	2.8–9.6
Surgical site related (post-operative)	54[a]	2.7	2.0–3.5	9	4.5	2.1–8.4

([a]N = 1996)

Table 4 Reported complications associated with surgery presented in major and minor subclasses

Complication	Group A 24 h (N = 1998)		Group B 4-day (N = 200)	
	Number	Percent	Number	Percent
a) Surgery related complications				
Major complications				
Postoperative mortality	1	(0.1)	0	(0.0)
Anaesthetic death	2	(0.1)	0	(0.0)
Scrotal ablation required	4	(0.2)	1	(0.5)
Surgical intervention	4	(0.2)	0	(0.0)
Anaesthetic intervention	10	(0.5)	0	(0.0)
Antibiotic treatment	10	(0.5)	0	(0.0)
Pyometra	11	(0.6)	0	(0.0)
Surgical wound flushing	17	(0.9)	2	(1.0)
Minor complications				
Hypothermia	4	(0.2)	1	(0.5)
Incisional discharge	5	(0.3)	3	(1.5)
Incision wound swelling	6	(0.3)	0	(0.0)
Moderate blood loss	7	(0.4)	0	(0.0)
Moderate scrotal swelling	8	(0.4)	3	(1.5)
Diarrhoea	8	(0.4)	3	(1.5)
Cardiac rhythm abnormalities	8	(0.4)	0	(0.0)
Procedure related	10	(0.5)	1	(0.5)

the proportion of dogs with of wound scores greater than 1, and pain scores greater than 0.

The statistical model examined the study group (group A or group B), age, weight, and surgery-time:sex interaction, against the three classifications of complications as an outcome. There was no evidence of an association between the number of major, minor, surgery site specific, or total complications seen, and the study group, age, sex or weight. There was an association between all complications and longer surgery time (effect size = 1.01, p = 0.02), as well as major complications and longer surgery time in males (effect size 1.03, p = 0.03).

Discussion

This study demonstrated that dogs can be sterilised with a low level of surgical complications in a low-income setting without the use of routine post-operative antibiotics. The incidence of post-operative surgical site complications was similar to that seen in teaching hospitals in developed countries (Fig. 2), as well as to field high-volume sterilisation campaigns [9, 19]. Nevertheless variation will exist in the definition of complications between the studies, so direct comparisons should be interpreted with caution. Ovariohysterectomy and castration are classified as clean surgeries, and previous studies indicate a wound infection rate of 0.0–4.9% in clean surgeries and 4.5–5.9% in clean-contaminated surgery [20–25]. In private practice, Pollari and Bonnett, (1996) [26] saw that major surgical site complications ranged from 1 to 4% for dogs and cats undergoing ovariohysterectomy, castration and onychectomy, but this varied widely between surgeons and between practices. Unfortunately the follow-up period in this study was too short to specifically investigate the development of infection which could take weeks to manifest. The total complication rates seen in this study were nevertheless comparable to other studies [19, 27, 28].

In this population with a high proportion of feral dogs, long term follow is not possible without extensive cost and housing facilities. Additionally, hospitalisation may be a marked change from their natural environment, limiting their movement, possibly decreasing territorial behaviours, providing differing nutrition, and added

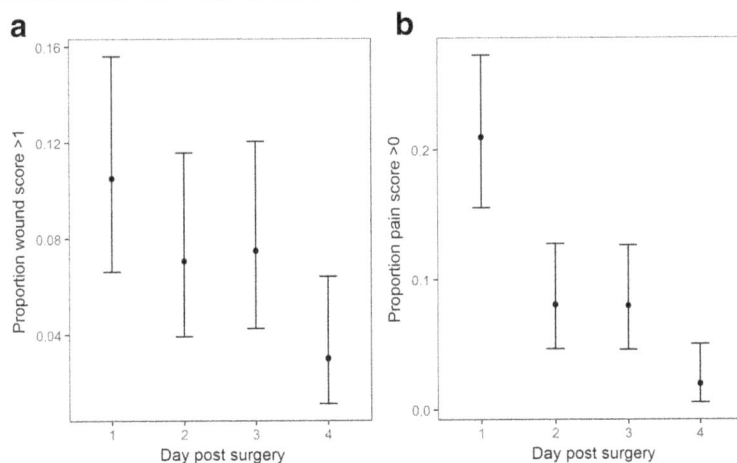

Fig. 1 Wound and pain scores for the 4-day follow up study group B (N = 200). (**a**) The proportion of dogs with a wound score > 1, and (**b**) the proportion of dogs with a pain score > 0, with 95% confidence intervals

Study	Surgery type	N	Cases (%)
Berzon (1979)	OHE (<50 lbs)	290	2.1
Vasseur (1988)	OHE, Orchidectomy	478	2.7
Pollari (1996)	OHE, Orchidectomy	1016	3.1
Levy (2008)	Orchidectomy	58	3.4
Burrow (2005)	OHE	142	3.5
Reece (2012) (Retro.)	OHE	1246	4.6
Reece (2012) (Prosp.)	OHE	114	5.3
This study (Group A)	OHE, Orchidectomy	1996	2.7
This study (Group B)	OHE, Orchidectomy	200	4.5

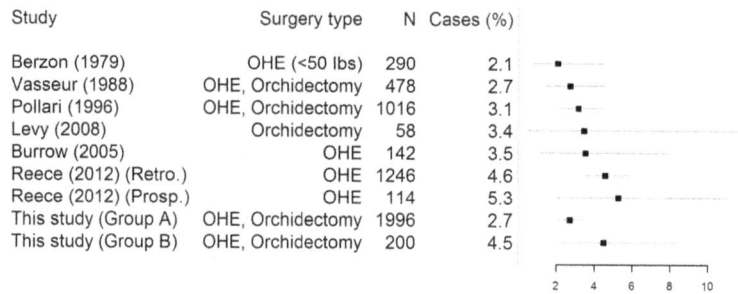

Fig. 2 Comparative plot of reported incidence of surgical site specific infection and/or complications. Data shown as percentage of cases with 95% confidence intervals

stress from close human and animal contact. Therefore, long periods of hospitalisation both for research and as standard practice, were ethically difficult to justify for this population. Keeping healthy dogs longer than needed is an additional drain on clinic resources, limiting capacity, and is often not logistically feasible in high volume clinics. Totton et al., (2011) [29] suggested that the close contact of animals in kennels may aid in the spread of infectious diseases, including ectoparasites. Moreover, Eugster et al., (2004) [25] found an association between a longer hospitalisation period and increased surgical wound infection rates. Minimising the time spent in the hospital is therefore likely to be beneficial for the free-roaming dogs, as the added stress of confinement may further negatively impact wound healing [30].

In a study by Burrow, Batchelor and Cripps, (2005) [28], major post-surgery complications, such as haemorrhage, were usually seen within 24 h after surgery, and Pearson (1973) [31] found haemorrhage to be the most common cause of death following an ovariohysterectomy. Our study did not see an elevated proportion of major complications in the 4-day follow up compared to the 24 h follow up. Although there was a higher level of minor complications, and those related to the surgical site, this difference was not statistically supported ($p = 0.18$ and $p = 0.10$). This similarity of complication rates between groups shows some evidence that short follow-up times may not be detrimental to the welfare of free-roaming or feral dogs, provided surgical and sterile technique is of a high standard. It is possible that animals released from the clinic early develop post-surgical complications that go undocumented, and could account for the higher complication rate in the dogs studied for a longer period of time. The WVS ITC sterilises owned dogs daily under the same standards as the free-roaming dogs and internal reports (unpublished) indicate a low incidence of complications in owned animals although a formal comparison with free-roaming animals was beyond the scope of this study.

Under-reporting is an inherent bias in this type of study, especially for minor or incidental complications, and record keeping differs between individuals. Additional bias may have been introduced in the selection of the prospective study participants as randomisation was not possible for logistical reasons. This is no reason to believe that patients included in the prospective cohort were different to the retrospective cohort, as origin populations and surgical protocols were similar. However, a difference in monitoring and record keeping of the prospective cohort was plausible. Veterinarians and students were not directly responsible for the research aspects of the study, only clinical duties, and did not have any incentive to report or handle these cases beyond standard care. Though it is possible the veterinarians were influenced by the study in their clinical decision making and reporting, even though standard protocols exist.

Longer anaesthetic and surgery times, were previously associated with an increase in postoperative surgical site infections [21–25, 28]. This study showed no evidence of a relationship between surgery time and surgical site complications, when taking study type, age, weight and sex into account. This may be due to the effectiveness of short-acting, pre-operative antibiotic use in all animals, or the short follow up time. The use of antibiotics before surgery was justified because student surgeries were often expected to take longer than 90 min and Vasseur et al., (1988) [21] saw a 1.6 times increase in infection in student surgeries without prophylactic antibiotic use. Burke, (1961, 1973) [32, 33] showed that antimicrobials given roughly one hour before surgery to maximise the MIC in the blood during the procedure had a favourable effect on wound infection outcomes. However, post-operative administration did not influence wound outcomes in the same study.

A particularly controversial area of surgical sterilisation programmes relates to the use of antimicrobials. Whilst it may seem intuitively sensible to administer a longer course of antibiotics to dogs sterilised in low income settings where ensuring high levels of sterility can be challenging, there are increasing concerns over antimicrobial resistance linked to inappropriate and excessive use of antibiotics. The British Small Animal Veterinary Association (BSAVA), and the Association of Shelter Veterinarians in the USA, advise against antimicrobial use in castrations and ovariohysterectomy, unless the surgery is expected to be prolonged or contaminated [20, 21, 34, 35]. In contrast, the current guidelines for animal birth control (ABC) programmes in India advise 3–5 days of broad-spectrum postoperative antibiotics [15]. Antimicrobial use has been increasing in recent years in India, and isolated studies have shown high levels of resistance in human health care settings [36]. This has stimulated a review of policies within the Indian government on antimicrobial use, including within the veterinary sector, for which the controls are currently limited. Unnecessary use of antimicrobials have other disadvantages including increasing the cost of neutering programmes, causing host microbiome disruption, and drug reactions [37]. In light of these disadvantages, the minimal use of antimicrobials would therefore be beneficial, but there is a paucity of studies which have assessed whether the guidelines from developed countries can be safely applied to low resource sterilisation clinics. In the UK setting, antimicrobials have been administered post-operatively to compensate for poor aseptic technique during surgery [38, 39]. This may also provide the foundation for their use post-operatively in low resource settings. However, this study maintained high aseptic standards under these conditions, precluding the need for additional post-operative antimicrobials. Limiting unnecessary antimicrobial use in these settings reduces costs, could improve compliance to recommended usage, and follows responsible use guidelines to prevent antimicrobial resistance.

In this study, a wound scoring system was used as an objective measure of wound appearance to gauge whether animals were ready for release. The majority of animals, had evidence of acceptable wound healing within 2 days post-surgery. Cases showed a higher proportion of wounds scores > 1 and pain scores > 0, but a higher score did not necessarily imply that an intervention was needed. The scoring may be a helpful tool in assessing whether an animal should be released or requires monitoring, and needs further validation. In this setting, the wound scoring does provide a documented check of each individual animal, necessary when a large volume of patients are seen by a team of veterinarians, ensuring good practice in follow-up care.

This study showed low postoperative pain scores in the majority of animals, with no animals showing severe pain. Poor pain management can contribute to delays in wound healing [40] or result in self-inflicted trauma which also delays healing [14]. The generally accepted multimodal, pre-emptive analgesic approach [41] used in this study may contribute to the good post-operative recovery seen and is an essential factor to consider in sterilisation clinic protocols.

Conclusions

This study demonstrated that high volume, low-resource sterilisation of dogs can be performed with a low incidence of surgical complications and low mortality. Importantly, we have shown that this can be achieved without the administration of postoperative antibiotics, provided high aseptic and surgical standards are followed and individual assessment takes place for antimicrobial and monitoring requirements with longer hospitalisation as needed, without compromising the welfare of the patients.

Abbreviations.
WVS: Worldwide Veterinary Service; ITC: International Training Centre; ABC: Animal Birth Control; OHE: ovariohysterectomy.

Acknowledgements
The surgeries performed in the WVS ITC by the trainee veterinarians were supervised by the WVS ITC team of teaching veterinarians, Ilona Airikkala-Otter, Maiju Tamminen, Dr. Vinay Bhagat, Dr. Jawahar Kolliyul, Dr. Aswin Alis, Dr. Sandeep Karna, Dr. Navas Shareef, Dr. Surya Prakash, Dr. Rahul Nair and Dr. Queenie Fernandes, who have for years with great dedication contributed to the WVS ITC work for improved surgical practices and humane dog population control. Thanks to Miceala Shocklee for assisting with data capture.

Funding
This study was performed in the WVS ITC, founded and run by the Worldwide Veterinary Service, sponsored by Dogs Trust, the Marchig Trust, and Brigitte Bardot Foundation, working in collaboration with two Indian registered animal charities, WVS India (www.wvsindia.org) and India Project for Animals and Nature (www.indiapan.org). NVM is supported by the Marchig Trust and Dogs Trust.

Authors' contributions
IA-O and LG designed the study and oversaw data collection. SM and NVM were involved in data gathering and analysis. RJM, IH, BMCB contributed to the planning and analysis. NVM, RJM and IA-O were responsible for the final manuscript with contributions from all authors. All authors read and approved the final manuscript.

Consent for publication
Not applicable.

Competing interests
The authors declare that they have no competing interests.

Author details
[1]Worldwide Veterinary Service, 4 Castle Street, Cranborne, Dorset BH21 5PZ, UK. [2]The Epidemiology, Economics and Risk Assessment (EERA) Group, The Roslin Institute and the Royal (Dick) School of Veterinary Studies (R(D)SVS), Easter Bush, Midlothian EH25 9RG, UK. [3]The Royal (Dick) School of Veterinary Studies (R(D)SVS) and the Roslin Institute, Hospital for Small Animals, Easter Bush Veterinary Centre, Midlothian EH25 9RG, UK.

References
1. ICAM. Humane Dog Population Management Guidance. 2007.
2. Dalla Villa P, Kahn S, Stuardo L, Iannetti L, Di Nardo A, Serpell JA. Free-roaming dog control among OIE-member countries. Prev. Vet. Med. Elsevier B.V. 2010;97:58–63.
3. Lunney M, Jones A, Stiles E, Waltner-Toews D. Assessing human-dog conflicts in Todos Santos, Guatemala: bite incidences and public perception. Prev. Vet. Med. Elsevier B.V. 2011;102:315–20.
4. Reece JF, Chawla SK, Hiby AR. Decline in human dog-bite cases during a street dog sterilisation programme in Jaipur, India. Vet. Rec. 2013;172:473.
5. Reece JF, Chawla SK. Control of rabies in Jaipur, India, by the sterilisation and vaccination of neighbourhood dogs. Vet. Rec. 2006;159:379–83.
6. Yoak AJ, Reece JF, Gehrt SD, Hamilton IM. Disease control through fertility control: secondary benefits of animal birth control in Indian street dogs. Prev Vet Med Elsevier BV. 2014;113:152–6.
7. Beran GW, Frith M. Domestic animal rabies control: an overview. Rev Infect Dis. 1988;10:S672–7.
8. Morters MK, Restif O, Hampson K, Cleaveland S, Wood JLN, Conlan AJK. Evidence-based control of canine rabies: a critical review of population density reduction. J Anim Ecol. 2013;82:6–14.
9. Levy JK, Crawford PC, Appel LD, Clifford EL. Comparison of intratesticular injection of zinc gluconate versus surgical castration to sterilize male dogs. Am J Vet Res. 2008;69:140–3.
10. Munks MW. Progress in development of immunocontraceptive vaccines for permanent non-surgical sterilization of cats and dogs. Reprod Domest Anim. 2012;47:223–7.
11. ACC&D. Contraception and fertility control in dogs and cats. 2013.
12. Lembo T. The blueprint for rabies prevention and control: a novel operational toolkit for rabies elimination. PLoS Negl Trop Dis. 2012;6:1–4.
13. Adin CA. Complications of ovariohysterectomy and orchiectomy in companion animals. Vet Clin North Am - Small Anim Pract Elsevier Inc. 2011;41:1023–39.
14. Berzon J. Complications of elective ovariohysterectomies in the dog and cat at a teaching institution: clinical review of 853 cases. Vet Surg. 1979;65:89–91.
15. AWBI. Standard Operating Procedures for sterilization of stray dogs under the Animal Birth Control programme. 2009. Available from: http://www.awbi.org/awbi-pdf/SOP.pdf
16. Howe LM. Surgical methods of contraception and sterilization. Theriogenology. 2006;66:500–9.
17. Mathews KA. Pain assessment and general approach to management. Vet. Clin. North Am. - Small Anim. Pract. Elsevier Inc.; 2000;30:729–55.
18. R Core Team. R: A language and environment for statistical computing. Vienna, Austria: R Foundation for Statistical Computing; 2016. Available from: https://www.r-project.org
19. Reece JF, Nimesh MK, Wyllie RE, Jones AK, Dennison AW. Description and evaluation of a right flank, mini-laparotomy approach to canine ovariohysterectomy. Vet Rec 2012;171:248–248.
20. Vasseur PB, Paul HA, Enos LR, Hirsh DC. Infection rates in clean surgical procedures: a comparison of ampicillin prophylaxis vs a placebo. J Am Vet Med Assoc. 1985;187:825–7.
21. Vasseur PB, Levy J, Dowd E, Eliot J. Surgical wound infection rates in dogs and cats. Data from a teaching hospital. Vet Surg. 1988;17:60–4.
22. Brown DC, Conzemius MG, Shofer F, Swann H. Epidemiologic evaluation of postoperative wound infections in dogs and cats. J Am Vet Med Assoc. 1997;210:1302–6.
23. Beal MW, Brown DC, Shofer FS. The effects of perioperative hypothermia and the duration of anesthesia on postoperative wound infection rate in clean wounds: a retrospective study. Vet Surg. 2000;29:123–7.
24. Nicholson M, Beal M, Shofer F, Brown DC. Epidemiologic evaluation of postoperative wound infection in clean-contaminated wounds: a retrospective study of 239 dogs and cats. Vet Surg. 2002;31:577–81.
25. Eugster S, Schawalder P, Gaschen F, Boerlin P. A prospective study of postoperative surgical site infections in dogs and cats. Vet Surg. 2004;33:542–50.
26. Pollari FL, Bonnett BN. Evaluation of postoperative complications following elective surgeries of dogs and cats at private practices using computer records. Can Vet J. 1996;37:672–8.
27. Howe LM. Short-term results and complications of prepubertal gonadectomy in cats and dogs. J Am Vet Med Assoc. 1997;211:57–62.
28. Burrow R, Batchelor D, Cripps P. Complications observed during and after ovariohysterectomy of 142 bitches at a veterinary teaching hospital. Vet. Rec. 2005;157:829–33.
29. Totton SC, Wandeler AI, Ribble CS, Rosatte RC, McEwen SA. Stray dog population health in jodhpur, India in the wake of an animal birth control (ABC) program. Prev. Vet. Med. Elsevier B.V. 2011;98:215–20.
30. Padgett DA, Marucha PT, Sheridan JF. Restraint stress slows cutaneous wound healing in mice. Brain Behav Immun. 1998;12:64–73.
31. Pearson H. The complications of ovariohysterectomy in the bitch. J Small Anim Pract. 1973;14:257–66.
32. Burke JF. The effective period of preventive antibiotic action in experimental incisions and dermal lesions. Surgery. 1961;50:161–8.
33. Burke JF. Preventive antibiotic management in surgery. Annu Rev Med. 1973;24:289–94.
34. Looney AL, Bohling MW, Bushby PA, Howe LM, Griffin B, Levy JK, et al. The Association of Shelter Veterinarians veterinary medical care guidelines for spay-neuter programs. J Am Vet Med Assoc. 2008;233:74–86.
35. BSAVA. BSAVA Guide to the use of veterinary medicines 2nd edition. 2016.
36. GARP. Rationalizing Antibiotic use to limit antibiotic resistance in India. Indian J Med Res. 2011;134:3193708.
37. Iragüen D, Urcelay S, San Martín B. Pharmacovigilance in veterinary medicine in Chile: a pilot study. J Vet Pharmacol Ther. 2010;34:108–15.
38. Knights CB, Mateus A, Baines SJ. Current British veterinary attitudes to the use of perioperative antimicrobials in small animal surgery. Vet. Rec. 2012;170:646.
39. Mateus ALP, Brodbelt DC, Barber N, Stark KDC. Qualitative study of factors associated with antimicrobial usage in seven small animal veterinary practices in the UK. Prev. Vet. Med. Elsevier B.V. 2014;117:68–78.
40. McGuire L, Heffner K, Glaser R, Needleman B, Malarkey W, Dickinson S, et al. Pain and wound healing in surgical patients. Ann Behav Med. 2006;31:165–72.
41. Lamont LA. Multimodal pain management in veterinary medicine: the physiologic basis of pharmacologic therapies. Vet Clin North Am - Small Anim Pract Elsevier Ltd. 2008;38:1173–86.

A large animal model for standardized testing of bone regeneration strategies

James C. Ferguson[1,2†], Stefan Tangl[3,4*†] (iD), Dirk Barnewitz[5], Antje Genzel[5], Patrick Heimel[1,2,4], Veronika Hruschka[1,2], Heinz Redl[1,2] and Thomas Nau[1,2]

Abstract

Background: The need for bone graft substitutes including those being developed to be applied together with new strategies of bone regeneration such as tissue engineering and cell-based approaches is growing. No large animal model of bone regeneration has been accepted as a standard testing model. Standardization may be the key to moving systematically towards better bone regeneration. This study aimed to establish a model of bone regeneration in the sheep that lends itself to strict standardization and in which a number of substances can be tested within the same animal. To this end the caudal border of the ovine scapula was used as a consistent bed of mineralized tissue that provided sufficient room for a serial alignment of multiple experimental drill holes.

Results: The findings show that for the sake of standardization, surgery should be restricted to the middle part of the caudal margin, an area at least 80 mm proximal from the Glenoid cavity, but not more than 140 mm away from it, in the adult female Land Merino sheep. A distance of 5 mm from the caudal margin should also be observed.

Conclusions: This standardized model with defined uniform defects and defect sites results in predictable and reproducible bone regeneration processes. Defects are placed unilaterally in only one limb of the animal, avoiding morbidity in multiple limbs. The fact that five defects per animal can be evaluated is conducive to intra-animal comparisons and reduces the number of animals that have to be subject to experimentation.

Background

Bone grafting takes place in over 100 000 procedures annually in the US [1]. Where autograft material is limited or inadequate, or when donor-site morbidity is to be avoided [2, 3], substitute materials are required. The market for bone graft substitute materials exceeds 2 billion dollars in a group of 10 major countries [4].

This need for bone graft substitutes also motivates the development of new methods to improve bone regeneration; increasingly, these novel treatment techniques include tissue engineering and cell-based approaches. Proof of concept in bone regeneration studies can only be shown with the help of animal models; no in vitro method can mimic the complexity of an in vivo environment sufficiently or predict clinical efficacy. Whereas initial screening and feasibility testing are popularly carried out in rodent models, large animal models whose bone regeneration is closer to the same processes in humans are essential to provide translational proof of concept.

The FDA, for example, often requires the testing of bone therapies in both a small and large animal model before accepting an agent for clinical trials [5, 6]. Rodent models cannot adequately mimic human bone regeneration for a number of reasons, among them a lack of cortical remodeling and the fact that cessation of growth occurs much later than in other mammals [7, 8]. The biomechanical conditions of human skeletal loading can obviously not be simulated in small animal models with their lower body mass. The mechanisms of bone regeneration depend on the size of the defect, because a mass transport of oxygen and nutrients, cell migration and vascular invasion into and the removal of degradation

* Correspondence: stefan.tangl@univie.ac.at
†James C. Ferguson and Stefan Tangl contributed equally to this work.
³Department of Evolutionary Anthropology, Faculty of Life Sciences, University of Vienna, Vienna, Austria
⁴Karl Donath Laboratory for Hard Tissue and Biomaterial Research, Department of Oral Surgery, School of Dentistry, Medical University of Vienna, Vienna, Austria
Full list of author information is available at the end of the article

products out of the defect area are strongly influenced by the distances that have to be overcome [9, 10]. This constitutes a need to create large defects that can only be set in large animals [7]. Also the fact that the immune system of large animals is more similar to humans than that of rodents is especially important when the influence of immunogeneic substances and (allogeneic) cells on bone regeneration is studied [11–16].

Although many studies have been carried out already [17, 18], no final consensus on the standardization of large animal models has been reached so far. Factors that potentially influence the outcome like defect size, time points of evaluation or the species of test animal continue to be controversially discussed.

One important requirement is that the model should not be too rigid in its application. When new experimental needs and different indications arise it should be adaptable enough to meet these new demands. However a standardized animal model where the quality and quantity of bone regeneration and its ability to integrate bone substitute material are known in detail could be of great value. The most important factor to achieve this standardization is the fact that several defects can be evaluated in the same narrow anatomical region of the same individual animal. Uniform surgical technique is paramount to facilitate comparability in animal models and the exact location of a bone defect has a profound influence on the bone regeneration properties being tested. Hopefully the sum of this could lead to a wider acceptance of this model as a standard method in testing bone graft substitute materials and thereby improve comparability between studies. Standardization may be the key to moving systematically towards better bone regeneration therapies in the future.

In the following study, we aimed to establish an orthotopic model of bone regeneration in the sheep that allows stringent standardization and in which several test substances can be analyzed within the same animal. The products or substances that are about to be tested in the defects should be subjected to identical physiological influences by being implanted in the same narrow anatomical region where conditions are constant. We describe here the establishment of this standardized model from selection of animals to surgery to the histologic and morphometric evaluation as it has been proven in a recently published study on the preclinical testing of hydroxyapatite biomaterials [19].

Results

All animals tolerated the surgery well, no lameness or other clinically relevant findings were seen after the immediate postoperative period and the animals returned to free pasture after sutures were removed 10 days after surgery.

All samples from all animals were available for CT analysis although two defects were not analyzed due to CT reconstruction problems. One defect site was not available for histological analysis because of faulty drilling.

Anatomical and histological characteristics of the experimental site

The caudal border of the ovine scapula is a thick bony structure that provides a bone volume that is sufficient for placing several drill hole defects in a row parallel to the caudal margin (Fig. 1). While the main body of the shoulder blade is flat and thin, the caudal border shows a bulge or thickening on the medial aspect. This bulge or torus is predominantly semi-circular in cross-section and is surrounded by cortical bone of the plexiform type (Fig. 2d), while the center is filled with lamellar cancellous bone and fatty marrow. The overall height of the semi-circular bulge (Fig. 3a-1) is on average 10.9 +/− 1.2 mm and its width (Figs. 3a-4) is 16.9 +/− 2.5 mm. There are topographic differences: closer to the Glenoid cavity the ridge is higher and narrower, but it flattens out in the proximal direction, i.e. it becomes lower and wider (Figs. 1, 4).

The cortical wall of the bulge is thickest on the medial face (Fig. 3a-2) with a mean value of 3.2 +/− 0.9 mm. Again, the dimensions show a gradient, because the bone is thicker close to the joint and thinner farther away from it. In the cortical bone of the lateral face (Fig. 3a-3) where the defects are placed, no such change in dimension can be observed. It shows an almost constant thickness of about 1.3 +/− 0.3 mm over the whole area. A demarcation of the bulge in the cranial direction is difficult to make, as it gradually becomes thinner. In some cases, the medial and lateral cortical plate fuse with one another, forming one unified cortical plate (Fig. 3a). In other cases, the two plates run parallel to each other, separated by a thin layer of cancellous bone (Fig. 3c). For the purposes of this study, the cranial border of the bulge was per definition placed at the point where the lateral cortical bone wall together plus the marrow space were at least 5 mm high (Fig. 3a-4). This demarcates the area where the drill holes can be optimally placed and constitutes the relevant experimental space available for the placement of the drill hole and the test substances (green area in Fig. 3a). This experimental space shows little variation in its height in the proximodistal direction (Fig. 4) while its width increases in the proximal direction.

The minimum necessary distance of the drill hole to the caudal margin (Fig. 3a-5) was measured on histological specimens. This distance was important to guarantee a minimal height of the experimental space of 5 mm and to securely place the defect in the marrow space without impinging on the caudal cortical bone. On average this minimal necessary distance from the caudal margin was 3.4 ± 0.7 mm (Fig. 4). The absolute largest value was 5.1 mm.

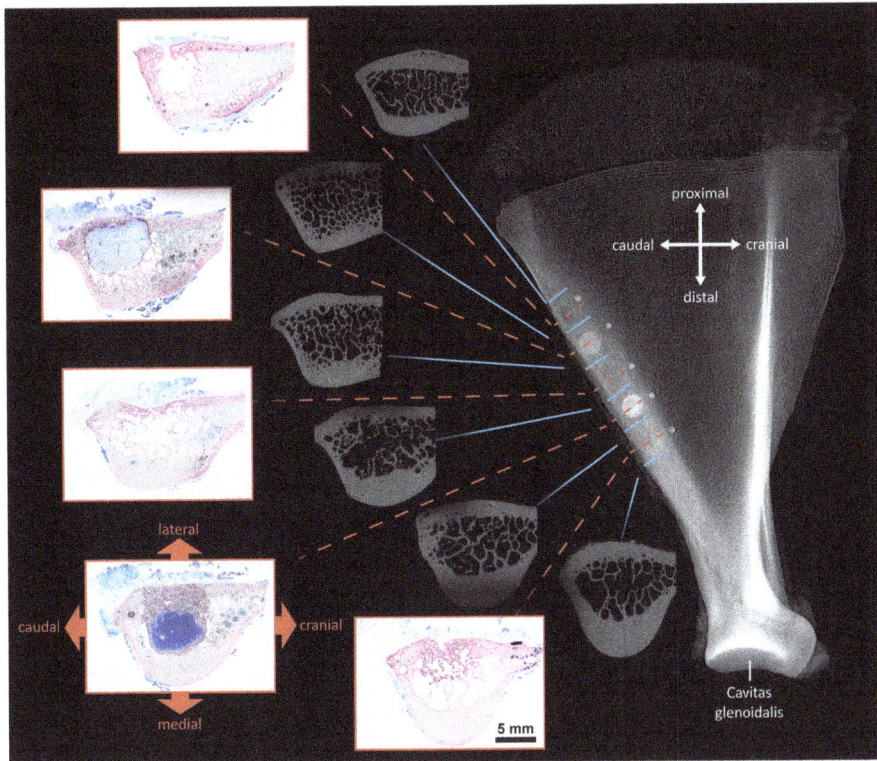

Fig. 1 Anatomical and histological characteristics of the ovine scapula model. On the right a radiographic presentation of the scapula in lateral view with 5 drill holes in the caudal margin. On the left the histologic specimens through the center of the defects (red lines) filled with different bone substitute materials showing the regional differences from proximal to distal. In the center μCT images depicting the regions between the drill holes (blue lines). The medial bulge decreases in height from distal to proximal while its width increases

Histologic and histomorphometric healing characteristics

Not all of the defects had fully healed after 6 months. In the empty control group only 27% of the drill holes and 17% of the autologous bone group were completely bridged. Discontinuities in the cortical region left deep depressions that penetrated into the marrow space (Figs. 2c and 5a).

The bone tissue that filled the drill holes was a mixture of lamellar bone in the form of secondary osteons and interspersed remnants of plexiform bone (Fig. 2b). Plexiform bone, which consists of woven bone and parallel fibered bone (Fig. 2e), is formed in the early stages of bone healing [20, 21]. It initially fills the gaps and stabilizes the defect. After mechanical stability is achieved, this primary bone is resorbed by osteoclasts and replaced by more mature secondary lamellar bone, formed by osteoblasts. At 6 months, this process of remodeling had already progressed far in our model. In most cases, more than half of the primary plexiform bone in the cortical region had already been replaced by secondary osteons. This process of remodeling was still going on at a very high rate, as proven by the presence of many large secondary osteons in all active stages of formation (Fig. 2b). In the cancellous region of the defect, trabecular bone filled the space and was also a mixture of primary plexiform and secondary lamellar bone, but remodeling activity was far lower than in the cortex. Only a few hemiosteonal remodeling sites could be observed on the surface of the trabeculae. In the autochthonous bone surrounding the drill hole, pre-existing trabeculae were compacted and thickened by layers of bone that had been added posttraumatically. A similar effect was seen at the periosteal surface surrounding the defects, where often large quantities of bone tissue had been laid down.

After 12 months, the findings were not remarkably different. In the empty control group 33% showed continuous bony bridging while in the autologous bone group the rate was 25%. Histologically, the tendencies detectable at 6 months had simply continued and progressed. More, but not all, of the primary bone had been converted by remodeling into secondary osteons. The most striking difference was the lower rate of ongoing remodeling. Far fewer active remodeling sites were seen than at the 6 month time point.

These qualitative histologic findings were not significantly different between drill holes filled with autologous bone and those left completely empty. Autologous bone graft had obviously been resorbed rapidly; only small traces of it were still detectable after 6 months.

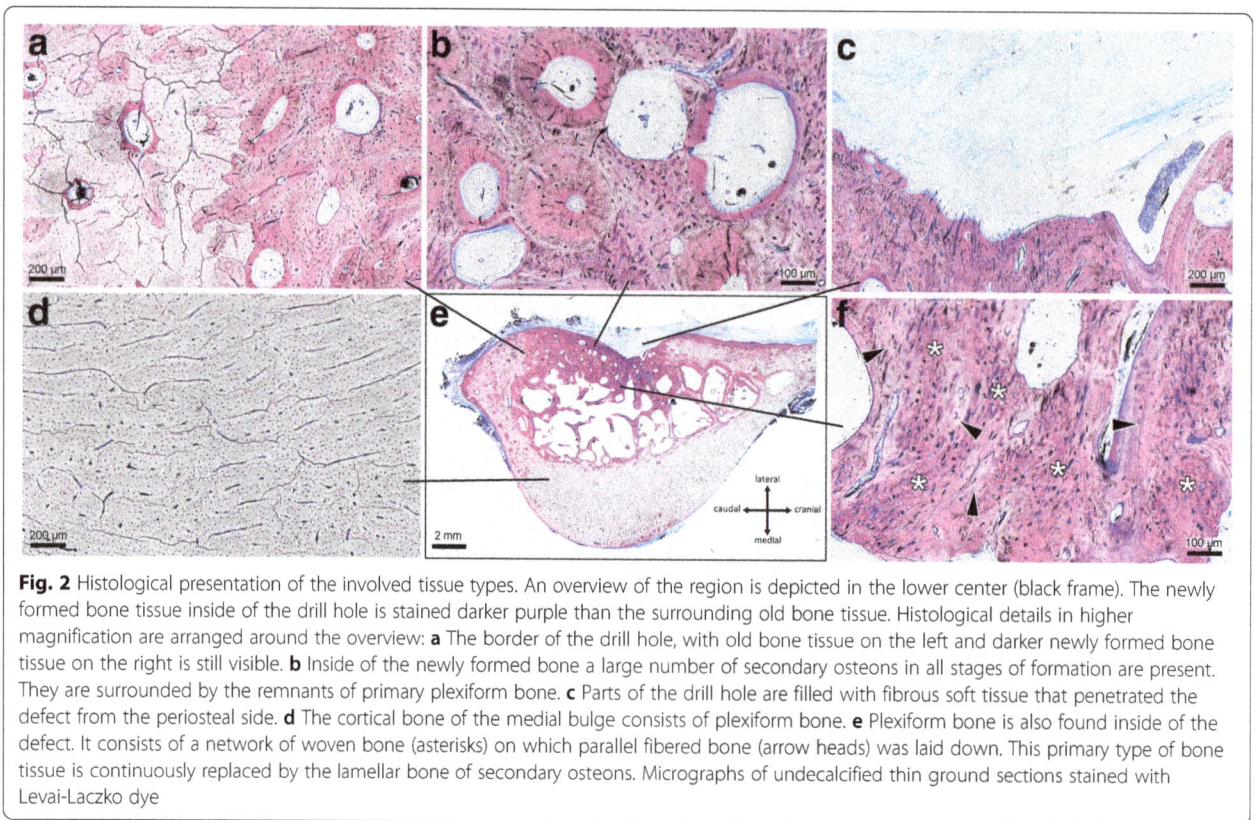

Fig. 2 Histological presentation of the involved tissue types. An overview of the region is depicted in the lower center (black frame). The newly formed bone tissue inside of the drill hole is stained darker purple than the surrounding old bone tissue. Histological details in higher magnification are arranged around the overview: **a** The border of the drill hole, with old bone tissue on the left and darker newly formed bone tissue on the right is still visible. **b** Inside of the newly formed bone a large number of secondary osteons in all stages of formation are present. They are surrounded by the remnants of primary plexiform bone. **c** Parts of the drill hole are filled with fibrous soft tissue that penetrated the defect from the periosteal side. **d** The cortical bone of the medial bulge consists of plexiform bone. **e** Plexiform bone is also found inside of the defect. It consists of a network of woven bone (asterisks) on which parallel fibered bone (arrow heads) was laid down. This primary type of bone tissue is continuously replaced by the lamellar bone of secondary osteons. Micrographs of undecalcified thin ground sections stained with Levai-Laczko dye

Histomorphometry

After 6 months, the mean percentage of newly formed bone (nBV/TV) in the cortical region was $54.39 \pm 21.71\%$ for the empty control while it was $60.36 \pm 18.34\%$ in the autologous bone group, i.e. the defects were about half filled, with a large degree of variation. In the medullary areas, nBV/TV for the empty control was $28.52 \pm 14.20\%$ and that for autologous bone $18.34 \pm 13.82\%$. Bone regeneration was only about half as strong as in the cortical environment. There were no significant differences between the two treatment groups.

After twelve months, the percentage of newly formed bone in the cortical region was not greatly different from that at 6 months. The drill hole in the empty control group was filled to $56.34 \pm 25.92\%$ with new bone and that of the autologous bone group to $59.83 \pm 27.98\%$. The situation in the medullary space was not as unambiguous. The empty control group showed higher values for nBV/TV of $40.56 \pm 15.85\%$ while in the autologous bone group they were with 32.41 ± 13. Again, there were no significant differences between the treatment groups.

To characterize the completeness of bone regeneration in a cortical defect, it is important to measure the fraction of the area that was not filled with bone, but with soft tissues that invaded from the periosteal region and impaired bone formation. The percentage of these soft tissues in areas were only cortical bone should be was $35.06 \pm$ 25.67% for the empty control and $29.72 \pm 22.55\%$ for autologous bone after 6 months. After a period of 12 months, the values were $37.26 \pm 30.69\%$ and $32.67 \pm 33.39\%$ respectively. Variation was conspicuously high.

These results for nBV/TV have been used in the publication by Hruschka et al. [19] as control groups in comparison to several bone substitute materials but were not described in greater detail. They are presented here more extensively in order to illustrate the quantitative healing properties of the experimental model.

Description of technical problems with the model

The exact placement of the drill holes proved to be the most severe problem. The planned ideal defect, which should cut through the lateral cortical wall and then penetrate the medullary space with bone marrow surrounding it on all sides (Fig. 3a) could not always be established in the in vivo scenario. In some cases the drilling was placed too close to the caudal margin and the caudal cortical bone was penetrated leading to stronger bone formation due to the greater regenerative potential of this cortical region (see histomorphometric results). A drill hole placed too far caudally was subjected to disproportionately high bone formation (Fig. 3c). If the drill hole is located too far cranially, there is a risk of cutting through the entire bone thickness, which is thinner in these regions (Fig. 3b).

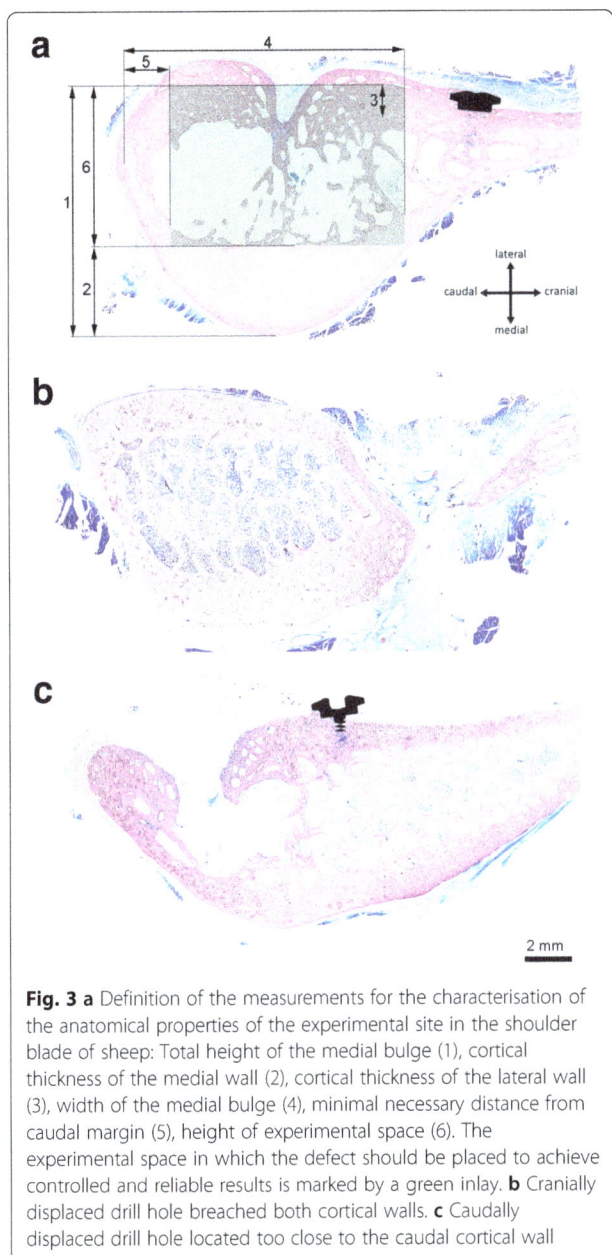

Fig. 3 a Definition of the measurements for the characterisation of the anatomical properties of the experimental site in the shoulder blade of sheep: Total height of the medial bulge (1), cortical thickness of the medial wall (2), cortical thickness of the lateral wall (3), width of the medial bulge (4), minimal necessary distance from caudal margin (5), height of experimental space (6). The experimental space in which the defect should be placed to achieve controlled and reliable results is marked by a green inlay. **b** Cranially displaced drill hole breached both cortical walls. **c** Caudally displaced drill hole located too close to the caudal cortical wall

The titanium pins marking the centre of the defects proved to be unnecessary. Even after long observation periods, the empty drill holes were clearly visible on x-rays. Degradation of bone graft substitute material was easily followed over periods up to one year. A critical size model could not be established. Bone growth after one year in the empty defects was much higher than the 10% that stipulates a critical size defect [22] but healing was severely impaired.

Discussion

In the adult sheep a 60 mm long area of the caudal border of the scapula shows a bone architecture and

quality constant enough for a standardized serial alignment of multiple test drill holes. To uphold and improve standardization, surgery should be restricted to the middle part of the caudal margin because of the regional differences in the height and width of the bulge mentioned above. A reasonable recommendation is to use an area beginning at least 80 mm from the Glenoid cavity, but not more than 140 mm away from it (Fig. 4). The narrower the chosen region is, the more similar the anatomical and histological characteristics will be. Nevertheless, there should be at least 5 mm distance from the margins of one drill hole to the next, so that the healing processes of the individual defects will not interfere with one another. These measurements apply to the adult female Land Merino breed and will differ in other breeds and in male sheep.

Precision operating technique is needed in this model and is perhaps the most challenging aspect with the greatest influence on standardization. That a true critical size defect is not possible in this anatomical site is, indeed, an admitted weakness.

The immediate milieu and environment of drill hole test sites consists of well vascularized muscle tissue on one side and bone marrow on the other side providing a plethora of progenitor cells and factors necessary for defect healing. Because of this, the region facilitates substantial new bone growth and, in longer observation periods, allows the evaluation of remodeling and degradation of bone substitutes. The sharp dissection of the muscle tissue adjacent to the scapula test area also does, to a certain extent, mimic the soft tissue damage seen in the vicinity of a typical traumatic wound/defect.

Sheep are compliant and docile animals [23] and are a less controversial test subject in the public opinion than, for example, the dog. The body weight of sheep and the size of its long bones are roughly similar to those of humans. Their remodeling rate, lamellar bone structure and primary bone healing characteristics are similar to humans [11]. Monitoring and delivery techniques can be the same as those used in humans. The ability to use young, aged or ovariectomized ewes as well as male animals means that the influences of age, sex and pathologies such as osteopenia/osteoporosis can be simulated in sheep models. When biomechanical testing is important, large animals such as the sheep have an advantage over rodent models [24] as they more readily approximate human anatomy.

A number of models have been developed, also in the sheep and also utilizing drill hole defects, to test bone graft substitutes [12, 23–25], some placing the drill holes in the long bones of the extremities, others using a combination of femur drill holes and a slot defect in the tibia [26–28]. The comparison of different variants or different dosages of bioactive substances is best achieved when

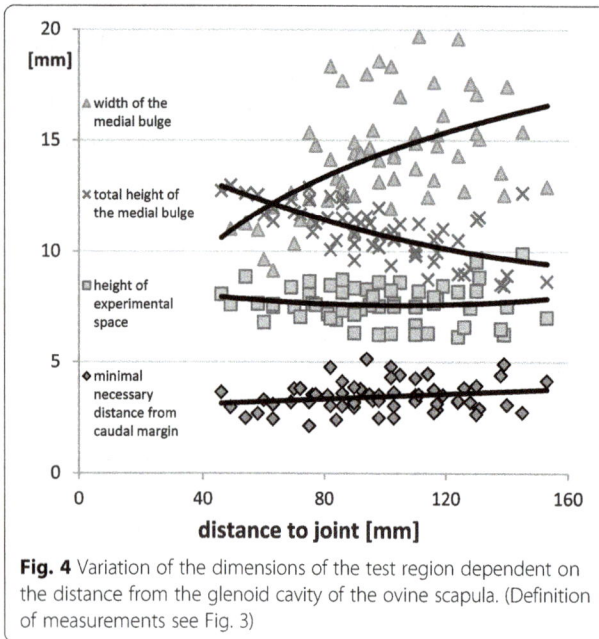

Fig. 4 Variation of the dimensions of the test region dependent on the distance from the glenoid cavity of the ovine scapula. (Definition of measurements see Fig. 3)

comparisons of all can be made in a single animal. Nuss et al. and others [17, 25] proposed a sheep model with 8 bilateral drill hole sites in both the femur and humerus. Van der Pol achieved a higher degree of standardization [29] by using customized drilling jigs but in sites in two different bones (the tibia and femur). Gisep et al. tested non-loaded bone regeneration in a drill hole model combined with a loaded tibia slot defect [27]. The use of different anatomical bone sites are not, however, comparable with regards to loading boundaries and amount and quality of new bone growth and bone densities [24].

The site of a bone defect has a large influence on its properties of regeneration. The density of bone in various anatomic sites varies widely [24]. When multiple defects are drilled in the epiphysis, their differing proximity to the metaphysis can directly influence growth and tissue characteristics. Defects placed in the metaphysis and the neighboring diaphysis differ starkly in new bone growth [30]. Bone regeneration is site specific; in our model, all graft samples and controls are placed in the same osteologically homogenous anatomical region. Different bone sites are also influenced by the type of tissue in its immediate vicinity (i.e. muscle) and may suffer from lack of uniform bone growth environments.

The use of bilateral defects, in which limbs on both sides of the animal are affected, are discouraged due to animal welfare reasons [7].

A model in which all test substances can be implanted in a single animal can keep animal numbers down [31]. The assessment of multiple defects in one animal provides for control of variation between animals and thus limits the number of animals needed [7]. Indeed, the

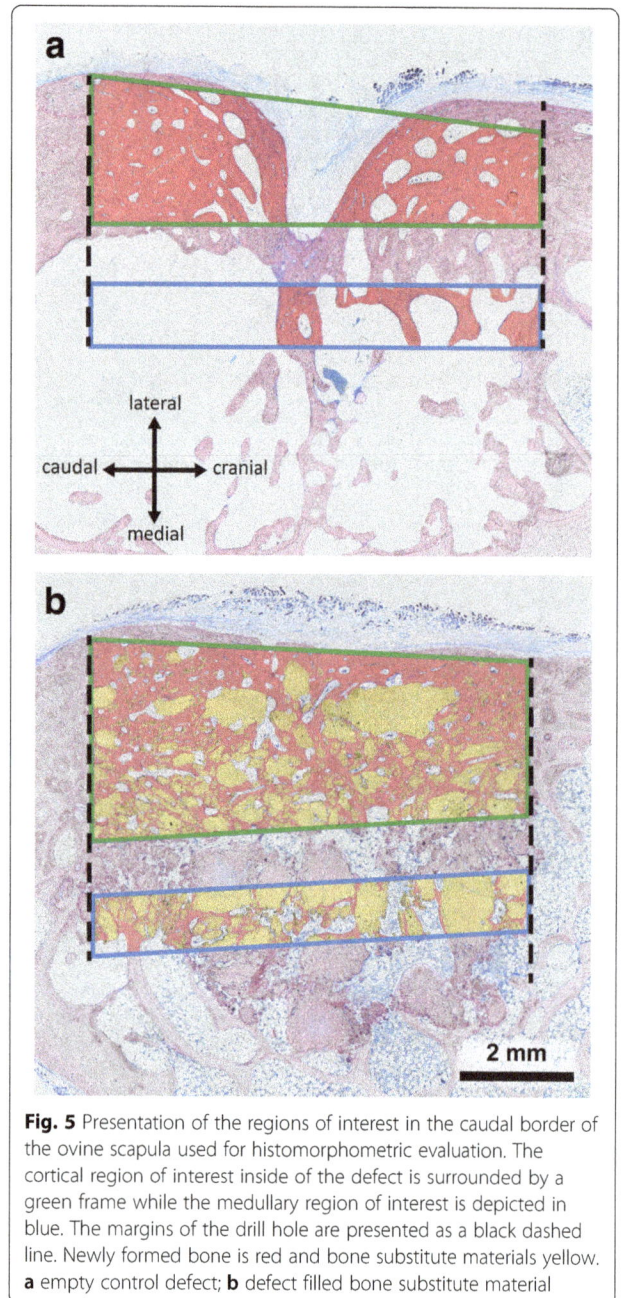

Fig. 5 Presentation of the regions of interest in the caudal border of the ovine scapula used for histomorphometric evaluation. The cortical region of interest inside of the defect is surrounded by a green frame while the medullary region of interest is depicted in blue. The margins of the drill hole are presented as a black dashed line. Newly formed bone is red and bone substitute materials yellow. **a** empty control defect; **b** defect filled bone substitute material

main advantage of this model is the possibility of implanting 5 different test items or allowing 5 treatment groups in a single large animal while refraining from setting a bilateral defect.

This model allows for implantation biocompatibility testing of new bone graft substitutes as well as efficacy testing, although short term evaluations maybe more efficient in, or in combination with, a rodent model. Short term observation periods would allow for the tracking of inflammatory reactions, osteofibrosis or osteonecrosis. The model lends itself particularly well to following and comparing the degradation characteristics of bone graft substitutes and their replacement with new bone over longer periods of time.

Clearly, no animal model matches human physiology perfectly. Sheep do tend to have higher trabecular bone densities than humans, depending on site [32, 33]. Although some breeds cycle all year round, sheep are seasonal breeders that have varying oestrogen levels over the course of the year and this must be taken into account during the study design phase and season of the year of any interventions reported [18, 34].

This model also allows for the use of autologous graft that is comparable to the cancellous graft applied in clinical human use – something that is not possible in rodents in which typically only bone marrow with cortical bone and periosteum is available for grafting and in which osteogenic colony forming units in grafts are much lower than in humans [7].

Aside from the practicalities and the mechanical factors that speak for the use of large animals in bone regenerative medicine, there are other biological reasons as well. An example of this is the difference in bone regeneration between small animals and large animals as can be seen in the fact that calcium phosphate scaffolds rarely show osteoinduction in rodent models while successfully inducing bone growth in large animals [35]. Also the immune system of large animals is more similar to humans than that of rodents [11–16].

One of the largest obstacles in the study of regenerative medicine is the host/graft reaction against human cells in animal models. No immunodeficient sheep model is available for cell transplantation, although protocols of sheep immunosuppression have been developed [36]. Looking towards the future, induced pluripotent stem cells have been recently produced from sheep cells [37, 38] and may find their way into preclinical testing methods.

Conclusion

We have presented here a large animal model for the study of bone regeneration that is relatively easy to perform and provides a strictly standardized testing assay from surgery to quantitative evaluation. It has defined uniform defects and defect sites with uniform regeneration and allows up to 5 defects per animal, conducive to intra-animal comparisons and to reducing animal numbers. Defects are placed unilaterally in only one limb of the animal, avoiding the morbidity associated with the use of multiple limbs seen in other models.

Methods
Animals
This study was approved by the local ethics committee ("Thüringer Landesamt für Verbraucherschutz")

and was consistent with the Guide for the Care and Use of Laboratory Animals of the National Institute of Health (revised 2011) and the European directive 2010/63/EU.

The model was tested in a study by Hruschka et al. [19] using 24 adult (aged 2–3 years) female Land Merino sheep. Empty ewes which had experienced at least one lactation period were purchased by the research institute from an agricultural company prior to the study. The animals were fed with hay and allowed to drink water ad libitum and housed in a free stall barn in the immediate postoperative period, then transferred to free ranging pasture.

General anaesthesia was induced by an intravenous administration of xylazine (Rompun, Bayer GmbH), diazepam (Gewacalm, Takeda GmbH) and ketamine (Ketamidor, Richter pharma AG) (0.1 mg/kg, 0.1 mg/kg, 4.4 mg/kg). After induction, the animals were intubated and anesthesia was maintained with isoflurane at 1.0–1.5 vol% and oxygen. The animals received both a pre-emptive analgesic, carprofen (Rimadyl, Pfizer Inc.; 1.4 mg/ kg intravenous) and a systemic antibiotic (Veracin-Compositum, Albrecht GmbH, 3 ml/50 kg intramuscular). Haematological and parasitological examinations were performed prior to the study and animals were operated on in late autumn.

Surgery
The animal was laid in lateral recumbency. The region of the left shoulder blade was clipped, shaved and disinfected and the animal was draped. A longitudinal skin incision approximately 15 cm long and parallel to the caudal border of the left scapula was made using the acromion and caudal angle of the scapula as landmarks. The caudal margin of the scapula was exposed by sharp dissection of the musculature. All soft tissue was separated from the bone with a periosteal elevator. Using a trephine drill, five defects with a diameter and depth of 8 mm were created, leaving a 5 mm bony bridge in between each defect. The defects were irrigated with saline solution during drilling. The longitudinal axis of the drill holes was oriented perpendicular to the lateral face of the scapula and included the lateral cortical layer and the trabecular layer down to the medial corticalis (Fig. 1).

The cylinders from the drill holes were preserved for autologous bone grafting. Titanium pins (3 mm long, 0.7 mm in diameter) were placed close to the defects to mark their exact location. The five drill hole defects were randomized to either an empty control, autologous graft or test article group. Autologous cancellous material was mixed together as a rough paste before implantation. The surgical incision was closed in multiple layers using absorbable Monocryl 3–0 (Ethicon Inc.) suture material with the skin closure using everting horizontal mattress sutures and nonabsorbable material. The animals received carprofen subcutaneously for five days post-operatively.

Animals were euthanised under general anaesthesia as described above. T61, a commercial euthanasia solution based on embutramide, mebozonium, iodide and tetracaine hydrochloride (Merck Animal Health, Munich, Germany), was administered by a trained veterinarian by slow intravenous injection at a dosage of 0.1 ml/kg body weight. Sampling was carried out at 6 months and 12 months after treatment.

Histology and sample preparation

The left shoulder blades were removed from the animals and fixed in buffered formalin. An overview radiograph was produced of each sample to ascertain the exact location of the augmentation sites. Blocks containing each one of the defects were cut using a diamond coated band saw (EXAKT Apparatebau, Norderstedt, Germany) separating them precisely in between the drill holes as visible on the radiograph (Fig. 1). These blocks were scanned after 14 days of fixation with a SCANCO µCT 50 (SCANCO Medical AG, Bruttisellen, Switzerland) micro-CT (µ CT) at 90 kV/200 µA with an isotropic resolution of 17.2 µm and an integration time of 500 ms. The scans were exported as 16 bit DICOM image stacks. Three-dimensional reconstruction of the data was performed using the visualization software Amira 6.2 (Thermo Fisher Scientific, Waltham, USA).

After µCT scanning, blocks were dehydrated and embedded in plastic (Technovit 7200 VLC + BPO; Kulzer & Co., Wehrheim, Germany). Undecalcified, thin ground sections were made using a method established by Donath [39]. These histologic specimens were stained with Levai-Laczko dye, a variant of the Giemsa dye that allows to distinguish reliably between old bone, new bone and bone substitute materials [40].

This model allows qualitative and descriptive histological evaluations of bone regeneration as well as a histomorphometric analysis. Histologic thin ground sections were segmented histomorphometrically using Definiens Developer XD 2.1 (Definiens AG, Munich, Germany) and corrected manually using Photoshop CS 4 (Adobe Systems Inc., San Jose, CA, USA). The corrected images were then measured in Definiens Developer XD 2.1.

Two specific regions of interest were defined to allow a differentiated evaluation of bone growth and test substance degradation. The cortical region of interest was defined as the area between the boundaries of the drill hole inside the cortical bone and the periosteal and endosteal margins of the neighboring bone. A medullary region of interest was set at a location 1 mm beneath the cortical region of interest and had a height of 1 mm (Fig. 5). This medullary region of interest included the

marrow space within the whole breadth of the drill hole. The corrected images then were measured using the Definiens software. Examples of evaluation parameters that can be measured include: areas of newly formed bone, areas of soft tissue, amount of residue substitute material and the complete region of interest (tissue volume). Also, the sizes of individual graft substitute particle agglomerates and their number can be determined. From these primary measurements the following parameters can be calculated: The percentage of bone substitute material in the regions of interest, the average size of particle agglomerates in mm^2, the number of bone substitute particle agglomerates per mm^2, the percentage of newly formed bone in the regions of interest (BV/TV), the percentage of the composite of newly formed bone plus bone substitute material, the percentage of the region of interest filled with soft tissue that had grown from the periosteal region into the defect area (Periosteal void volume). An example of the model that used these parameters of evaluation has been published [19].

For the purposes of this study, only the bone healing of the empty control group and the autologous bone group were histomorphometrically characterized. These two treatment regimens are commonly used as a control and in comparison with newly developed test substances. The amount of newly formed bone tissue (nBV) was divided by the size of the complete region of interest (TV), resulting in the percentage of new bone tissue inside of the region of interest (nBV/TV).

Statistical evaluation

Descriptive statistics were performed calculating means and standard deviations. Multiple linear mixed models for all independent variables were constructed, where treatment was used as an independent variable and animal ID as a random factor. Tukey-type post-hoc tests were calculated for treatment effect [19].

All computations were done using R version 3.2.3 [41].

Micro-CT

We scanned samples at 90 kV with an isotropic resolution of 17.2 µm. We evaluated the closure of defects and categorised them either as "non-bridging" (leaving a continuous opening in the cortical bone which allowed communication of the medullary cavity with the periosteal area) or "bridging" when the continuity of the cortical bone was completely restored.

Abbreviations
BPO: Benzoyl peroxide; nBV/TV: New bone volume per tissue volume; µCT: Microcomputed tomography

Acknowledgements
We would like to thank Julia Drnek and Amin Rezakhani for their technical help with the production of thin ground sections and the histomorphometric classification.

Funding
Not applicable.

Authors' contributions
JCF and ST contributed equally to this publication. HR and VH conceived, designed and supervised the study. DB and AG developed the animal model and participated in the surgery. TN and JCF performed the experimental surgery. ST performed the histological evaluation and histomorphometry. PH carried out the μCT-scans and was involved in the histomorphometric measurements. JCF and ST drafted the manuscript and produced the figures. HR, TN and VH were involved in the critical revision of the manuscript. All authors read and approved the final manuscript.

Consent for publication
Not applicable.

Competing interests
The authors declare that they have no competing interests.

Author details
[1]Ludwig Boltzmann Institute for Experimental and Clinical Traumatology in AUVA research center, Vienna, Austria. [2]Austrian Cluster for Tissue Regeneration, Vienna, Austria. [3]Department of Evolutionary Anthropology, Faculty of Life Sciences, University of Vienna, Vienna, Austria. [4]Karl Donath Laboratory for Hard Tissue and Biomaterial Research, Department of Oral Surgery, School of Dentistry, Medical University of Vienna, Vienna, Austria. [5]Research Centre of Medical Technology and Biotechnology, fzmb GmbH, Bad Langensalza, Germany.

References
1. Kinaci A, Neuhaus V, Ring DC. Trends in bone graft use in the United States. Orthopedics. 2014;37:e783–8.
2. Matsa S, Murugan S, Kannadasan K. Evaluation of morbidity associated with iliac crest harvest for alveolar cleft bone grafting. J Maxillofac Oral Surg. 2012;11:91–5.
3. Jäger M, Westhoff B, Wild A, Krauspe R. Knochenspanentnahme am Becken. Techniken und Probleme. Orthopade 2005;34:976–82, 984, 986–90, 992–4.
4. North American bone grafts and substitutes market to hit $2.1 billion by 2023. GlobalData Plc. 2017. https://www.globaldata.com/north-american-bone-grafts-substitutes-market-hit-2-1-billion-2023/. Accessed 15 Apr 2017.
5. Thompson DD, Simmons HA, Pirie CM, Ke HZ. FDA guidelines and animal models for osteoporosis. Bone. 1995;17(4 Suppl):125S–33S.
6. Osteoporosis: Nonclinical evaluation of drugs intended for treatment; draft guidance for industry; availability. Federal Register. 2016. https://www.federalregister.gov/documents/2016/06/14/2016-13988/osteoporosis-nonclinical-evaluation-of-drugs-intended-for-treatment-draft-guidance-for-industry. Accessed 15 Apr 2017.
7. Muschler GF, Raut VP, Patterson TE, Wenke JC, Hollinger JO. The design and use of animal models for translational research in bone tissue engineering and regenerative medicine. Tissue Eng Part B Rev. 2010;16:123–45.
8. Kilborn SH, Trudel G, Uhthoff H. Review of growth plate closure compared with age at sexual maturity and lifespan in laboratory animals. Contemp Top Lab Anim Sci. 2002;41:21–6.
9. Muschler GF, Nakamoto C, Griffith LG. Engineering principles of clinical cell-based tissue engineering. J Bone Joint Surg Am. 2004;86-A:1541–58.
10. Knothe Tate ML, Steck R, Forwood MR, Niederer P. In vivo demonstration of load-induced fluid flow in the rat tibia and its potential implications for processes associated with functional adaptation. J Exp Biol. 2000;203(Pt 18): 2737–45.
11. von Rechenberg B. Experiences with sheep models in musculoskeletal research at the MSRU. Eur Cell Mater. 2008;16(SUPPL. 4):31.
12. Harding J, Roberts RM, Mirochnitchenko O. Large animal models for stem cell therapy. Stem Cell Res Ther. 2013;4:23.
13. Cibelli J, Emborg ME, Prockop DJ, Roberts M, Schatten G, Rao M, et al. Strategies for improving animal models for regenerative medicine. Cell Stem Cell. 2013;12:271–4.
14. Gibson AJ, Coffey TJ, Werling D. Of creatures great and small: the advantages of farm animal models in immunology research. Front Immunol. 2013;4:124.
15. Hein WR, Griebel PJ. A road less travelled: large animal models in immunological research. Nat Rev Immunol. 2003;3:79–84.
16. Yuan H, van Blitterswijk CA, de Groot K, de Bruijn JD. Cross-species comparison of ectopic bone formation in biphasic calcium phosphate (BCP) and hydroxyapatite (HA) scaffolds. Tissue Eng. 2006;12:1607–15.
17. Nuss KM, Auer JA, Boos A, von Rechenberg B. An animal model in sheep for biocompatibility testing of biomaterials in cancellous bones. BMC Musculoskelet Disord. 2006;7:67.
18. Oheim R, Amling M, Ignatius A, Pogoda P. Large animal model for osteoporosis in humans: the ewe. Eur Cell Mater. 2012;24:372–85.
19. Hruschka V, Tangl S, Ryabenkova Y, Heimel P, Barnewitz D, Möbus G, et al. Comparison of nanoparticular hydroxyapatite pastes of different particle content and size in a novel scapula defect model. Sci Rep. 2017;7:43425.
20. Schenk RK. Bone regeneration: biologic basis. In: Buser D, Dahlin C, Schenk RK, editors. Guided bone regeneration in implant dentistry. London: Quientessence; 1995. p. 49–100.
21. Martin RB, Burr DB. Structure, function, and adaptation of compact bone. New York: Raven Press; 1989.
22. Spicer PP, Kretlow JD, Young S, Jansen JA, Kasper FK, Mikos AG. Evaluation of bone regeneration using the rat critical size calvarial defect. Nat Protoc. 2012;7:1918–29.
23. Turner AS. Animal models of osteoporosis-necessity and limitations. Eur Cell Mater. 2001;1:66–81.
24. Liebschner MAK. Biomechanical considerations of animal models used in tissue engineering of bone. Biomaterials. 2004;25:1697–714.
25. Hannink G, Wolke JGC, Schreurs BW, Buma P. In vivo behavior of a novel injectable calcium phosphate cement compared with two other commercially available calcium phosphate cements. J Biomed Mater Res B Appl Biomater. 2008;85B:478–88.
26. von Rechenberg B, Génot OR, Nuss K, Galuppo L, Fulmer M, Jacobson E, et al. Evaluation of four biodegradable, injectable bone cements in an experimental drill hole model in sheep. Eur J Pharm Biopharm. 2013;85:130–8.
27. Gisep A, Wieling R, Bohner M, Matter S, Schneider E, Rahn B. Resorption patterns of calcium-phosphate cements in bone. J Biomed Mater Res A. 2003;66:532–40.
28. Theiss F, Apelt D, Brand B, Kutter A, Zlinszky K, Bohner M, et al. Biocompatibility and resorption of a brushite calcium phosphate cement. Biomaterials. 2005;26:4383–94.
29. van der Pol U, Mathieu L, Zeiter S, Bourban P-E, Zambelli P-Y, Pearce SG, et al. Augmentation of bone defect healing using a new biocomposite scaffold: an in vivo study in sheep. Acta Biomater. 2010;6:3755–62.
30. Takigami H, Kumagai K, Latson L, Togawa D, Bauer T, Powell K, et al. Bone formation following OP-1 implantation is improved by addition of autogenous bone marrow cells in a canine femur defect model. J Orthop Res Off Publ Orthop Res Soc. 2007;25:1333–42.
31. Campion CR, Chander C, Buckland T, Hing K. Increasing strut porosity in silicate-substituted calcium-phosphate bone graft substitutes enhances osteogenesis. J Biomed Mater Res B Appl Biomater. 2011;97:245–54.
32. Pearce AI, Richards RG, Milz S, Schneider E, Pearce SG. Animal models for implant biomaterial research in bone: a review. Eur Cell Mater. 2007;13:1–10.
33. Nafei A, Kabel J, Odgaard A, Linde F, Hvid I. Properties of growing trabecular ovine bone. Part II: architectural and mechanical properties. J Bone Joint Surg Br. 2000;82:921–7.
34. Kilkenny C, Browne W, Cuthill IC, Emerson M, Altman DG. Animal research: reporting in vivo experiments: the ARRIVE guidelines. Br J Pharmacol. 2010; 160:1577–9.
35. Barradas AMC, Yuan H, van Blitterswijk CA, Habibovic P. Osteoinductive biomaterials: current knowledge of properties, experimental models and biological mechanisms. Eur Cell Mater. 2011;21:407–29 discussion 429.
36. Wei L, Xue T, Yang H, Zhao G-Y, Zhang G, Lu Z-H, et al. Modified uterine allotransplantation and immunosuppression procedure in the sheep model. PLoS One. 2013;8:e81300.
37. Li Y, Cang M, Lee AS, Zhang K, Liu D. Reprogramming of sheep fibroblasts into pluripotency under a drug-inducible expression of mouse-derived defined factors. PLoS One. 2011;6:e15947.
38. Kumar D, Talluri TR, Anand T, Kues WA. Induced pluripotent stem cells: mechanisms, achievements and perspectives in farm animals. World J Stem Cells. 2015;7:315–28.

39. Donath K. Die Trenn-Dünnschliff-Technik zur Herstellung histologischer
    Präparate von nicht schneidbaren Geweben und Materialien. Der Präparator.
    1988;34:197–206.
40. Laczko J, Levai G. a simple differential staining method for semi-thin
    sections of ossifying cartilage and bone tissues embedded in epoxy resin.
    Mikroskopie. 1975;31:1–4.
41. R Core Team. R: A language and environment for statistical Computing R
    Foundation for Statistical Computing, Vienna, Austria. ISBN 3-900051-07-0,
    URL http://www.R-project.org. 2012.

Tiludronate and clodronate do not affect bone structure or remodeling kinetics over a 60 day randomized trial

Heather A. Richbourg[1,2], Colin F. Mitchell[3*], Ashley N. Gillett[2] and Margaret A. McNulty[2,4]

Abstract

Background: Tiludronate and clodronate are FDA-approved bisphosphonate drug therapies for navicular disease in horses. Although clinical studies have determined their ability to reduce lameness associated with skeletal disorders in horses, data regarding the effect on bone structure and remodeling is lacking. Additionally, due to off-label use of these drugs in young performance horses, effects on bone in young horses need to be investigated. Therefore, the purpose of this randomized, experimental pilot study was to determine the effect of tiludronate and clodronate on normal bone cells, structure and remodeling after 60 days in clinically normal, young horses. Additionally, the effect of clodronate on bone healing 60 days after an induced defect was investigated.

Results: All horses tolerated surgery well, with no post-surgery lameness and all acquired biopsies being adequate for analyses. Overall, tiludronate and clodronate did not significantly alter any bone structure or remodeling parameters, as evaluated by microCT and dynamic histomorphometry. Tiludronate did not extensively impact bone formation or resorption parameters as evaluated by static histomorphometry. Similarly, clodronate did not affect bone formation or resorption after 60 days. Sixty days post-defect, healing was minimally affected by clodronate.

Conclusions: Tiludronate and clodronate do not appear to significantly impact bone tissue on a structural or cellular level using standard dose and administration schedules.

Keywords: Horse, Bone, Bisphosphonate, Clodronate, Tiludronate, Micro-computed tomography, Histomorphometry, Biopsy

Background

Tiludronate disodium (Tildren, Ceva Animal Health LLC, Lenexa, KS, USA) and Clodronate disodium (Osphos, Dechra, Ltd., Staffordshire, UK) are bisphosphonate drugs that are licensed for use in horses to reduce lameness associated with navicular disease [1, 2]. Tiludronate and clodronate are non-nitrogen containing bisphosphonates that reduce osteoclastic bone resorption by causing osteoclast apoptosis [3]. Tiludronate has been used to treat conditions associated with bone remodeling, such as navicular disease [4, 5] and tarsal osteoarthritis [6]; however, none of these studies have evaluated the effect of tiludronate on bony tissue and have only evaluated the effects on lameness outcomes.

Clodronate is similar to tiludronate in drug properties and has been shown to have an analgesic effect by acting on glutamate and/or adenosine triphosphate-related pain transmission pathways [7]. Tiludronate has not been shown to have such analgesic properties. The Freedom of Information (FOI) Summary for both clodronate and tiludronate report on the clinical outcome in a group of horses diagnosed with navicular disease. Treated horses displayed clinical improvements in their degree of lameness; however, neither FOI Summary study discerns whether the reduction in lameness associated with either drug is due to the effect on bone remodeling, analgesic potential (specifically in regards to clodronate), or other mechanisms.

The FOI summary for clodronate describes the effects on bone mineral content, cortical bone strength and bone marrow evaluation evaluated by radiographic photometry, mechanical testing and histopathology, respectively, in

* Correspondence: cmitchel@lsu.edu
[3]Department of Veterinary Clinical Sciences, Louisiana State University School of Veterinary Medicine, Baton Rouge, LA 70803, USA
Full list of author information is available at the end of the article

normal horses. No difference were reported in these parameters between treated and saline controls at 6 months [1]. However, the methods regarding how bone density data were obtained were not stated, and given the poor sensitivity of radiographs to determine bone density [8], it is uncertain whether there was or was not a true effect on bone in this cohort. The FOI summary for tiludronate evaluated the 3rd metatarsal and metacarpal, 3rd carpal and navicular bone in 30 horses for pathological bone lesions using histopathology and found no abnormal bone tissue or resorption sites [2]. However, given the little details provided on how these assessments were performed, these outcomes may not be sensitive or reliable enough to determine bony effects.

Despite its known effect on bone remodeling rates in other species, the effect of clodronate on bone healing, especially in the horse, is unclear. In animal models, clodronate has been found to not alter endochondral bone formation within the fracture callus or epiphyseal plate of rats [9, 10]. However, reports regarding effects of clodronate are conflicting, including no changes in bone mineral density in a callus [11], 30% increase in bone mineral density [10], increased calcium content within the callus [12], and decreased healing callus strength [13]. Recently, it has been shown that osteoclasts are a necessary component of efficient endochondral ossification during fracture repair in mice [14]; therefore, it is possible that clodronate may impair normal bone healing in horses, which calls for careful consideration when used in a clinical setting.

The gold standard for bone analyses are histomorphometry [15] and micro-computed tomography (microCT) [16], both of which require bone biopsies. The tuber coxae has been reported to be the easiest site for bone biopsy acquisition in the horse [17, 18] and is a region that was found to have consistently higher levels of tiludronate in comparison to other bones [19]. A study published by the authors has shown the tuber coxae as a site to obtain reliable bony samples in a non-terminal equine model that are consistent in size and of adequate quality to evaluate trabecular bone using both histomorphometry and microCT [17].

Therefore, the purpose of this study is to evaluate the effect of clodronate and tiludronate on bone morphology, bony cells and bone remodeling in young horses. Additionally, the effect of clodronate on bone healing after an induced defect was also investigated. These evaluations were performed by obtaining bone biopsies of the tuber coxae using an established technique [17], and evaluated through histomorphometry and microCT. To evaluate bone healing, subsequent biopsies were taken from the initial biopsy site, which served as a novel bone defect model in the horse. We hypothesized that tiludronate and clodronate would reduce osteoclast number and function, resulting in increased bone volume and increased bone apposition when compared to baseline biopsies and untreated horses, as well as increased bone formation after injury in clodronate treated horses.

Methods
Study design
The experimental protocol was approved by the Louisiana State University Institutional Animal Care and Use Committee (IACUC). Nineteen Thoroughbred horses, between 2 and 5 years of age were obtained via donation to the Louisiana State University Equine Health Studies Program Herd. Medical history of the horses was unknown at the time of donation; however, all horses underwent at least a two-week isolation and washout period following donation prior to enrollment in the current study. Horses were randomly assigned, via a coin flip, to either a treatment (TIL: n = 5, CLO: n = 5) or control group (SAL: n = 9) (Table 1). Two separate studies were completed, individually assessing the impact of TIL or CLO respectively, resulting in slightly different study designs (i.e., inclusion of the re-biopsy outlined below in the CLO study). No significant differences in control groups were found, therefore they were

Table 1 Age (years), treatment and biopsies collected from study subjects. Day 0 biopsies were baseline biopsies collected on Day 0, Day 60 biopsies were collected from the contralateral side 60 days post-treatment, and Day 60R biopsies were collected from the ipsilateral side 60 days post- defect and post-treatment. Summary Information for Study Subjects

ID	Age (yrs)	Treatment	Biopsies collected
1	5	Saline	Day 0, Day 60, Day 60R
2	4	Saline	Day 0, Day 60, Day 60R
3	3	Saline	Day 0, Day 60, Day 60R
4	4	Saline	Day 0, Day 60, Day 60R
5	3	Saline	Day 0, Day 60
6	5	Saline	Day 0, Day 60
7	2	Saline	Day 0, Day 60
8	3	Saline	Day 0, Day 60
9	4	Saline	Day 0, Day 60
10	5	Tiludronate	Day 0, Day 60
11	3	Tiludronate	Day 0, Day 60
12	3	Tiludronate	Day 0, Day 60
13	5	Tiludronate	Day 0, Day 60
14	2	Tiludronate	Day 0, Day 60
15	5	Clodronate	Day 0, Day 60, Day 60R
16	4	Clodronate	Day 0, Day 60, Day 60R
17	4	Clodronate	Day 0, Day 60, Day 60R
18	3	Clodronate	Day 0, Day 60, Day 60R
19	3	Clodronate	Day 0, Day 60, Day 60R

combined into a single control group. Because this is a novel pilot study, sample sizes were calculated based on available data for tiludronate in another species using the same endpoints (microCT & histomorphometry) [20], which found that $n = 5$ was sufficient to identify bony changes. Additionally, horses served as their own control, as bilateral biopsies were taken from each animal, thereby eliminating the need for additional horses. The surgeon, who was not involved in subsequent analyses, was not masked to treatment groups.

Bone biopsies were taken from each subject; a baseline biopsy at Day 0, a contralateral biopsy 60 days post-treatment (Day 60) (Fig. 1). Additionally, a re-biopsy of the initial biopsy site was taken from clodronate-treated horses and a subset of control horses 60 days post-treatment (Day 60R). This 60-day time frame was determined based on data in previous studies that showed a positive effect of tiludronate administration on various skeletal disorders in horses 60 days post initiation of treatment [5, 6, 21]. The right or left tuber coxae was randomly selected, via coin flip, for the first biopsy (outlined below in "Surgical Procedure"). Immediately following the initial biopsy surgery (Day 0), each horse was either administered 1 L of 0.9% saline IV (tiludronate control), 1 mg/kg of tiludronate dissolved in 1 L of 0.9% saline IV, or 1.8 mg/kg of clodronate IM (dose was divided into three injection locations) or a similar volume of 0.9% saline IM (clodronate control). Saline and tiludronate were infused intravenously over 90 min using an IV fluid pump. The horses stood in the stocks during drug administration and were monitored for signs of colic. Sixty days later, the contralateral tuber coxae was biopsied in the same manner. Additionally, clodronate treated horses ($n = 5$) and half of the control horses ($n = 4$) were evaluated for bone healing after a defect. Therefore, an additional biopsy (60R Day) was obtained from these horses only by taking a re-biopsy of the initial biopsy site, 60 days post- defect (i.e., the original biopsy collection). Prior to the 60 day biopsies, oxytetracycline (Vetrimycin 100, VetOne, Boise, ID, USA) was administered at Day 47 and Day 57 as a fluorochrome label. Biopsies were evaluated with microCT and histomorphometry for changes in bone morphology and remodeling rates, as outlined below under "Biopsy handling and imaging".

Study subjects

Thoroughbred horses, as outlined above under "Study Design", were included if they were free from outward musculoskeletal disease as assessed by a boarded veterinary surgeon during a physical exam, and were between two to five years of age. A coin flip was used to randomly assign horses to a treatment group (e.g., treated or saline) and only the surgeon (CFM) knew group assignments until subsequent statistical analyses on data collected were ready to be performed. Throughout the study, they were housed in individual stalls following the biopsies and then turned out in groups in pastures. They were fed free choice hay and water, with grain being provided twice daily.

Surgical Procedure & Treatment

Horses were restrained in stocks and sedated with IV xylazine (Xylamed, Bimeda, Cambridge, ON, Canada) (0.35 to 0.5 mg/kg). The surgical method has been previously published in detail [17]. In short, the biopsy site was centered on the proximal palpable protuberance of the tuber coxae. A rectangular region (approximately 10 cm X 10 cm) was clipped around the tuber coxae and then aseptically prepared. Lidocaine (Lidocaine 2%, VetOne, Boise, ID, USA) was injected subcutaneously 4 cm proximal and distal to the palpable tuber coxae, and then deeply to the periosteum of the tuber coxae. The horse was further sedated with detomidine (Dormosedan, Zoetis, Kalamazoo, MI, USA) (3 to 5 mg IV) and butorphanol tartrate (Torbugesic, Fort Dodge, New York, NY, USA) (3 to 5 mg IV) prior to making the skin incision [17].

A vertical incision was made over the tuber coxae, and dissected to expose the cranial, caudal, proximal and axial margins. The lateral periosteum was incised using a scalpel blade, and then an oscillating saw was used to transect the proximal portion of the tuber coxae. In order to limit thermal damage, the saw blade was continuously lavaged with saline. The surgery site was lavaged, and then the subcutaneous tissue and skin were sutured separately. An aluminium based bandage spray (Aluspray, Neogen Corporation, Lexington, KY, USA) was applied to the surgery site and a lidocaine patch (Lidocaine Patch 5%, Qualitest, Huntsville, AL, USA) was then applied over the incision [17].

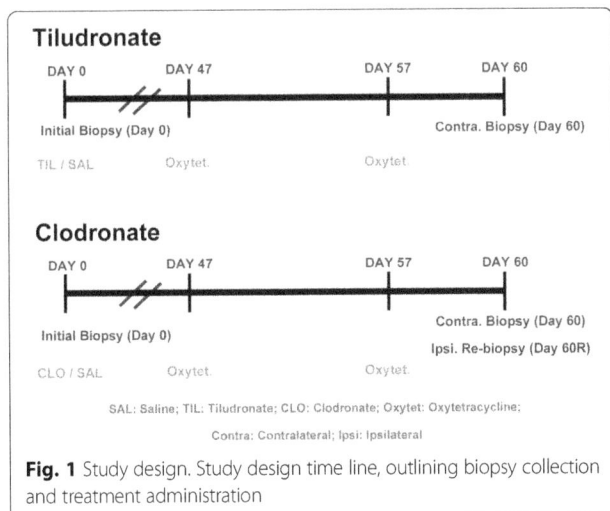

Fig. 1 Study design. Study design time line, outlining biopsy collection and treatment administration

Following the initial biopsy (Day 0 Biopsy), horses were stalled for at least 24 h and monitored every 2 h over the first 24-h period using a visual pain score [22]. After 24 h, horses were returned to their respective pastures and checked daily for signs of lameness or incisional complications until suture removal at 14 days post biopsy. At Day 47 and 57 post-biopsy, the horses were treated with 25 mg/kg of oxytetracycline administered slowly IV [17, 23]. Sixty days after the initial biopsy, the contralateral tuber coxae was biopsied (Day 60 biopsy), and the ipsilateral tuber coxae was re-biopsies in a subset of horses (Day 60R biopsy) using the same surgical methods as described above. Careful consideration was made when placing the oscillating saw for the re-biopsy (60R) to ensure an adequately-sized biopsy of the tuber coxae was obtained without cutting into the pelvis. In addition to aforementioned post-surgical care for the initial biopsy, after surgery to obtain the 60R biopsy, horses were administered flunixin meglumine (Prevail, Bimeda, Cambridge, ON, Canada) (1.1 mg/kg IV) for an additional analgesic. Surgical aftercare was then identical following this repeat biopsy to the care following the initial biopsy from the post-surgery period to 14 days later when the sutures were removed.

MicroCT

Following biopsy, tuber coxae samples were dissected free from tissue and fixed in 10% non-buffered formalin for 7 days, then transferred to and stored in 70% ethanol at 20 °C. Samples were placed in holders with 70% ethanol for scanning by microCT (Scanco model 40, Scanco Medical AG, Basserdorf, Switzerland). Biopsies were scanned at 55 kV, 0.3-s integration time, with a 30 µm voxel size in plane and a 30 µm slice thickness. MicroCT data for two Day 0 biopsies from clodronate-treated samples were not obtained because motion artifact occurred during the scan, and this issue was not identified until the samples had been decalcified for histology. The region of interest was determined for trabecular bone. The proper threshold for image segmentation was tested, with the same threshold being used throughout the experiment to ensure consistency and accuracy in measurements between samples. Trabecular bone was evaluated for bone volume (BV), total volume (TV), BV/TV, tissue mineral density, trabecular number (TbN), trabecular thickness (TbTh), trabecular separation (TbSp), connectivity density (ConnD), and structural model index (SMI) based on established procedures and nomenclature [24]. A detailed list of these parameters, including definitions, has been previously published by Bouxsein, et al. (Table 2 within reference [24]).

Histology

Following microCT evaluation, biopsies were prepared for histology. Day 0 and Day 60R biopsies were prepared for decalcified histology, and Day 60 biopsies were prepared for plastic-embedded undecalcified histology using standard methods so visualization of fluorochrome labels was possible. Due to differences in preparation techniques between decalcified and undecalcified histology, and size of slides used for each, histological preparation of both sets of biopsies differed slightly. However, care was taken to ensure sections from each biopsy were taken in the same location and plane of section, regardless of preparation method. Day 0 and Day 60R biopsies were decalcified with 10% ethylenediaminetetraacetic acid (EDTA) and prepared for routine paraffin embedding. In order to fit on glass histological slides, Day 0 biopsies were split in half and embedded separately. This resulted in 6–8, 4 µm thick sections per biopsy that were stained with hematoxylin and eosin (H&E). Day 60 biopsies were prepared intact for undecalcified histology and two, 45–60 µm thick sections were produced. The first was stained with Stevenel's Blue and Van Gieson's picrofuchsin for evaluation by static histomorphometry, and the second section was left unstained for evaluation by dynamic histomorphometry. Although histological slides for Day 0 and Day 60 biopsies were prepared differently for ease of handling, all bony features were easily discernable and comparable [25, 26] in both sets of slides, as outlined in Fig. 2.

All bone histomorphometry evaluations were performed by an individual (HAR) using histomorphometry software (Osteomeasure© Bone Histomorphometry System, Osteometrics, Inc., Decatur, GA, USA) following standard procedures and nomenclature [26]. Measurements were taken per standardized and published protocols [26]. Static histomorphometry parameters included direct measurements of: tissue area (TA), BV, marrow volume (MaV), bone perimeter (BPm), osteoblast perimeter (ObPm), bone surface (BS), eroded surface (ES), reversal surface (RevS), osteoblast number (NOb), osteoblast surface (ObS), osteoclast number (NOc), osteoclast surface (OcS). Indirect measurements included: TbN, TbTh, TbSp, and the aforementioned direct measurements standardized to respective areas and volumes. Osteoblasts and osteoclasts were identified by their unique morphologic characteristics [27, 28]. A detailed list of these parameters, including definitions, has been previously published by Dempster, et al. (Tables 3 & 5 within reference [26]). However, due to normal variation in biopsy sizes, only parameters normalized to areas and volumes were evaluated statistically. Dynamic histomorphometry included mineralizing surface per bone surface (MS/BS), mineral apposition rate (MAR) and the bone formation rate per total volume (BFR/TV). A detailed

Table 2 Summary data (mean ± SD) of bone structure and remodeling parameters from Day 0, Day 60 and Day 60R biopsies for micro-computed tomography (MicroCT), static and dynamic histomorphometry (histo) analyses. Groups are separated based on treatment received

Saline

MicroCT	Day 0 (n = 9)	Day 60 (n = 9)	Day 60R (n = 4)	Static histomorphometry	Day 0 (n = 9)	Day 60 (n = 9)	Day 60R (n = 9)	Dynamic histomorphometry	Day 60 (n = 9)
BV/TV (%)	29.4 ± 5.0	32.0 ± 6.4	35.7 ± 17.1	BV/TV (%)	29.6 ± 10.9	24.7 ± 10.6	33.0 ± 15.7	sLS/BS (%)	26.2 ± 5.4
TbTh (mm)	0.16 ± 0.02	0.17 ± 0.02	0.20 ± 0.07	ES/BS (%)	1.96 ± 2.55[a]	0.19 ± 0.17[b]	0.12 ± 0.05[a]	dLS/BS (%)	4.21 ± 2.17
TbN (/mm)	1.73 ± 0.22	1.72 ± 0.28	1.9 ± 0.4	NOb/TA (/mm²)	75.9 ± 58.1	63.6 ± 27.0[c]	72.5 ± 22.1	MAR (μm/d)	1.16 ± 0.23
ConnD (/mm³)	7.84 ± 1.88	7.90 ± 2.79	9.1 ± 3.4	NOc/TA (/mm²)	0.45 ± 0.38	0.01 ± 0.02	1.00 ± 0.75	BFR/TV (%/yr)	26.2 ± 7.4

Tiludronate

MicroCT	Day 0 (n = 5)	Day 60 (n = 5)	Static Histo	Day 0 (n = 5)	Day 60 (n = 5)	Dynamic Histo	Day 60 (n = 5)
BV/TV (%)	28.1 ± 3.9	31.1 ± 5.0	BV/TV (%)	24.1 ± 7.2	30.8 ± 6.8	sLS/BS (%)	24.4 ± 7.0
TbTh (mm)	0.16 ± 0.01	0.16 ± 0.02	ES/BS (%)	2.86 ± 1.38	1.49 ± 0.65[b]	dLS/BS (%)	6.33 ± 4.59
TbN (/mm)	1.65 ± 0.17	1.81 ± 0.24	NOb/TA (/mm²)	29.7 ± 17.6	17.8 ± 11.3[c]	MAR (μm/d)	1.16 ± 0.21
ConnD (/mm³)	7.46 ± 1.28	9.39 ± 3.17	NOc/TA (/mm²)	0.61 ± 0.41	0.06 ± 0.11	BFR/TV (%/yr)	29.8 ± 12.6

Clodronate

MicroCT	Day 0 (n = 3)	Day 60 (n = 5)	Day 60R (n = 5)	Static Histo	Day 0 (n = 5)	Day 60 (n = 5)	Day 60R (n = 5)	Dynamic Histo	Day 60 (n = 5)
BV/TV (%)	32.3 ± 3.6	31.7 ± 2.9	39.2 ± 10.6	BV/TV (%)	30.7 ± 3.9	23.4 ± 4.8	34.5 ± 9.4	sLS/BS (%)	28.4 ± 19.0
TbTh (mm)	0.15 ± 0.02	0.16 ± 0.01	0.20 ± 0.04	ES/BS (%)	0.02 ± 0.03[d]	0.14 ± 0.13	0.13 ± 0.06[d]	dLS/BS (%)	4.3 ± 4.6
TbN (/mm)	1.95 ± 0.11	1.87 ± 0.18	2.22 ± 0.25	NOb/TA (/mm²)	88.3 ± 32.5	49.6 ± 16.0	63.4 ± 17.6	MAR (μm/d)	1.02 ± 0.29
ConnD (/mm³)	9.75 ± 1.02	8.85 ± 1.80	13.50 ± 2.96	NOc/TA (/mm²)	0.44 ± 0.61	0.04 ± 0.05	0.84 ± 0.40	BFR/TV (%/yr)	25.5 ± 15.2

Abbreviations: BV/TV, bone volume per total volume; TbTh, trabecular thickness; TbN trabecular number; ConnD, connectivity density; ES/BS, eroded surface per bone surface; NOb/TA, number of osteoblasts per tissue area; NOc/TA, number of osteoclasts per tissue area; sLS/BS, single label surface per bone surface; dLS/BS, double label surface per bone surface; MAR, mineral apposition rate; BFR/TV, bone formation rate per total volume

Superscripts designate a significant difference of $P < 0.05$ between the same letters. Summary of bone analyses for treatment groups

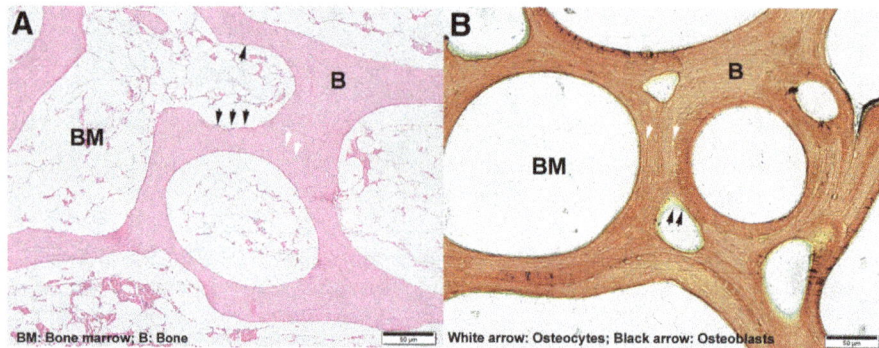

Fig. 2 Overview of bony features for different histological preparations. Representative histologic sections of (**a**) decalcified Day 0 biopsy and (**b**) un-decalcified Day 60 biopsy, highlighting similar trabecular bone features. Abbreviations: B, bone; BM, bone marrow. Black arrows = osteoblasts; white arrows = osteocytes

list of these parameters, including definitions, has been previously published by Dempster, et al (Tables 4 & 5 within reference [26]).

Statistics

Data were tested for normality using the Shapiro-Wilk test, and depending on normality, either parametric or non-parametric analyses were used. If data were parametric, microCT and histomorphometry data were analyzed using one-way ANOVA analysis to determine the effect of treatment within Day 0 or Day 60 biopsy. If significance was found, a Tukey post-hoc analysis was evaluated. If data were nonparametric, microCT and histomorphometry data was analyzed using an Independent Samples Mann-Whitney U Test, comparing TIL or CLO to SAL. A Student's t-test was performed to determine the effect of clodronate on bone healing parameters, comparing CLO to SAL within Day 60R biopsy. Additionally, a related-sample test was used to evaluate changes from Day 0 biopsy to Day 60R biopsy, within the SAL or CLO horses. Statistical analyses were performed using commercially-available software (SPSS, version 22, IBM Corporation, Armonk, NY, USA), and p-values of < 0.05 were considered significant. Due to the aforementioned issues with obtaining microCT data from two Day 0 biopsies, all data from those horses were excluded from dependent analyses.

Results

Surgical technique

All surgeries were successful in obtaining adequately sized bone biopsies during each attempt, with only one horse experiencing incisional dehiscence. However, this complication resolved with minimal medical intervention. No horses displayed any rear limb lameness or ratable discomfort at any time over the duration of this study. Day 0, Day 60 and Day 60R biopsies had a mean

($\pm$ SD) volume of 1632 ± 785, 1347 ± 622 and 1080 ± 646 mm^3, respectively.

Bone morphology

Select results are outlined in Table 2. When comparing microCT data between three treatment (saline, clodronate, tiludronate) groups within Day 0 biopsy or within Day 60 biopsy, there was no significant effect of treatment on any of the 19 bone morphology parameters as evaluated by microCT. Similarly, there were no significant changes in bone morphology parameters between Day 0 and Day 60 biopsies within treated horses as evaluated by microCT. However, when evaluating bone morphology using static histomorphometry, TIL-treated horses had a significant increase in BS/TV after 60 days when compared to control ($p = 0.02$).

Cellular structure

Select results are outlined in Table 2. There were minor differences when evaluating bone formation parameters. When comparing TIL-treated horses to control horses within the Day 60 biopsy, there was a significant decrease in NOb/TA ($p = 0.004$) and NOb/BPm ($p = 0.003$), and a significant increase in NOb/ObPm ($p < 0.000$). When making the similar comparison within Day 60 biopsy, CLO-treated horses did not have significantly different bone formation parameters when compared to control. Overall, TIL significantly altered three of four normalized bone formation parameters, while CLO did not have an effect.

There were also minor differences when evaluating bone resorption parameters. When comparing TIL-treated horses to control horses, there was a significant increase in ES/BS ($p = 0.001$) and RevS/BS (p = 0.001) after 60 days. There were no significant changes in bone resorption parameters within CLO-treated horses compared to control horses after 60 days. Overall, TIL significantly altered two of six normalized bone resorption parameters, while CLO did not have an effect.

Bone remodeling kinetics

Select results are outlined in Table 2. After 60 days, there was no effect of either treatment on any of the 14 bone remodeling parameters evaluated via dynamic histomorphometry.

Bone healing

When comparing CLO-treated horses to control horses within the Day 60R biopsy, there was no significant effect on any of the 19 bone morphology parameters, as evaluated by microCT (Table 2). When comparing changes from baseline biopsy to Day 60R biopsy within CLO-treated and SAL-treated horses, there were no significant differences in any of the 19 bone morphology parameters evaluated via microCT. Comparing CLO-treated horses to control horses within the Day 60R biopsy using histomorphometry, treated horses had significantly higher BS/TV ($p = 0.02$) and TbN (p = 0.02). However, as outlined above, these results were not confirmed with microCT analyses, and overall, this accounts for two out of 20 bone morphology parameters that were significantly affected.

When evaluating changes from baseline to Day 60R within CLO-treated horses, there was significantly higher ES/BS ($p = 0.03$), as evaluated by static histomorphometry. However, the same effect was seen in the control horses after 60 days (ES/BS; $p = 0.049$). Comparing CLO-treated horses to control horses within the Day 60R biopsy, CLO-treated horses had significantly less ObS/BS (p = 0.04). Overall, this accounts for one of four bone formation parameters, with no bone resorption parameters affected.

While few significant changes were identified in bone morphology parameters following re-biopsy in the control horses, there were areas identified within the re-biopsy samples that clearly demonstrated reconstitution and maturation of trabecular structure (Fig. 3). This indicates that the Day 60R samples were composed at least in part of non-native bone.

Discussion

This report describes the effect of a single administration, consistent with clinical dosages and administration, of tiludronate or clodronate on bony cells, trabecular bone morphology, bone remodeling, and bone regeneration in ten healthy, young horses. A previous study utilizing a bone biopsy model attempted to elucidate changes in bone morphology secondary to tiludronate treatment in horses [19]. Unfortunately, the samples obtained in that study were inadequate for evaluation of bone morphology and remodeling; therefore, the current study provides these missing data, and includes preliminary data demonstrating no effect on bone regeneration following re-biopsy of the original biopsy site. Additionally, there have been no studies attempting to evaluate the effect of clodronate, despite its prolific use in veterinary clinics. A barrier to the veterinary field is that there is currently no data regarding whether tiludronate or clodronate affects bone remodeling in the horse at the recommended dosage and route of administration. Therefore, the current study provides these preliminary data indicating that there may be little to no effect on bone remodeling at this timepoint. To our knowledge, this is also the first study evaluating the cellular and structural effect of tiludronate and clodronate in horses of any age, as no published studies have evaluated these changes in either skeletally mature or immature horses. There were no significant effects of tiludronate or clodronate on bony cells or bone structure and remodeling parameters after 60 days in young horses, nor any significant differences in treatment groups following

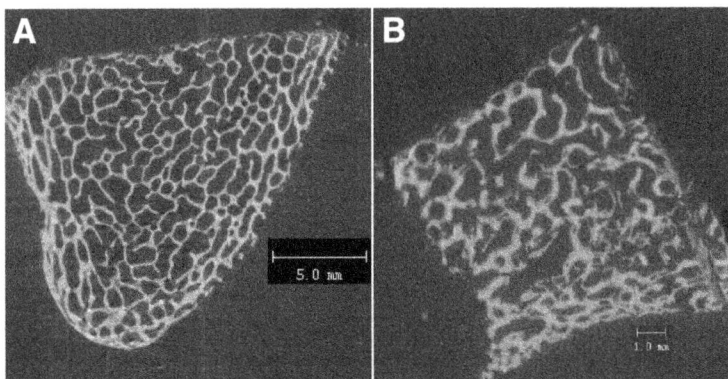

Fig. 3 MicroCT slices demonstrating morphological evidence of trabecular remodeling. Two dimensional microCT slices representing a 30 μm thick section of an original biopsy (**a**) and re-biopsy (**b**) from the tuber coxae. Evidence of reconstitution and maturation of the trabecular structure is evident in (**b**), indicating active bone remodeling following the original biopsy

induction of an injury (re-biopsy of the original biopsy site). Treatment success in the previous study [1] may have been based on clodronate's pain-minimizing properties, and not due to changes in bone remodeling. This would explain the treatment success demonstrated in that clinical trial [1], but support the lack of bony changes shown in this study.

Overall, there were no effects on bone resorption or bone remodeling kinetics, and only slight alterations in bone formation parameters. Bisphosphonates, in general, are widely known to affect bone remodeling kinetics, specifically suppressing bone remodeling, as measured by dynamic histomorphometry using fluorochrome labeling [29]. In the present study, there were bone morphology changes found during static histomorphometric evaluations that were not confirmed in microCT results. Therefore, they were not considered in overall conclusions, as microCT is a 3D measurement that accounts for the entire biopsy, and has greater sensitivity to bony measurements [24] when compared to histomorphometry. Additionally, when considering only a couple of bone formation parameters were affected out of over 20 parameters evaluated, including both directly measured and calculated, the minor changes to bone formation in the TIL-treated group is not considered a significant conclusion.

A limitation of the current study is a low sample size of 5 horses per group; therefore, it is possible that a small effect of tiludronate or clodronate on bone remodeling and structure may not have been apparent, or that the minor changes in bone formation parameters may indicate true changes that would be more apparent using a larger study population. However, it is well known that bisphosphonates are powerful modifiers of the bone remodeling process, including in normal bone [30]. Therefore, it was hypothesized that if there were a systemic effect of tiludronate or clodronate administration in the horse at the routine clinical dose administered, it would have been detected in the current study. In addition, a recent study evaluating the effect of the bone resorption inhibitor cathepsin K, which does not fully prevent osteoclastic resorption as bisphosphonates have been shown to do [31], was performed with groups of 6 horses, with significant differences found [32]. Therefore, we conclude that the lack of changes identified in the current study, especially related to the re-biopsy results and effects on a model of bone healing, are truly reflective of an overall lack of influence of these drugs on bone remodeling kinetics in the horse. The authors are currently unsure of why a lack of effect was found in these studies, and if horses have a different response to these drugs than other species. Ongoing work is being conducted to evaluate the effectiveness of these drugs to bind to equine bone and the effect on the tissue and bony cells in vitro. In addition, we are exploring whether more modern bisphosphonates and/or other drugs used to modify bone remodeling in other species have an effect in the horse.

It is possible that the time frame (60 days) evaluated in this study was not appropriate to evaluate overall changes in bone remodeling. As outlined in the methods, this time frame was selected based on the only published data regarding the effect of tiludronate and clodronate on horses, which found significant clinical improvements in horses diagnosed with navicular disease, distal tarsal osteoarthritis and osteoarthritis in the axial skeleton after 60 days [1, 2, 5, 6, 21]. In addition, a study evaluating bone remodeling in horses following treatment with phenylbutazone, which, unlike tiludronate, is not utilized as a treatment for diseases of bone remodeling, found significant changes in MAR using similar sample sizes after only 30 days [33]. Therefore, it would be expected that normal bone apposition rates in horses should be affected by tiludronate and clodronate within the study timeframe. However, future studies including additional time points post-treatment would be required to confirm whether tiludronate or clodronate has a significant impact on bone morphology. Similar work would need to be done to fully characterize intramembranous and/or endochondral bone regeneration and remodeling process following injury (i.e., re-biopsy) at this location in order to determine an optimal time point to evaluate potential effects of these drugs on bone regeneration in the horse. As such, more recent data evaluating effectiveness of tiludronate administration on lameness associated with navicular disease as evaluated by more objective force platform analyses found significant improvements 120 and 200 days post treatment, but not after 60 days [4]. Ideally, the studies presented herein would be based on known timeframes regarding bone remodeling kinetics in the horse as opposed to strictly clinical outcomes data; however, the authors are not aware such data exists.

Tiludronate and clodronate therapies are widely used in the clinical setting to treat disorders involving abnormal bone remodeling, including distal tarsal joint osteoarthritis [6], thoracic & lumbar vertebral arthritis [21], and dorsal metacarpal disease [34]. Evaluations of tiludronate on skeletally immature rats and baboons has been reported [35, 36], and showed a reduction of trabecular bone resorption adjacent to growth plates and increased bone density. Tiludronate and clodronate have been previously evaluated for pathological bone changes in horses aged 4 years and older [1, 2]; however, clinicians are administrating these drugs to horses that are younger than 4 years of age, including off-label use for treatment of dorsal metacarpal disease [34]. It is well known that younger horses undergo more rapid bone remodeling than skeletally mature adults [37], and these differences would be reflected in the chosen biopsy site, so this study aimed to also evaluate the effect of tiludronate and clodronate administration in young horses, where negative impacts on normal bone remodeling could result in detrimental clinical outcomes in young equine athletes. As outlined above, we saw minimal, if any, influence on bone remodeling or morphology in this young population, and we would hypothesize to see similar results in skeletally mature horses. However, due to the smaller sample size for each age included the study and the known effect of age on bone remodeling parameters, there cannot be definitive conclusions based on age. In addition to a larger number of subjects, a smaller range of ages in subjects may have resulted in a significant effect in other bone morphology parameters.

The iliac biopsy location utilized in the study was chosen for multiple reasons. First, it has been shown that bisphosphonates accumulate at the highest density in the tuber coxae when compared to the 3rd metacarpal, rib, and fourth tarsal bone in the horse [19]. Secondly, it is an easily accessible location that allowed for a non-terminal model. Thirdly, it has been shown that the tuber coxae accurately predicts the effect of alendronate, another form of bisphosphonate, on non-homogenous skeletal locations in the body (i.e., vertebral column) [38]. Bisphosphonates have been repeatedly shown to have systemic effects on bone [39], especially trabecular bone [40], so it can be reasonably argued that any changes that would occur secondary to treatment with clodronate would be identified in the selected biopsy location. The anatomical location of the biopsy does have a few limitations, including the lack of compressive forces upon it as one would see in bony tissue of the distal limb; however, the benefits of this biopsy method (e.g., ease of obtaining a sample, large size, presence of both trabecular and cortical bone) far outweigh the negatives [17]. However, care must also be taken when evaluating the re-biopsy results, as this model is novel and the exact timeline of intramembranous and/or endochondral ossification at this location in the horse has yet to be explored in detail. The morphology of the samples (Fig. 3) indicates that at least part of the re-biopsies contained non-native bone and therefore would have been subjected to extensive remodeling during the study timeframe. Given the relatively large biopsy size, this study was able to utilize multiple study endpoints, including both static and dynamic histomorphometry. The second biopsy was prepared for un-decalcified histology in order to preserve the fluorescent label, which required different preparation than the initial biopsy received. Although preparation methods varied, methods of analyses and outcome measures were identical for both preparation methods of static histomorphometry sections [26]. In addition, recent work has identified that outcomes of evaluations of bony tissue and cells do not differ between the two preparation techniques [25].

Conclusions

In conclusion, this study utilized several established methods to evaluate bone morphology and remodeling secondary to treatment with either tiludronate or clodronate from a non-terminal bone biopsy method of the equine tuber coxae. These data demonstrate that tiludronate and clodronate do not have a substantial impact on normal bone remodeling kinetics, morphology or bony cells in young horses 60 days post-treatment. With the lack of alteration of any expected bone remodeling parameters in these horses, the authors are unsure if clinical improvement in lameness is due to effects on bone remodeling or the analgesic effect of clodronate or other effects secondary to bisphosphonate administration in the horse. More studies are warranted to further explore these negative findings, including the investigation of clinically diseased horses.

Abbreviations
AAEP: American Association of Equine Practitioner; BFR: Bone formation rate; BPm: Bone perimeter; BS: Bone surface; BV: Bone volume; CLO: Clodronate; ConnD: Connectivity density; dLS: Double label surface; EDTA: Ethylenediaminetetraacetic acid; ER: Eroded surface; FOI: Freedom of Information; H&E: Hematoxylin and eosin; IACUC: Institutional Animal Care and Use Committee; IM: Intramuscular; IV: Intraveneous; MAR: Mineral apposition rate; MaV: Marrow volume; microCT: Micro-computed tomography; NOb: Osteoblast number; NOc: Osteoclast number; ObPm: Osteoblast perimeter; ObS: Osteoblast surface; OcS: Osteoclast surface; RevS: Reversal surface; SAL: Saline; sLS: Single label surface; SMI: Structural model index; TA: Tissue area; TbN: Trabecular number; TbSp: Trabecular separation; TbTh: Trabecular thickness; TIL: Tiludronate; TV: Total volume

Acknowledgements
We would like to thank the Hard Tissue Research Laboratory at the University of Minnesota School of Dentistry and Dr. Cathy Carlson and her laboratory at the University of Minnesota College of Veterinary Medicine for performing histological preparations. We would also like to thank the hospital technicians and veterinary students of the Louisiana State University School of Veterinary Medicine for their assistance in biopsy collections.

Funding
Funding for this study was provided by the Louisiana State University Equine Health Studies Program.

Authors' contributions
HAR performed surgical procedures, data analysis, interpretation, preparation of the manuscript and gave final approval of the manuscript. CFM contributed to the study design, surgical procedures, data analysis, preparation of manuscript and gave final approval of the manuscript. ANG contributed to data analysis and gave final approval of the manuscript. MAM contributed to the study design, data analysis, interpretation, preparation of manuscript and gave final approval of the manuscript.

Consent for publication

Not applicable

Competing interests

The authors declare that they have no competing interests.

Author details

[1]Department of Orthopaedic Surgery, University of California San Francisco, San Francisco, CA, USA. [2]Department of Comparative Biomedical Sciences, Louisiana State University School of Veterinary Medicine, Baton Rouge, LA, USA. [3]Department of Veterinary Clinical Sciences, Louisiana State University School of Veterinary Medicine, Baton Rouge, LA 70803, USA. [4]Department of Anatomy and Cell Biology, Indiana University School of Medicine, Indianapolis, IN, USA.

References

1. Freedom of Information Summary: For the control of clinical signs associated with navicular syndrome in horses. [https://animaldrugsatfda.fda.gov/adafda/app/search/public/document/downloadFoi/923].

2. Freedom of Information Summary: For the control of clinical signs associated with navicular syndrome in horses [https://animaldrugsatfda.fda.gov/adafda/app/search/public/document/downloadFoi/918].

3. Lehenkari PP, Kellinsalmi M, Näpänkangas JP, Ylitalo KV, Mönkkönen J, Rogers MJ, Azhayev A, Väänänen KH, Hassinen IE. Further insight into mechanism of action of clodronate: inhibition of mitochondrial ADP/ATP translocase by a nonhydrolyzable, adenine-containing metabolite. Mol Pharmacol. 2002;61(5):1255–62.

4. Whitfield CT, Schoonover MJ, Holbrook TC, Payton ME, Sippel KM. Quantitative assessment of two methods of tiludronate administration for the treatment of lameness caused by navicular syndrome in horses. Am J Vet Res. 2016;77(2):167–73.

5. Denoix JM, Thibaud D, Riccio B. Tiludronate as a new therapeutic agent in the treatment of navicular disease: a double-blind placebo-controlled clinical trial. Equine Vet J. 2003;34(4):407–13.

6. Gough MR, Thibaud D, Smith RKW. Tiludronate infusion in the treatment of bone spavin: a double blind placebo-controlled trial. Equine Vet J. 2010;42(5):381–7.

7. Shima K, Nemoto W, Tsuchiya M, Tan-No K, Takano-Yamamoto T, Sugawara S, Endo Y. The bisphosphonates Clodronate and Etidronate exert analgesic effects by acting on glutamate- and/or ATP-related pain transmission pathways. Biol Pharm Bull. 2016;39(5):770–7.

8. Moyad MA. Osteoporosis: a rapid review of risk factors and screening methods. Urol Oncol. 2003;21:375–9.

9. Nyman MT, Gao T, Lindholm TC. Healing of a tibial double osteotomy is modified by clodronate administration. Arch Orthop Trauma Surg. 1996;115:111–4.

10. Madsen JE, Berg-larsen T, Kirkeby OJ, Falch JA, Nordsletten L. No adverse effects of clodronate on fracture healing in rats. Acta Orthop Scand. 1998;69(5):532–6.

11. Koivukangas A, Tuukkanen J, Kippo K, Jamsa T, Hannuniemi R, Pasanen I, Vaananen K, Jalovaara P. Long-term administration of clodronate does not prevent fracture healing in rats. Clin Orthop Relat Res. 2003;408:268–78.

12. Nyman MT, Paavolainen P, Lindholm TS. Clodronate increases the calcium content in fracture callus. An experimental study in rats. Arch Orthop Trauma Surg. 1993;112(5):228–31.

13. Tarvainen R, Olkkonen H, Nevalainen T, Hyvonen P, Arnala I, Alhava E. Effect of clodronate on fracture healing in denervated rats. Bone. 1994;15(6):701–5.

14. Lin HN, O' Connor JP. Osteoclast depletion with clodronate liposomes delays fracture healing in mice. J Orthop Res. 2017;35(8):1699–706.

15. Müller R, Campenhout VH, Damme VB, Perre GVD, Dequeker J, Hildebrand T, Ruegsegger P. Morphometric analysis of human bone biopsies: a quantitative structural comparison of histological sections and micro-computed tomography. Bone. 1998;23(1):59–66.

16. MacNeil JA, Boyd SK. Accuracy of high-resolution peripheral quantitative computed tomography for measurement of bone quality. Med Eng Phys. 2007;29:1096–105.

17. Mitchell CF, Richbourg HA, Goupil BA, Gillett AN, McNulty MA. Assessment of tuber coxae bone biopsy in the standing horse. Vet Surg. 2017;46(3):396–402.

18. Steiger RH, Geyer H, Provencher A, Perron-Lepage MF, von Salis B, Lepage OM. Equine bone core biopsy: evaluation of collection sites using a new electric drilling machine. Equine Practice. 1999;21:14–21.

19. Delguste C, Doucet M, Gabriel A, Guyonnet J, Lepage OM, Amory H. Assessment of a bone biopsy technique for measuring tiludronate in horses: a preliminary study. Can J Vet Res. 2011;75(2):128–33.

20. Barou O, Lafage-Proust MH, Martel C, Thomas T, Tirode F, Laroche N, Barbier A, Alexandre C, Vico L. Bisphosphonate effects in rat unloaded hindlimb bone loss model: three-dimensional microcomputed tomographic, histomorphometric, and densitometric analyses. J Pharmacol Exp Ther. 1999;291(1):321–8.

21. Coudry V, Thibaud D, Riccio B, Audigié F, Didierlaurent D, Denoix J-M. Efficacy of tiludronate in the treatment of horses with signs of pain associated with osteoarthritic lesions of the thoracolumbar vertebral column. Am J Vet Res. 2007;68(3):329–37.

22. Wilson DV. Recognition of pain. In: Doherty T, Valverde A, editors. Manual of Equine Anesthesia and Analgesia. Iowa: Wiley; 2008. p.300–02.

23. Jenner F, Kirker-Head C. Core decompression of the equine navicular bone: an in vivo study in healthy horses. Vet Surg. 2011;40(2):151–62.

24. Bouxsein ML, Boyd SK, Christiansen BA, Guldberg RE, Jepsen KJ, Müller R. Guidelines for assessment of bone microstructure in rodents using micro-computed tomography. J Bone Min Res. 2010;25(7):1468–86.

25. Sangchay N, Felts P, Cunningham C. A comparison of histomorphometric parameters in decalcified and non-decalcified porcine and bovine bone. J Anat. 2017; In press

26. Dempster DW, Compston JE, Drezner MK, Glorieux FH, Kanis JA, Malluche H, Meunier PJ, Ott SM, Recker RR, Parfitt AM. Standardized nomenclature, symbols, and units for bone histomorphometry: a 2012 update of the report of the ASBMR Histomorphometry nomenclature committee. J Bone Miner Res. 2013;28(1):1–16.

27. Florencio-Silva R, GRdS S, Sasso-Cerri E, Simões MJ, Cerri PS. Biology of bone tissue: structure, function, and factors that influence bone cells. Biomed Res Int. 2015;2015:421746.

28. Nakamura H. Morphology, function, and differentiation of bone cells. J Hard Tissue Biol. 2007;16(1):15–22.

29. Allen MR, Burr DB. Bisphosphonate effects on bone turnover, microdamage, and mechanical properties: what we think we know and what we know that we don't know. Bone. 2011;49(1):56–65.

30. Mashiba T, Mori S, Burr DB, Komatsubara S, Cao Y, Manabe T, Norimatsu H. The effects of suppressed bone remodeling by bisphosphonates on microdamage accumulation and degree of mineralization in the cortical bone of dog rib. J Bone Miner Metab. 2005;23(1):36–42.

31. Duong LT. Therapeutic inhibition of cathepsin K-reducing bone resorption while maintaining bone formation. Bonekey Rep. 2012;1:67. https://doi.org/10.1038/bonekey.2012.67.

32. Hussein I, Dulin J, Smanik L, Drost W, Russell D, Wellman M, Bertone A. Repeated oral administration of a cathepsin K inhibitor significantly suppresses bone resorption in exercising horses with evidence of increased bone formation and maintained bone turnover. J Vet Pharmacol Ther. 2016;40(4):327–34.

33. Rhode C, Anderson DE, Bertone AL, Weisbrode SE. Effects of phenylbutazone on bone activity and formation in horses. Am J Vet Res. 2000;61(5):537–43.

34. Carpenter R. How to treat dorsal metacarpal disease with regional tiludronate and extracorporeal shock wave therapies in thoroughbred racehorses. In: AAEP Annual Convention. 2012;2012:546–9.

35. Geusens P, Nijs J, Van der Perre G, Van Audekercke R, Lowet G, Goovaerts S, Barbier A, Lacheretz F, Remandet B, Jiang Y. Longitudinal effect of tiludronate on bone mineral density, resonant frequency, and strength in monkeys. J Bone Min Res. 1992;7(6):599–609.

36. Murakami H, Nakamura T, Tsurukami H, Abe M, Barbier A, Suzuki K. Effects of tiludronate on bone mass, structure, and turnover at the epiphyseal, primary, and secondary spongiosa in the proximal tibia of growing rats after sciatic neurectomy. J Bone Miner Res. 1994;9(9):1355–64.

37. Goyal H, MacCallum F, Brown M, Delack J. Growth rates at the extremities of limb bones in young horses. Can Vet J. 1981;22(2):31.

38. Mashiba T, Hui S, Turner CH, Mori S, Johnston CC, Burr DB. Bone remodeling at the iliac crest can predict the changes in remodeling dynamics, Microdamage accumulation, and mechanical properties in the lumbar vertebrae of dogs. Calcif Tissue Int. 2005;77(3):180–5.

39. Drake MT, Cremers S. Bisphosphonate therapeutics in bone disease: the hard and soft data on osteoclast inhibition. Mol Interv. 2010;10(3):141.

Comparison of three imaging modalities used to evaluate bone healing after tibial tuberosity advancement in cranial cruciate ligament-deficient dogs and comparison of the effect of a gelatinous matrix and a demineralized bone matrix mix on bone healing

Marije Risselada[1,2]*[iD], Matthew D. Winter[1], Daniel D. Lewis[1], Emily Griffith[3] and Antonio Pozzi[1,4]

Abstract

Background: Bone healing and assessment of the state of bone bridging is an important part of clinical orthopedics, whether for fracture healing or for follow up of osteotomy procedures. Tibial tuberosity advancement (TTA) is designed to restore stability in cruciate deficient stifle joints by advancing the tuberosity while creating an osteotomy gap. The current study aims to: 1) compare three different imaging modalities to assess bone healing: ultrasound, radiographs and computed tomography (CT) and, to 2) compare the effect of a gelatinous matrix (GM) versus a demineralized bone matrix mix (DBM mix) on bone healing and bridging of this osteotomy gap in 10 otherwise healthy client-owned dogs with cranial cruciate ligament insufficiency. Osseous union of the osteotomy gap was evaluated with ultrasound, radiographs and CT at one, two, and 3 months postoperatively. Dogs were randomly selected to receive GM or DBM mix to fill the osteotomy gap created during the TTA procedure. Bone healing was assessed subjectively on all modalities as well as scored on radiographs and measured using Hounsfield units (HUs) on CT. Time to heal based on ultrasound, radiographs and CT were statistically compared between groups with significance set at $p < 0.05$.

(Continued on next page)

* Correspondence: mrissela@purdue.edu
[1]Department of Small Animal Clinical Sciences, College of Veterinary Medicine, University of Florida, Gainesville, FL 32610-0126, USA
[2]Present address: Department of Veterinary Clinical Sciences, College of Veterinary Medicine, Purdue University, Lynn Hall, 625 Harrison Street, West Lafayette, IN 47907, USA
Full list of author information is available at the end of the article

(Continued from previous page)

Results: All osteotomy gaps were bridged with bone within 3 months for all modalities. Bridging bone was diagnosed in 5.6 weeks, 10.4 weeks and 9.6 weeks based on ultrasound, radiographs, and CT, respectively, in dogs treated with DBM mix. In dogs treated with GM osseous union was diagnosed in a mean of 4.0 weeks, 9.6 weeks and 7.2 weeks based on ultrasound, radiographs and CT. Ultrasound diagnosed osseous union significantly faster than both CT and radiographs ($p < 0.001$). The dimensions of the newly formed bone differed between treatment groups with the central portion of the bone only providing a small bridge in GM cases. Although bridging of the osteotomy gap occurred earlier in the group that received GM, no significant statistical difference was found between the two groups.

Conclusions: Radiographs overestimate the time needed for osseous union of the osteotomy gap. All osteotomy sites healed radiographically within 3 months.

Keywords: Osteotomy, Bone healing, Ultrasound, CT, TTA

Background

The tibial tuberosity advancement (TTA) procedure aims to restore stability in the cranial cruciate ligament deficient stifle by advancing the patellar ligament cranially. The resulting decrease in patellar tendon angle causes a caudal shift in the femorotibial shear force, which has been shown to eliminate the cranial subluxation of the tibia in cadaveric ex vivo models [1, 2]. Clinically the TTA procedure has gained acceptance as a surgical option to address stifle instability in cranial cruciate ligament-deficient stifles, and the efficacy of this procedure has been documented in several studies [3–8]. During the TTA (Kyon, Technopark-strasse 1, Zurich, Switzerland) procedure, a cage ranging in size from three to 15 mm is inserted to maintain the tibial tuberosity in the advanced position. This advancement creates a wedge shaped osteotomy gap. Recommendations for managing the gap caused by cranial advancement of the tibial tuberosity include filling the osseous defect with autogenous cancellous bone [3–5, 9] or allogenic bone graft substitutes such as demineralized bone matrix mixed with allogenic corticocancellous bone (DBM mix: Freeze dried Cancellous Demineralized Standard mix ($1cm^3$) Veterinary Transplant Services, Inc. (Kent WA, USA)) [3]. Use of a cancellous bovine bone graft material (bovine xenoimplant) has been recently described [9]. Other authors have suggested that filling the gap with autologous cancellous bone or suitable graft substitute may not be necessary [8, 10, 11]. At the time of this study gelatinous matrix (GM)(TRMatrix™, IMEX™ Veterinary Inc., Longview, TX) was a commercially available bone graft substitute that resembles tertiary embryonic connective tissue. This material was purported to have osteopromotive properties [12, 13] but the clinical efficacy of this GM has not been previously described in a case series or prospective study. It is currently not available for purchase, and was discontinued for the veterinary market due to limited volume [14].

Traditionally, radiographs have been used to assess bone formation following fracture repair or osteotomy procedures [1, 3–6, 8–11]. Several definitions of radiographic union have been reported, generally using cortical bridging as an indication for a healed osteotomy [8–11]. Other imaging modalities available to assess bone healing include ultrasonography (US) [15–17] and computed tomography (CT) [18, 19]. Ultrasonography has been used to detect (occult) fractures, evaluate bone production in limb-lengthening procedures and to evaluate fracture healing [15–17, 20–26]. Based on several studies, US detects tissue bridging earlier than radiography [15–17, 20–26]. Ultrasonographic union has been defined as a complete hyperoechic bridge with acoustic shadowing and validated using histology [15–17]. Although CT is rarely used to diagnose fracture healing with only two prospective studies published [18], it has been extensively used to follow up bone osteogenesis [27–30]. Furthermore, it can quantify bone healing by measuring Hounsfield units (HUs) [19, 27], which could make it an excellent method to evaluate an osteotomy union objectively. The current study was designed to compare utility of these three different imaging modalities for assessing new bone formation in a standardized clinical osteotomy gap model. Our first objective was to compare the time to osteotomy union using US, radiography and CT based on previously reported definitions of union [8–11, 15–18]. As a second objective, we wanted to compare the osseous response induced by placing two different bone graft subsites in the TTA osteotomy site. Our hypotheses were that: 1) all osteotomy gaps would be bridged by bone based on all three imaging modalities by the end of the study (3 months), 2) US would substantiate osteotomy union earlier than the other two imaging modalities, and that 3) GM would promote faster healing than DBM mix.

Methods

Animals

Ten healthy middle aged, medium or large breed client owned dogs with naturally occurring unilateral cranial cruciate ligament insufficiency were enrolled in the study. Five of the enrolled dogs were randomly assigned to the GM treatment group (TRMatrix™, IMEX™ Veterinary Inc., Longview, TX) and the other 5 dogs were assigned to the DBM mix treatment group (Freeze dried Cancellous Demineralized Standard mix (1cm³); Freeze-Dried Osteo-Allograft (1cm³) Veterinary Transplant Services, Inc. (Kent WA, USA). Approval for the study was granted by the University of Florida Institutional Animal Care and Use Committee (#200801191) according to the guidelines by the Animal welfare act and US Government principles for the utilization and care of vertebrate animals. Written informed owner consent was obtained according to the guidelines of and with approval of the University of Florida, College of Veterinary Medicine Clinical Research Review Committee.

Surgery

The required tuberosity advancement and cage size were determined prior to surgery according to overlay templates (Kyon, Technoparkstrasse 1, Zurich, Switzerland) [3]. Prior to performing the osteotomy, an arthrotomy or arthroscopy was performed to assess the integrity of the cruciate ligaments, menisci and articular cartilage. Remaining fibers of the cranial cruciate ligament were debrided. Cranial cruciate ligaments with only minor fiber pathology resulting in that stifle having minimal cranial tibial thrust and drawer were classified as partial ruptures and the cranial cruciate ligament was not debrided. Menisci with gross parenchymal pathology were treated appropriately by performing a caudal pole hemi-meniscectomy or partial meniscectomy. The decision to perform a meniscal release was based on surgeon preference and was documented in the medical record.

The osteotomy was performed using an oscillating saw, with continuous saline irrigation. An appropriately sized fork-plate combination was used and an appropriately sized cage was placed in the osteotomy gap [3, 4]. The osteotomy gap was lavaged copiously with sterile saline before placing either GM (1 vial of 1 cm³) or DBM mix (1 cm³) in the defect. One vial of GM was used to fill the defect, making sure not to place any product outside the osteotomy gap. One cc of DBM mix was used to fill the osteotomy gap. Closure of the surgery site was performed routinely. All surgeries were performed by the same surgeon (MR). Appropriate advancement of the tuberosity and position of the implants was assessed on orthogonal view radiographs obtained under anesthesia prior to recovering the dog.

All dogs had a modified Robert Jones bandage placed on the limb for 24 h following surgery. This bandage was removed the day after surgery. The bandage was not reapplied in some dogs or was reapplied and subsequently removed within 5 days after surgery. Owners were instructed to perform passive range of motion exercises for the first four to 6 weeks after surgery. All dogs received opioid analgesia: either methadone hydrochloride (Methadone, 10 mg/ml, Mylan Institutional LLC, Rockford, IL) 0.1–0.2 mg/kg IV q4-6 h or hydromorphone hydrochloride (Dilaudid, 2 mg/ml, West-Ward Pharmaceuticals, Eatontown, NJ) 0.05–0.1 mg/kg IV q6-8 h for the first 24 h after surgery, followed by tramadol hydrochloride (Ultram, Janssen Pharmaceuticals, Titusville, NJ) 2.2 mg/kg PO q8-12 h for five to 10 days. All dogs received additional non-steroidal anti-inflammatory drug (NSAID) analgesia at an appropriate dose unless contra-indicated as judged on a chemistry panel. Drugs administered were: deracoxib (Deramaxx© Novartis Animal Health, Greensboro, NC) or carprofen (Rimadyl® Pfizer Animal Health, Lincoln, NE) daily for the first 4 weeks and on an as needed basis thereafter, as judged on a day to day basis by the owner.

All dogs were confined to a crate or cage when unattended and restricted to leash walks when outdoors for the first 3 months following surgery. Owners were instructed to return their dogs to be re-evaluated and imaged at four, eight and 12 weeks following surgery.

Imaging modalities
Radiographs
Orthogonal view radiographs (CR) were obtained immediately postoperatively and at the four, eight, and 12 week re-evaluations using a computed radiography system (Kodak/Carestream, Directview, Carestream Health, Inc., Rochester, NY). All lateral projection radiographs were obtained with the stifle positioned in an approximate flexion angle of 135°.

Radiographic evidence of healing included progressive increase in mineral opacity in the osteotomy gap, with bridging of the osteotomy margins and confluence of the osteotomy segments. The lateral view radiographs were also scored on a scale from '0–4' using a previously published semi-quantitative scoring system [4] (Hoffman scores): '0' = no bone healing in any area; '1' = early bone healing, no bridging between the tibial tuberosity and tibial shaft; '2' = bridging bone at one site; '3' = bridging bone at two sites; '4' = bridging bone at three sites (proximal to the cage, between cage and plate, distal to the plate) [4]. These scores were used for temporal comparisons in individual dogs and between treatment groups. A 12-step metal stepwedge was placed in the primary beam and adjacent to the limb when obtaining the lateral view radiographs as an objective evaluation method to assess the radiographic opacity of the tissue in the osteotomy gap. The opacity of the tissue in the osteotomy gap at the aforementioned three sites (proximal to the cage, between cage and plate, distal to the plate) was compared to the steps. The tissue was assigned the step number of which the radiographic appearance most closely matched the radiographic appearance of the evaluated tissue in the osteotomy site by visual overlay. Visualization of the cortical chips in the DBM mix treatment group in the osteotomy gap was noted as visible or non-visible.

Computed tomography

CT examinations were performed immediately postoperatively and at the four, eight, and 12 week re-evaluations using an 8 slice multi-detector row computed tomography unit (Toshiba Acquilion 8, Toshiba America Medical Systems, Tustin, CA). Dogs were positioned in dorsal recumbency with the hind limbs extended to position both stifles at approximate a 135° angle. Contiguous 2 mm axial slices of both hind limbs were obtained from the mid femur to the distal tibia. The volume data was stored on disks and the rendered studies were stored on a picture archive and communication system (PACS) (AMICAS PACS™ Merge® Healthcare, Morrisville, NC). Measurements were performed using software proprietary to the PACS. Healing of the osteotomy on CT studies was subjectively assessed based upon volume and progression of mineral attenuating tissue within the osteotomy gap, bridging of the osteotomy margins and continuity of the osteotomy segments. Attenuation within the osteotomy gap was objectively assessed by measuring the CT numbers within a best fit oval region of interest (ROI) that only included the tissue within the osteotomy gap, drawn on all axial slices, starting immediately distal to the cage and continuing to the distal most portion of the osteotomy gap. The mean of these measurements was calculated for every CT examination and these values were used for temporal comparisons in individual dogs and between treatment groups. The minimal width of the osseous bridge in the osteotomy gap distal to the cage was measured using a digital caliper, with the points placed at the medial and lateral margins of the bone-soft tissue interface. To account for size differences between dogs, a ratio of the following measurements was used: 1) the width of the osteotomy line at the narrowest point, 2) width at the cut edge of the tibial tuberosity on the same axial slice, and 3) the width at the cut edge of the tibial diaphysis was on the same axial slice. The ratio was calculated as follows:

$$ratio = \frac{width\ of\ new\ bone\ formation}{(width\ of\ tibial\ tuberosity + width\ of\ tibial\ diapysis)/2}$$

Ultrasonography

B-mode ultrasonography was performed at four, eight and 12 week re-evaluations through a medial and lateral window centered over the osteotomy gap using a 5–17 MHz linear broadband transducer (Philips iU22, Philips Healthcare, Andover, MA). No ultrasound was performed immediately after surgery due to expected interference with air in the surgery site. Ultrasonographic criteria that were used to assess healing were taken from prior work [15–17, 21]. The following criteria were used: 1) the tissue in the osteotomy gap had a hyperechoic interface with presence of distal acoustic shadowing indicating mineralization of the tissue and consistent with new bone formation, 2) the hyperechoic tissue in the osteotomy gap was continuous with the tibial tuberosity cranially and the tibial shaft caudally indicating bridging of the osteotomy gap. Ultrasonographic studies were scored subjectively as sonographically healed or non-healed.

Comparisons

The two treatment groups were assessed independently for time until bony bridging for each individual modality. A diagnosis of a healed osteotomy gap by bridging bone for each individual modality was determined as defined by the parameters outlined above. This time point was used for comparison between the modalities. For this comparison, the two treatment groups were combined into one patient group.

Statistical analysis

The mean number of weeks until bony bridging was identified for each of the different imaging modalities (CR, CT and US). These values were used to compare the subjective assessment of osteotomy union between imaging modalities. The specific criteria outlined above were used to define healing. Both surgical treatment groups were combined in this assessment to provide a more robust group. The comparison was performed using the Cochran-Mantel-Haenzel tests for a difference in row mean scores. Within each imaging group the effect of imaging modalities and treatment (GM v. DBM mix) were tested using the same methodology. The radiographic scores based on the Hoffman grading system were also analyzed using Cochran-Mantel-Haenzel tests for a difference in row mean scores between treatments (GM v. DBM mix) at each time point. The HUs on the CT images were analyzed using a repeated-measures linear model to test for treatment and time effect.

A Kruskal-Wallace nonparametric test was used to compare the ratio of the width of new bone growth to the tibial width between the two treatments. Significance was defined as values of $p < 0.05$. All statistical analyses were performed by use of computer software (SAS, version 9.3; SAS Institute Inc., Cary, NC).

Results
Animals & surgery
The mean age of the dogs was 71 ± 15.8 months and the bodyweight 34.4 ± 8.2 kg. No significant differences were found between the two treatment groups

for age ($p = 0.18$), bodyweight ($p = 0.18$), or cage size ($p = 0.18$). All patient parameters are summarized in Table 1. Seven dogs received daily NSAIDs until the first recheck at 4 weeks, two dogs did not receive NSAIDs (one in each treatment group) and the remaining dog received daily NSAIDs for 8 weeks (DBM group).

Imaging
Radiographic assessment
Air was seen in the osteotomy gap in all immediate postoperative radiographs. Cortical bone chips were easily identified immediately postoperatively in the DBM mix treatment group (Fig. 1). The tissue in the osteotomy gap in the GM treatment group had a radiographic appearance similar to soft tissue (Fig. 2). No complications associated with the implants were seen at any of the recheck radiographs. Bone chips could still be identified at 3 months postoperatively in two of five DBM mix dogs (Fig. 1). The bridging bone at final recheck had a smooth trabecular pattern in all GM cases. All of the TTAs had achieved complete radiographic union at 3 months. Healing times are summarized in Table 2.

The median Hoffman [4] score was '0' immediately after surgery and progressed to a median score of '3' at 3 months in both groups (Table 3). The median stepwedge number associated with the tissue in the osteotomy gap was scored as a '1' for all four time points for both treatment groups (Table 4).

Computed tomographic assessment
On the immediate postoperative studies, air could be seen dissecting along the fascial planes in all cases, and along the caudal cortex of the femur at the level of the fabellae in eight out of 10 dogs. Bone chips were easily

identified in the DBM mix group in the immediate postoperative CT (Fig. 3). Transverse CT images showed progressive alterations of the bone graft substitutes in the osteotomy gap characterized by progressive increase in mineral attenuation in both groups. This increase was heterogenous and irregular in the DBM mix group. The mineralization in the GM group was smooth, and while bridging of the osteotomy gap was achieved, this process was (subjectively) less exuberant than the DBM mix group with a distinctive hourglass shape, resulting in less complete filling of the osteotomy gap (Fig. 4). Complete healing, or bony bridging on CT, of the osteotomy gap as defined by the volume and mineral attenuating nature of the tissue in the osteotomy gap, was diagnosed at 2 months postoperatively in three dogs and 3 months postoperatively in two dogs in the DBM mix treatment group. In the GM treatment group, complete bony bridging of the osteotomy gap on CT was diagnosed at 1 month postoperatively in one dog and at 2 months in the other four dogs (Table 2).

The width of the bone at the thinnest point of the bridge was significantly smaller in the GM group ($p = 0.03$) The mean of the ratios for the GM treatment group was 0.48 (range 0.28–0.78) whereas the mean for the DBM mix treatment group was 0.79 (range 0.6–0.93) (Table 5). For the width ratios, there was not a statistically significant difference at the 0.05 level ($p = 0.10$). The grouped measurements for the HUs increased sharply between imaging immediate postoperatively and at 4 weeks, but leveled off thereafter (Fig. 5, Table 6). There were no differences between treatment groups after the initial measurement ($p = 0.011$ at time 1, $p > 0.05$ for all other weeks), but there was a statistically significant increase in HUs over time for all dogs ($p = 0.047$).

Table 1 Breed, Age, Body weight (BW), MM (medial meniscal treatment) of dogs treated with DBM (D1–5) and dogs treated with GM (G1–5): CHM (caudal hemimeniscectomy), MR (meniscal release); cage size (in mm) and additive: DBM mix (demineralized bone matrix mix), or GM (gelatinous matrix) for the two treatment groups

	Breed	Age (months)	BW (kg)	CrCL	MM	Cage (mm)	Additive
D1	Mix	96	33.2	Partial	CHM	12	DBM
D2	Labr. R.	59	40	Complete	MR	9	DBM
D3	GSD	64	45	Complete	CHM	12	DBM
D4	Labr. R.	91	39	Complete	CHM	12	DBM
D5	Mix	69	27	Partial	None	12	DBM
Mean		75.8 ± 16.6	36.8 ± 6.9				
G1	Mix	48	30	Complete	CHM	9	GM
G2	Labr. R.	87	48	Complete	MR	12	GM
G3	Sharpei	56	23	Complete	CHM	9	GM
G4	Labr. R.	72	30	Complete	CHM	9	GM
G5	Mix	68	28.6	Partial	None	12	GM
Mean		66.2 ± 15	31.9 ± 9.4				
Total		71 ± 15.8	34.4 ± 8.2				

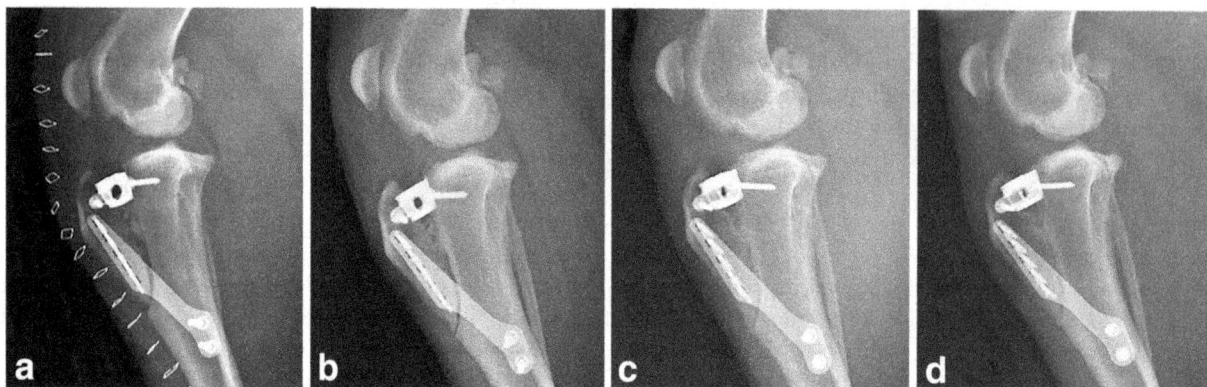

Fig. 1 Four mediolateral projections of the left stifle of a dog in the DBM mix group made with the stifle in 135° of flexion. (**a**) immediately postoperatively, (**b**) 1 month postoperatively, (**c**) 2 months postoperatively; (**d**) 3 months postoperatively. Note the progressive, heterogeneous increase in mineral opacity within the osteotomy gap over time, with progressive sclerosis of the osteotomy margins consistent with healing. On images (**b-d**), the patellar ligament is thickened. The increased soft tissue within the stifle joint and the moderate osteophyte production remain relatively static over time

Ultrasonographic assessment

The osteotomies were diagnosed as bridged with bone between one to 2 months postoperatively (Table 2). The bridging mineral present in osteotomy gaps of the GM treatment group had a smooth, but concave interface that was a feature of the hourglass shape noted on CT. The bridging mineral present in the osteotomy gaps of the DBM mix group was moderately irregular, without evidence of concavity, suggestive of the more complete filling noted on CT (Fig. 6). All five dogs in the GM treatment group were diagnosed as completely healed at their 4 week recheck (Fig. 7).

Comparisons

Imaging modalities

Subjective assessment of time until osseous union differed significantly between the three evaluation methods ($p = 0.001$). The time until osseous union was diagnosed

by CT and radiographs did not differ significantly ($p = 0.28$), but the time until ultrasonography diagnosed bone bridging with return of acoustic shadowing differed significantly from both an assessment of bone bridging on CT ($p = 0.005$) and on radiographs ($p < 0.0001$). When separated by imaging modality, the week that healing was first detected does not differ between the two treatment groups (radiographs, $p = 0.655$; CT, $p = 0.578$; ultrasonography, $p = 1.00$).

Comparison of treatment groups

No significant difference was found between treatment groups for time until a subjective assessment of radiographic healing was given ($p = 0.655$). There were no significant differences in Hoffman scores between the two treatment groups at any of the time points (1 month postoperatively ($p = 0.501$), and 2 months postoperatively ($p = 0.76$), and all but one dog had a score of '3' at 3 months postoperatively), nor was a significant difference

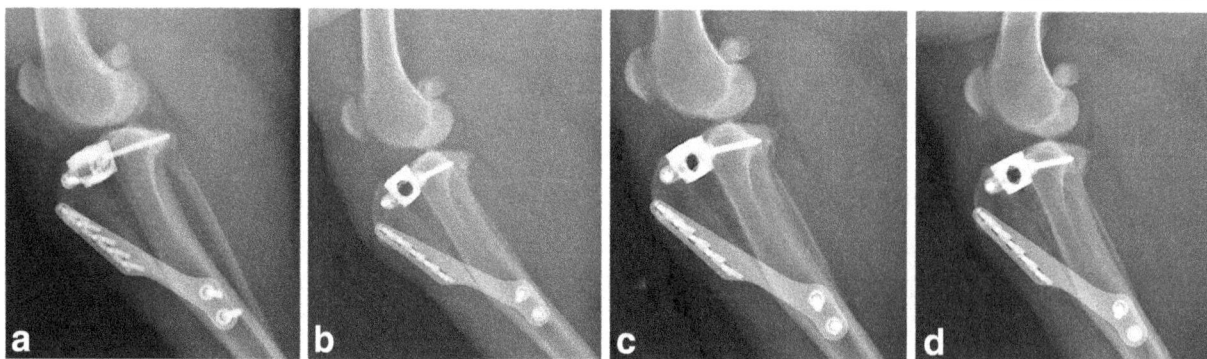

Fig. 2 Four mediolateral projections of the right stifle of a dog in the GM group made with the stifle in 135° of flexion. (**a**) immediately postoperatively, (**b**) 1 month postoperatively, (**c**) 2 months postoperatively; (**d**) 3 months postoperatively. Note the less pronounced, but still progressive increase in mineral opacity within the osteotomy gap over time. On images (**b-d**), the patellar ligament is thickened. The increased soft tissue within the stifle joint and the minimal osteophyte production remain static over time

Table 2 Outcomes of dogs treated with DBM mix (D1–5) and dogs treated with GM (G1–5). Healing diagnoses are listed subjectively as 'healed' or 'not-healed' and expressed as weeks postoperatively (i.e. the recheck in weeks postoperatively (PO) where the diagnosis was 'healed'. Individual cortical chips visible, qualitatively scored as yes or no, and expressed in months postoperatively. US: ultrasonography; CT: computed tomography; CR: computed radiography. The total healing time is expressed as mean [median]. There is a large difference between methods, but not between treatments by methods (for CR, $p = 0.655$; for CT, $p = 0.578$; for us, $p = 1.000$). * US healing times significantly different from both CT and CR ($p < 0.05$)

| | Complete Healing (weeks PO) | | | Visibility of bone chips (weeks PO) | |
	US	CT	CR	CT	CR
D1	8	12	12	12	12
D2	8	8	12	8	4
D3	4	8	8	4	4
D4	4	8	8	8	8
D5	4	12	12	12	12
DBM mix	5.6	9.6	10.4		
G1	4	8	12	n/a	n/a
G2	4	8	12	n/a	n/a
G3	4	8	8	n/a	n/a
G4	4	4	4	n/a	n/a
G5	4	8	12	n/a	n/a
GM	4	7.2	9.6		
Total	4.8*	8.4	10		

found in time until a score of '3' was obtained ($p = 0.259$). No significant differences were found between time points for the stepwedge number assigned at any time point. No significant difference was found between treatment groups for time until a subjective assessment of healing was given on CT ($p = 0.578$). There was a statistically significant increase in HUs over time (from 0 to 3 months) for all dogs ($p = 0.047$) (Table 6).There were no differences

Table 3 Presented are the healing outcomes of dogs treated with DBM (D1–5) and dogs treated with GM (G1–5), based on scores (0–4) on lateral radiographs, as previously described by Hoffman et al. [0 = no bone healing in any area; 1 = early bone healing, no bridging between the tibial tuberosity and tibial diaphysis; 2 = bridging bone at one site; 3 = bridging bone at two sites; 4 = bridging bone at 3 sites (proximal to the cage, between cage and plate, distal to the plate)] [4]. No significant differences were found between treatment groups at any time point or over time

| | Scores | | | |
	0w PO	4w PO	8w PO	12w PO
D1 (1)	0	1	2	3
D2 (5)	0	2	3	3
D3 (7)	0	1	3	4
D4 (9)	0	3	3	3
D5 (11)	0	1	–	3
Median	0	1	3	3
G1 (2)	0	3	3	3
G2 (4)	0	2	3	3
G3 (6)	0	1	3	3
G4 (8)	0	3	–	3
G5 (10)	0	1	3	3
Median	0	2	3	3

Table 4 Outcomes of dogs treated with DBM mix (D1–5) and dogs treated with GM (G1–5) based on stepwedge numbers. The stepwedge numbers ranged from 1 to 12, with one being the least dense and 12 the highest density possible. Comparisons were made at three sites: proximal to the cage, between cage and plate, distal to the plate, and the mean is reported. No significant differences were found between time points or treatment groups

| | Stepwedge numbers | | | |
	0w PO	4w PO	8w PO	12w PO
D1 (1)	1	1	1	1.67
D2 (5)	2	1	1	2
D3 (7)	1	1	1	1
D4 (9)	1	1	1	1
D5 (11)	1	1	–	1
G1 (2)	1	1	2	2
G2 (4)	1	1	1	2
G3 (6)	1	2	1	1
G4 (8)	1	1	–	1
G5 (10)	1	1	1	1

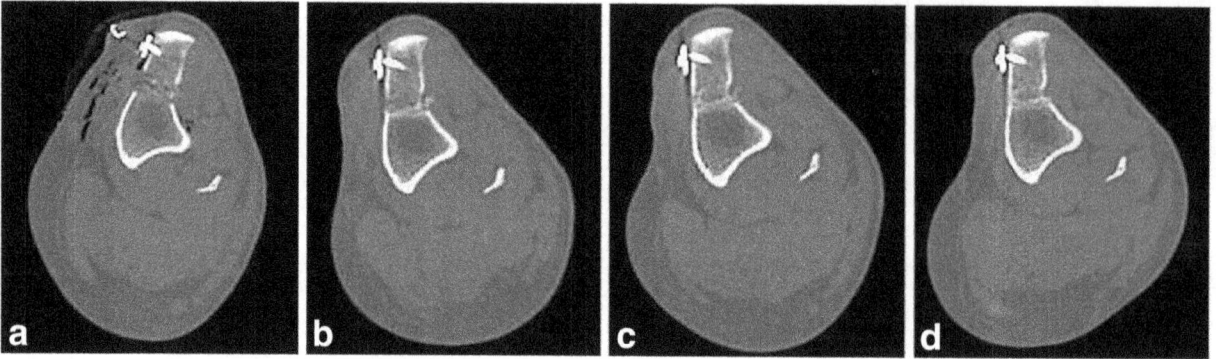

Fig. 3 Four axial computed tomographic (CT) images of the left stifle of the same dog in Fig. 1 (DBM mix group) made at the level of the first prong of the fork. (**a**) immediately postoperatively, (**b**) 1 month postoperatively, (**c**) 2 months postoperatively; (**d**) 3 months postoperatively. Note the progressive increase in heterogeneous mineral attenuation with near complete filling of the osteotomy gap. On image (**d**), there is smooth, contiguous bone at the medial aspect of the osteotomy

between treatment groups for measured HUs in the osteotomy on CT after the initial measurement ($p = 0.01$ at time 1, $p > 0.05$ for all other weeks). Complete bridging with return of acoustic shadowing (ultrasonographic diagnosis of healing) was not significantly statistically different between treatment groups ($p = 1.00$)(Table 2).

Discussion

The hypotheses tested during this study were that: 1) all osteotomy gaps would be bridged by bone based on all three imaging modalities by the end of the study (3 months), 2) US would substantiate osteotomy union earlier than the other two imaging modalities, and that 3) GM would promote faster healing than DBM mix. The results of this study showed that all of the osteotomy gaps in the dogs obtained osseous union without complications within 3 months, which validated our first hypothesis, that both treatment groups would progress

to complete union within the study time frame. Obtaining histological confirmation of osseous union would have strengthened this study, but was not deemed appropriate given the study population (client owned animals), and potential for surgical morbidity. A significant difference was found between CT, radiographs and ultrasound with ultrasound being able to provide a diagnosis of healing earlier than radiographs or CT, confirming our second hypothesis. No significant differences were found for healing times between the two treatment groups, rejecting our third hypothesis. A power analysis revealed that least 62 dogs would be needed to reach significance, based on the most sensitive modality (CT).

We elected to use a 3 month postoperative follow-up period in this study for all three imaging modalities as previously published reports have shown that the majority of TTA osteotomies have obtained union by 3 months following surgery [3, 4, 11]. In this study, we

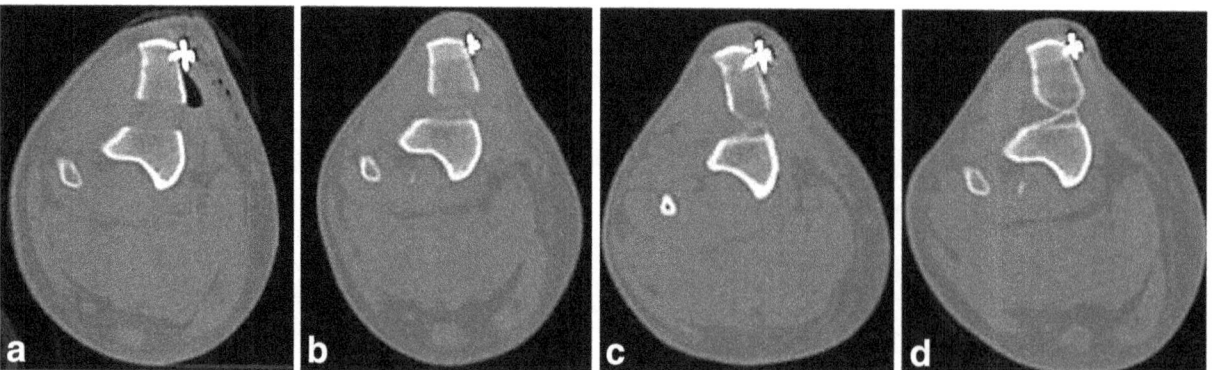

Fig. 4 Four axial computed tomographic images of the right stifle of the same dog in Fig. 2 (GM) made at the level of the first prong of the fork. (**a**) immediately postoperatively, (**b**) 1 m postoperatively, (**c**) 2 months postoperatively; (**d**) 3 months postoperatively. Note the slow progressive increase of smooth, more homogenous mineral attenuation that becomes more well-defined on Image (**d**), consistent with healing. This smooth bone production tapers toward the center of the osteotomy, forming an hourglass shape, and resulting in incomplete filling of the osteotomy gap

Table 5 Outcomes of dogs treated with DBM mix (D1–5) and dogs treated with GM (G1–5). Presented are the results based on Computed Tomographic imaging. 'Width bridge' is the width of the narrowest portion of the bony bridge in the osteotomy gap (in mm). [1]Ratio of the narrowest bridge and the original cut. No significant differences were found between the two treatment groups ($p = 0.1$)

	Width bridge (mm)	Ratio bridge to cut[1]
D1	8.1	0.86
D2	11.2	0.93
D3	8.9	0.83
D4	4.0	0.60
D5	5.7	0.71
Mean	7.58	0.79
G1	5.6	0.75
G2	3.6	0.33
G3	3.3	0.24
G4	4.9	0.78
G5	2.6	0.28
Mean	4.0	0.48

Table 6 Healing outcomes of dogs treated with DBM mix (D1–5) and dogs treated with GM (G1–5), measured in Hounsfield units (HUs) on a PACS, using a best fit elliptical fit on the osteotomy gap on all available axial slices and presented as a mean of all measurements. The HUs increased significantly over time ($p = 0.047$)

	Bone density on CT (HUs)			
	0w PO	4w PO	8w PO	12w PO
D1 (1)	147.54	213.33	395.37	384.13
D2 (5)	134.11	313.01	637.65	666.44
D3 (7)	58.83	354.22	445.02	370.69
D4 (9)	43.31	366.95	386.45	508.67
D5 (11)	261.19	186.14	–	125.24
G1 (2)	– 106.04	457.39	696.20	741.30
G2 (4)	– 42.64	267.09	470.10	501.85
G3 (6)	31.84	193.54	433.48	484.71
G4 (8)	−71.76	315.95	–	305.48
G5 (10)	−85.10	55.74	42.28	38.67

compared classic radiographic follow up (immediate postoperative and at one, two, and 3 months) with computed tomographic follow up (immediate postoperative and at one, two, and 3 months) and ultrasonographic follow up assessment (at one, two, and 3 months). Ultrasonography was able to reliably diagnose complete bridging of the osteotomy gap, and provided a subjective diagnosis of complete bony bridging of the osteotomy gap at 1 month in eight out of 10 dogs, which was significantly earlier than for CT or radiographs. The ultrasonographic diagnosis of confluent bridging bone in the osteotomy gap at 1 month provides further evidence that healing may be further advanced than radiographs show,

or rather that radiographic evidence of healing lags behind bone healing. This is similar to earlier reported studies investigating the use of ultrasonography in the follow up of fracture healing, where ultrasound reliably indicated bridging of the fracture gap with mineralized tissue at an earlier time point than radiographs [15, 16, 18, 21, 24–26]. One limitation is not obtaining a base line ultrasound image of the additives in the osteotomy gap immediately after surgery. The presence of air in the surgery site would have caused artifacts, limiting assessment of any tissues and structures deep to the air [31]. Ultrasonographic union was diagnosed on the appearance of a full bridge of mineralized tissue with acoustic shadowing deep to it, as defined during earlier studies assessing secondary fracture healing [15]. During secondary fracture

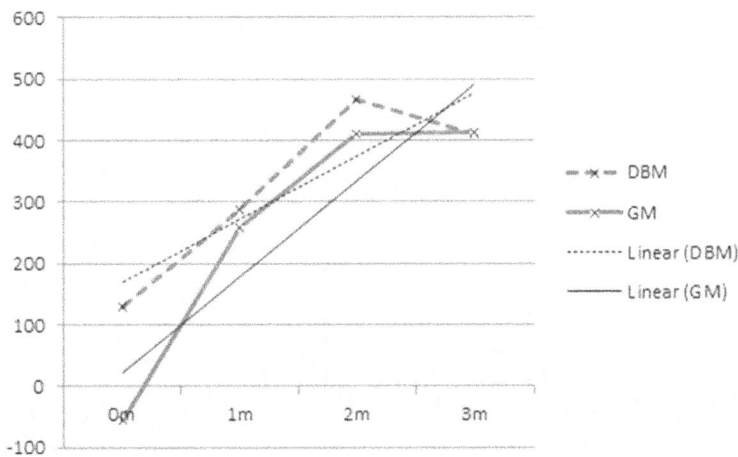

Fig. 5 The Y axis shows the density in Hounsfield units, and the time postoperatively is plotted on the X-axis. A trendline (thinner line) is shown for both the DBM mix and the GM

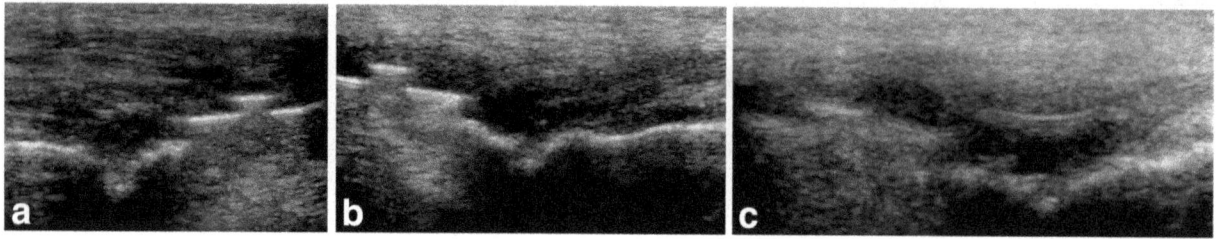

Fig. 6 Three ultrasonographic images made of the osteotomy site of the same dog in Figs. 1 & 3. (**a**) 1 m postoperatively, (**b**) 2 months postoperatively; (**c**) 3 months postoperatively. Note the presence of strongly reflective, irregular interfaces within the osteotomy gap indicative of bone production, and compatible with healing of the osteotomy in all images

healing, small areas of mineralization could be detected prior to formation of a full osseous bridge with return of acoustic shadowing [15]. Individual bone chips could have mimicked these foci of healing, but would not be visualized as a full osseous bridge.

Bone growth and regrowth are important clinical factors after orthopedic procedures involving osteotomies, ostectomies or after fracture stabilization. Using modalities that can diagnose healing reliably at an earlier stage could allow earlier rehabilitation and earlier return to full function postoperatively. Diagnosing or recognizing a delay in bone ingrowth or bone bridging will allow an earlier intervention to address the etiological cause for the delay in healing. Delayed healing of osteotomy sites will delay the return to normal function of the animal and healing complications after fracture treatment might be potentially devastating.

The CT studies provided more information than the radiographic studies, and could be performed during the same sedation with no need for general anesthesia. CT diagnosed complete healing by 2 months in eight out of the 10 dogs, which was not significantly earlier than the radiographic diagnosis. The current study found a significant increase in HUs over time, which is similar to a recently reported prospective study of antebrachial fractures [18]. However, using this objective method (quantifying the extent of mineralization in the developing osseous tissues by measuring HUs) did not provide a reliable method for diagnosing or predicting healing in this limited case series. One potential reason might be the continued presence of cortical chips in the DBM mix group in the earlier postoperative time, falsely increasing the HUs measurement. Another possible explanation might be the fact that for an accurate measurement only the tissues within the osteotomy gap should be included without capturing any adjacent soft tissues or bone, leaving only a very small area to be assessed. While using CT might not be indicated for routine follow up, it might provide additional information to the classic radiographic evaluations in selected cases.

Similarly, using the Hoffman radiographic scoring system did not add additional predictive value to the subjective healing assessment [4]. Only one dog in the current study had obtained a complete radiographic union by the end of the study (i.e. a score of '4'; bone bridging at all three sites). This is similar to the findings in the original paper by Hoffman et al. where five out 52 patients (10%) were given a score of '4' (at a mean of 11. 4 weeks postoperatively) [4]. The scores were not significantly different from the subjective healing assessment ($p = 0.052$) if we used bridging at two out of three sites as the definition of osseous union.

The Radiographic Union Score for Tibial fractures (RUST) described by Whelan et al. was also considered as a possible objective measurement to evaluate radiographic

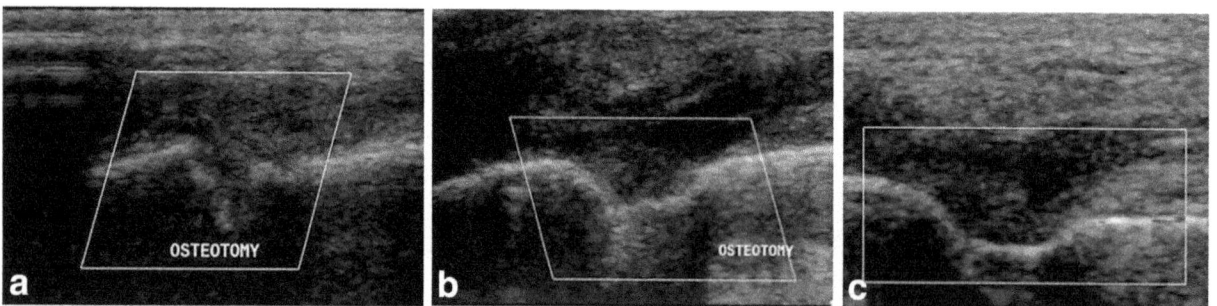

Fig. 7 Three ultrasonographic images made of the osteotomy site of the same dog in Figs. 2 & 4. (**a**) 1 m postoperatively, (**b**) 2 months postoperatively; (**c**) 3 months postoperatively. Note the presence of strongly reflective, smooth, concave (hourglass) interfaces within the osteotomy gap indicative of bone production, and compatible with healing of the osteotomy in all images

bone healing [32]. The RUST score was devised and tested specifically in tibial fractures treated with intramedullary fixation, allowing assessment of all four cortices. Using orthogonal radiographs, all four cortices are scored on a '1–3' system [fracture line, no callus (score = '1'), fracture line, visible callus (score = '2'); no fracture line, bridging callus (score = '3')] allowing for a total score ranging from '4' to '12'. While this system was proven to have substantial intra observer agreement, it relies heavily on the visibility of bridging callus and cortical margins across four cortices and given the anatomy of the tibial tuberosity, the wedge shape of the osteotomy gap, and gap healing at this site, the authors felt that the RUST scoring system was not an applicable tool for evaluating effective bone formation in this study.

The bridging bone which formed in the osteotomy gap was consistently thinner than the width of the original osteotomy. However, the width of the bone in the GM group was significantly thinner (as thin as 2.5 mm in one dog) than the bone in the DBM mix group. When we created an objective parameter (ratio of bridge to adjacent bone) for comparison of the bridge width this finding proved non-significant ($p = 0.10$), most likely due to small sample size (power 36%, with a sample size of eight needed, to obtain a significant difference). In addition, the clinical relevance of the smaller bone bridge is unknown.

In contrast to an earlier study reported by Barnes et al., that used an aluminum stepwedge converted to mm aluminum equivalent, we did not find a significant difference for the tissue in the osteotomy gap during the follow up recheck radiographs. We used a direct comparison of the tissue in the fracture gap with the closest corresponding step of the wedge, while Barnes et al. used a nonlinear regression analysis [11]. It therefore possible that our direct method of comparison was less sensitive than the model used by Barnes et al. [11].

The current study allowed for a direct comparison between two bone graft substitutes in an osteotomy gap model. The original TTA procedural description recommended placing an autogenous cancellous bone graft in the osteotomy gap; however, more recent studies have shown that a TTA osteotomy gap will progress to radiographic union without grafting [8, 10, 11]. We did not include a negative control group in which nothing was placed in the osteotomy gap, nor did we have a positive control group receiving an autogenous cancellous bone graft. Demineralized bone matrix had been and was routinely used when performing TTAs at our institution at the time that we initiated this study. We chose to compare the gelatinous matrix to the standard of care (DBM mix). The current study used the TTA osteotomy gap, in dogs with naturally occurring cranial cruciate ligament insufficiency that were otherwise healthy, to compare to commercially available bone graft substitutes' potential

for enhancing bone healing. While we did not find any significant differences between DBM mix and GM, most likely due to the small sample size, we did not observe any adverse effects in either treatment group. Due to its liquid form, GM may have a potential use in filling in smaller gaps, potentially through a key hole incision, in cases suspected to have, or at risk for, delayed bone healing.

Conclusions

Our results confirmed that ultrasonography reliably predicted osseous union earlier than the other imaging modalities evaluated and CT provided additional information in comparison to radiographs. Dogs in both treatment groups uniformly obtained complete union within the 3 month time frame, although the clinical implications of the bone bridging the osteotomy gap in the GM treatment being thinner than that in the DBM mix group warrants further evaluation.

Abbreviations
BW: Body weight; CR: Computed radiography; CT: Computed tomography; DBM mix: Demineralized bone matrix mix; GM: Gelatinous matrix; HM: Caudal hemimeniscectomy; HUs: Hounsfield units; MM: Medial meniscal treatment; MR: Meniscal release; NSAID: Non steroidal anti-inflammatory drug; PACS: Picture archive and communication system; PO: Postoperative; ROI: Region of interest; RUST: Radiographic union score for tibial fractures; TTA: Tibial tuberosity advancement; US: Ultrasonography

Acknowledgements
The author's acknowledge the patients enrolled in this study as well as their families for their participation in this study.

Funding
This study was funded by a 2008 University of Florida, College of Veterinary Medicine Spring Consolidated Research Development Award competition grant.

Authors' contributions
MR performed the surgeries and the follow up examination. MDW performed the interpretation of the diagnostic imaging. EG performed the statistical analyses. MR, MDW, DDL, EG and AP contributed to the writing of the manuscript. All authors read and approved the final version of the manuscript.

Competing interests
The authors declare that they have no competing interests.

Author details
[1]Department of Small Animal Clinical Sciences, College of Veterinary Medicine, University of Florida, Gainesville, FL 32610-0126, USA. [2]Present address: Department of Veterinary Clinical Sciences, College of Veterinary Medicine, Purdue University, Lynn Hall, 625 Harrison Street, West Lafayette, IN

47907, USA. ³Department of Statistics, College of Agriculture and Life Sciences, North Carolina State University, Raleigh, NC, USA. ⁴Present address: Department for Small Animals, Vetsuisse University of Zurich, Winterthurerstrasse 258c, 8057 Zurich, Switzerland.

References

1. Kipfer NM, Tepic S, Damur DM, Guerrero T, Hässig M, Montavon PM. Effect of tibial tuberosity advancement on femorotibial shear in cranial cruciate-deficient stifles. An in vitro study. Vet Comp Orthop Traumatol. 2008;21:385–90.

2. Kim SE, Pozzi A, Banks SA, Conrad BP, Lewis DD. Effect of tibial tuberosity advancement on femorotibial contact mechanics and stifle kinematics. Vet Surg. 2009;38:33–9.

3. Lafaver S, Miller NA, Stubbs WP, Taylor RA, Boudrieau RJ. Tibial tuberosity advancement for stabilization of the canine cranial cruciate ligament-deficient stifle joint: surgical technique, early results, and complications in 101 dogs. Vet Surg. 2007;36:573–86.

4. Hoffmann DE, Miller JM, Ober CP, Lanz OI, Martin RA, Shires PK. Tibial tuberosity advancement in 65 canine stifles. Vet Comp Orthop Traumatol. 2006;19:219–27.

5. Steinberg EJ, Prata RG, Palazzini K, Brown DC. Tibial tuberosity advancement for treatment of cranial cruciate ligament injury: complications and owner satisfaction. J Am Anim Hosp Assoc. 2011;47:250–7.

6. Burns CG, Boudrieau RJ. Modified tibial tuberosity advancement procedure with tuberosity advancement in excess of 12 mm in four large breed dogs with cranial cruciate ligament-deficient joints. Vet Comp Orthop Traumatol. 2008;21:250–5.

7. Voss K, Damur DM, Guerrero T, Haessig M, Montavon PM. Force plate gait analysis to assess limb function after tibial tuberosity advancement in dogs with cranial cruciate ligament disease. Vet Comp Orthop Traumatol. 2008; 21:243–9.

8. Guerrero TG, Makara MA, Katiofsky K, Fluckiger MA, Morgan JP, Haessig M, Montavon PM. Comparison of healing of the osteotomy gap after tibial tuberosity advancement with and without use of an autogenous cancellous bone graft. Vet Surg. 2011;40:27–33.

9. Kuipers von Lande RG, Worth AJ, Guerrero TG, Owen MC, Hartman A. Comparison between a novel bovine xenoimplant and autogenous cancellous Boe graft in tibial tuberosity advancement. Vet Surg. 2012;41:559–67.

10. Bisgard SK, Barnhart MD, Shiroma JT, Kennedy SC, Schertel ER. The effect of cancellous autograft and novel plate design on radiographic healing and postoperative complications in tibial tuberosity advancement for cranial cruciate-deficient canine stifles. Vet Surg. 2011;40:402–7.

11. Barnes K, Lanz O, Werre K, Clapp K, Gilley R. Comparison of autogenous cancellous bone grafting and extracorporeal shock wave therapy on osteotomy healing in the tibial tuberosity advancement procedure in dogs. Vet Comp Ortho Traumatol. 2015;28:207–14.

12. TR BioSurgical Commercializes Breakthrough Tissue Repair BioScaffold. Kellerman J. http://www.biospace.com/News/tr-biosurgical-commercializes-breakthrough-tissue/103082. Accessed 29 Nov 2017.

13. Update. A resource for Veterinary surgeons. April 2008. Griffin H. Kellerman J, Woods C

14. Personal communication, Hall Griffin, IMEX Veterinary, Inc. 18 april 2018.

15. Risselada M, Kramer M, de Rooster H, Taeymans O, Verleyen P, van Bree H. Ultrasonographic and radiographic assessment of uncomplicated secondary fracture healing of long bones in dogs and cats. Vet Surg. 2005;34:99–107.

16. Risselada M, van Bree H, Kramer M, Duchateau L, Verleyen P, Saunders JH. Ultrasonographic assessment of fracture healing after plate osteosynthesis. Vet Radiol Ultrasound. 2007;48:368–72.

17. Risselada M, van Bree H, Kramer M, Chiers K, Duchateau L, Verleyen P. Correlation of histology of healed fractures and tissue surrounding implants with ultrasonographic and radiographic appearance. J Small Anim Pract. 2008;49:226–32.

18. Ha AS, Lee AY, Hippe DS, Chou SH, Chew FS. Digital Tomosynthesis to evaluate fracture healing: prospective comparison with radiography and CT. Am J Roentgenol. 2015;205:136–41.

19. Ree JJ, Baltzer WI, Nemanic S. Randomized, controlled, prospective clinical trial of autologous greater omentum free graft versus autogenous cancellous bone graft in radial and ulnar fractures in minitiature breed dogs. Vet Surg. 2018:1–14.

20. Leitgeb N, Bodenteich A, Schweighofer F, Fellinger M. Ultrasonic diagnosis of fractures. Ultraschall Med. 1990;11:206–9.

21. Pozzi A, Risselada M, Winter MD. Assessment of fracture healing after minimally invasive plate osteosynthesis or open reduction and internal fixation of coexisting radius and ulna fractures in dogs via ultrasonography and radiography. J Am Vet Med Assoc. 2012;241:744–53.

22. Ricciardi L, Perissinotto A, Visentin E. Ultrasonography in the evaluation of osteogenesis in fractures treated with Hoffmann external fixation. Ital J Orthop Traumatol. 1986;12:185–9.

23. Ricciardi L, Perissinotto A, Dabala M. Mechanical monitoring of fracture healing using ultrasound imaging. Clin Orthop Relat Res. 1993;293:71–6.

24. Moed BR, Watson JT, Goldschmidt P, van Holsbeeck M. Ultrasound for the early diagnosis of fracture healing after interlocking nailing of the tibia without reaming. Clin Orthop Relat Res. 1995;310:137–44.

25. Moed BR, Subramanian S, van Holsbeeck M, Watson JT, Cramer KE, Karges DE, Craig JG, Bouffard JA. Ultrasound for the early diagnosis of tibial fracture healing after static interlocked nailing without reaming: clinical results. J Orthop Trauma. 1998;12:206–13.

26. Moed BR, Kim EC, van Holsbeeck M, Schaffler MB, Subramanian S, Bouffard JA, Craig JG. Ultrasound for the early diagnosis of tibial fracture healing after static interlocked nailing without reaming: histologic correlation using a canine model. J Orthop Trauma. 1998;12:200–5.

27. Jehn CT, Lewis DD, Farese JP, Ferrell EA, Conley WG, Ehrhart N. Transverse ulnar bone transport osteogenesis: a new technique for limb salvage for the treatment of distal radial osteosarcoma in dogs. Vet Surg. 2007;36:324–34.

28. Kahraman OE, Erdogan O, Namli H, Sencar L. Effects of local simvastatin on periosteal distraction osteogenesis in rabbits. Br J Oral Maxillofac Surg. 2015;53:18–22.

29. Casap N, Venezia NB, Wilensky A, Samuni Y. VEGF facilitates periosteal distraction-induced osteogenesis in rabbits: a micro-computerized tomography study. Tissue Eng Part A. 2008;14:247–153.

30. Cuijpers VM, Alghamdi HS, Van Dijk NW, Jaroszewicz J, Walboomers XF, Jansen JA. Osteogenesis around CaP-coated titanium implants visualized using 3D histology and micro-computed tomography. J Biomed Mater Res A. 2015;103:3463–73.

31. Nyland TG, Mattoon JS, Herrgesell EJ, Wisner ER. Physical principles, instrumentation, and safety of diagnostic ultrasound. In: Nyland TG, Mattoon JS, editors. Small animal diagnostic ultrasound. 2nd ed. Philadelphia: W.B. Saunders; 2002. p. 1–8.

32. Whelan DB, Bhandari M, Stephen D, Kreder H, McKee MD, Zdero R, Schemitsch EH. Development of the radiographic union score for tibial fracture healing after intramedullary fixation. J Trauma. 2010;68:629–32.

Exploring the behavioural drivers of veterinary surgeon antibiotic prescribing: a qualitative study of companion animal veterinary surgeons in the UK

C. King[1][*] [iD], M. Smith[1], K. Currie[1], A. Dickson[1], F. Smith[1], M. Davis[2] and P. Flowers[1]

Abstract

Background: Multi-drug resistant bacteria are an increasing concern in both human and veterinary medicine. Inappropriate prescribing and use of antibiotics within veterinary medicine may be a contributory factor to antimicrobial resistance (AMR). The 'One Health' Initiative aims to work across species and environments to reduce AMR, however; little is currently known about the factors which influence antibiotic prescribing among veterinary surgeons in companion animal practice.

This paper reports on qualitative data analysis of interviews with veterinary surgeons whose practice partially or wholly focuses on companion animals ($N = 16$). The objective of the research was to explore the drivers of companion animal veterinary surgeons' antibiotic prescribing behaviours. The veterinary surgeons interviewed were all practising within the UK (England ($n = 4$), Scotland ($n = 11$), Northern Ireland ($n = 1$)). A behavioural thematic analysis of the data was undertaken, which identified barriers and facilitators to specific prescribing-related behaviours.

Results: Five components of prescribing behaviours were identified: 1) confirming clinical need for antibiotics; 2) responding to clients; 3) confirming diagnosis; 4) determining dose, duration and type of antibiotic; and 5) preventing infection around surgery (with attendant appropriate and inappropriate antibiotic prescribing behaviours). Barriers to appropriate prescribing identified include: business, diagnostic, fear, habitual practice and pharmaceutical factors. Facilitators include: AMR awareness, infection prevention, professional learning and regulation and government factors.

Conclusion: This paper uses a behavioural lens to examine drivers which are an influence on veterinary surgeons' prescribing behaviours. The paper contributes new understandings about factors which influence antibiotic prescribing behaviours among companion animal veterinary surgeons. This analysis provides evidence to inform future interventions, which are focused on changing prescribing behaviours, in order to address the pressing public health concern of AMR.

Keywords: Antibiotics, Antimicrobial resistance, AMR, Antimicrobial stewardship, AMS, Prescribing behaviours, Companion animals, Veterinary surgeons, Qualitative

* Correspondence: Caroline.King@gcu.ac.uk
[1]Department of Nursing and Community Health, School of Health and Life Sciences, Glasgow Caledonian University, Cowcaddens Road, Glasgow G4 0BA, Scotland, UK
Full list of author information is available at the end of the article

Background

Inappropriate antibiotic use in companion animals (dogs, cats, rabbits that live in households) has been identified as potentially contributing to antimicrobial resistance (AMR) [1]. The extent of the contribution of antibiotic use within companion animal populations to AMR remains unknown. In the UK alone, it is estimated that 45% of all households have a pet with 26% of households in the UK owning a dog and 18% of households owning a cat [2]. While antibiotic prescribing for companion animals has been decreasing in recent years [1], there remains substantial potential for inappropriate antibiotic use in the companion animal population to drive AMR. The proximity of humans and companion animals in domestic environments means that there also is potential for the transfer of antibiotic resistant bacteria between species [3, 4]. This inter-species transmission of resistant bacteria has implications for both human and animal health [5].

The complexity of the relationships between AMR, human and animal health requires an inter-disciplinary approach that allows for the combination of a range of research methods and expertise. Until now, the focus within veterinary practice has been on identifying the reasons why antibiotics may be used indiscriminately in large-animal populations, for example, cattle and sheep [6]. To our knowledge, our study is the first UK-based AMR research to use a behavioural lens to analyse qualitative accounts of companion animal veterinary surgeons in order to understand antibiotic prescribing behaviours. A focus on understanding the behavioural components of prescribing is particularly relevant and useful in the context of AMR and antimicrobial stewardship (AMS) as it provides evidence for the development of behavioural interventions [7]. These interventions can provide policy-makers and practitioners with practical, focused and evidenced ways to implement AMS programmes aimed at reducing AMR. The behavioural approach taken in this study builds on a developing body of literature using qualitative methods to explore the drivers of antibiotic use in small animal veterinary practice [8]. It explores both the broad behavioural domain of prescribing (the clustering of specific behaviours that relate to prescribing) and the determinants, or antecedents, of such behaviours.

Research aim and questions

The aim of this study was to identify key companion animal veterinary antibiotic prescribing behaviours, which might be amenable to change, in order to reduce drivers of AMR.

Research questions

1. What are the component behaviours related to companion animal veterinary surgeon antibiotic prescribing?

2. What are the barriers and facilitators of appropriate antibiotic prescribing by companion animal veterinary surgeons?

Methods

The study was approved by the Ethics Committee at Glasgow Caledonian University (Reference: HLS/NCH/16/001). Participating veterinary surgeons were recruited voluntarily using email invitations circulated through professional networks and connections from Health Protection Scotland (HPS) and the Control of Antimicrobial Resistance Scotland (CARS) project steering group. Written information was provided and informed consent was obtained prior to interview.

Individual telephone or face-to-face interviews were conducted at a time convenient to the participant and lasted between 25 and 40 min. Three experienced members of the research team carried out the interviews (MS, FS, MD). Individual researcher's skills have been developed through advanced methods training, previous research, and interview and analysis practicums held by the Principal Investigator of the research, who is a leader in the field [9].

The semi-structured interview schedule was designed to provide a framework for the veterinary surgeons to express their views and experiences of antibiotic prescribing and resistance freely and in depth. Interview topics, with related questions, included: exploring veterinary surgeons use of antibiotics in practice; influences on their prescribing of antibiotics; understandings of AMR and AMS; barriers and facilitators of AMS; challenges and facilitators to using guidance for AMS; and their future use of antibiotics. In keeping with the exploratory, inductive focus of the research no a priori behavioural categories were imposed at this stage of the research to give the interviewees opportunity to respond freely and so that the interviewers could follow-up on important emergent themes.

All interviews were recorded and transcribed then imported into NVivo (Version 10) (Computer Software for Qualitative Data Analysis). Principles of thematic analysis (Braun & Clark 2006) [10] were applied to identify components of prescribing behaviour and to categorise associated barriers and facilitators to each aspect of the behaviour. The components of antibiotic prescribing behaviour outlined in Table 1 were generated through a two stage process: first, all behaviours relating to AMR and AMS were identified. Three key behaviours were identified: prescribing; the use of diagnostics; and interactions between veterinary surgeons and pet-owners (reported in Smith et al., 2018) [11]. Second, the overall category of prescribing behaviour was analysed further to identify distinct component behaviours. While it is recognised that these component behaviours overlap the

Table 1 Components of antibiotic prescribing behaviour

Component behaviour	Appropriate behaviour	Inappropriate behaviour
1. Confirming clinical need for antibiotic	Identified clinical need for antibiotic	Cautionary prescribing 'just in case' antibiotics are required
2. Responding to clients	Providing client education on antibiotic use	Responding to perceived client pressure
3. Confirming diagnosis	Use of diagnostic tests to confirm antibiotic need	Prescribing antibiotics without confirmed diagnosis
4. Dose, duration and type of antibiotic	Accurate prescribing: dose and duration of antibiotic use in line with guidelines	Inaccurate prescribing: prescribing too high or too low a dose of antibiotics or too short or long a course of antibiotics or the wrong type of antibiotic
5. Preventing infection around surgical interventions	Enhanced infection prevention and control measures around surgery	Prescribing antibiotics as a preventative measure related to surgical interventions

detailing of the five different components was felt by the research team to be useful in fully understanding the behaviour.

Rigour in analysis was ensured by peer review within the research team. This process involved initial coding of the data to identify a coding map (CK) which was reviewed independently by two other members of the research team (MS and PF). All three researchers then discussed the coding map, negotiated discrepancies and clarified the meanings of all the codes. The coded behaviours were then tabulated alongside their barriers and facilitators and reviewed by the full research team.

Results

Sixteen companion animal veterinary surgeons from across the UK (Scotland, England, Northern Ireland) took part in interviews. Areas of practice ranged from front-line services, consulting directly with members of the public, to secondary referral services in specialist centres. Nine of the participants were male and seven were female. Eleven of the veterinary surgeons were currently based and working in Scotland, four in England and one in Northern Ireland.

Within this paper we explore the behaviour of companion animal veterinary surgeons' antibiotic prescribing. First, we identify five specific components within prescribing-related behaviour. Second, we examine the factors that can act as either barriers or facilitators to these specific prescribing behaviours.

Understanding prescribing behaviour

In Table 1 the five distinct yet overlapping components of antibiotic prescribing behaviour that led to either appropriate or inappropriate prescribing in specific contexts are described.

Barriers and facilitators to appropriate prescribing behaviours

Veterinary surgeons' accounts suggest that prescribing is influenced by a range of barriers and facilitators which have a 'push-pull' effect on prescribing behaviour. Five drivers were found to act as barriers to appropriate prescribing. The barriers were: business, diagnostic, fear, habitual practice and pharmaceutical factors. Four drivers were found to facilitate appropriate prescribing. The facilitators were: AMR awareness, infection prevention, professional learning and regulation and government factors. The key barriers and facilitators influencing appropriate prescribing behaviours are described below and summarised in Figs. 1 and 2.

Barriers to appropriate prescribing:

Business factors

Veterinary surgeons talked about the tensions, which they experienced, between maintaining a viable business, client satisfaction and appropriate antibiotic prescribing:

... people are our customers and they are what keeps the business going, so if we annoy them and there is another veterinary surgeon practice they can go to where they may just be handed out antibiotics [they will potentially do that] (Veterinary surgeon 1)

Clients' desires for their pet to recover could, at times, be in conflict with the appropriate prescribing of antibiotics. Antibiotics were often seen as direct action and symbolic of a clear pathway to a pets' recovery compared to having to 'wait it out' while they recovered without medication:

... owners don't want to say that [they want an antibiotic], but they want their animal better. ... You want to make the animal better, therefore you think 'Oh sod it, I'll just give them a jag (Scottish version of the word injection)'. (Veterinary surgeon 13)

Although veterinary surgeons themselves identified that it was increasingly rare for a client to ask directly for an antibiotic the implicit assumption was that they would

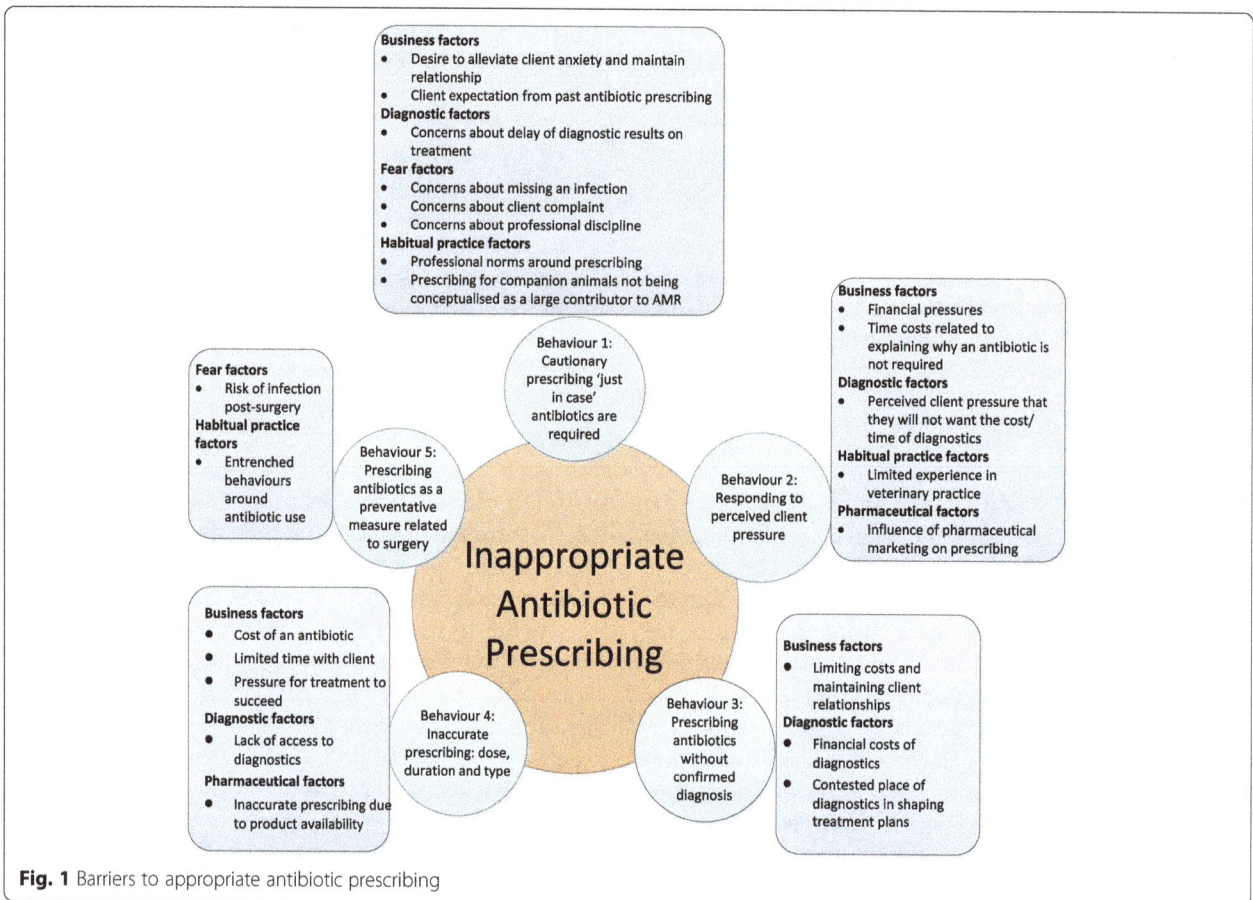

Fig. 1 Barriers to appropriate antibiotic prescribing

want the quickest and most effective treatment. Client satisfaction was identified by veterinary surgeons as important for business success and, as such, could drive inappropriate prescribing behaviour.

Diagnostic factors

The role of diagnostics in shaping treatment plans was contested in veterinary surgeons' accounts. Almost all of the veterinary surgeons talked about not using diagnostics as much as they felt that they should:

I will do culture and sensitivity but maybe nowhere near as often as I should. And I think most vets in the country would probably admit to that. (Veterinary surgeon 2)

Despite an expressed desire by veterinary surgeons to use diagnostics more to inform their prescribing, the barriers of cost and time often influenced their decision-making around whether they would decide to use a diagnostic test:

... the dog comes to the vet vaguely unwell and we can't find out what's wrong with it without spending money doing tests ... or you could just give them a

shot of antibiotics and see what it does (Veterinary surgeon 1)

Diagnostics, then, held a contested place in veterinary surgeons' accounts. They were recognised as an important facilitator of appropriate prescribing, yet their actual use in practice was inhibited by resource constraints.

Fear factors

A key driver of inappropriate prescribing discussed by veterinary surgeons related to feelings of fear. Fear related to concerns that if they did not diagnose and treat an infection this could have negative consequences for an animal and for themselves, professionally. Although veterinary surgeons were aware of AMR, the fear of not diagnosing an infection could still act as an over-riding influence on their antibiotic prescribing behaviour:

... fear, I think for the intra-operative, they're frightened not to use them [antibiotics] in case they get infections (Veterinary surgeon 15)

The fear of missing an infection, and potential professional consequences, were also magnified for veterinary surgeons with the forever present possibility of client

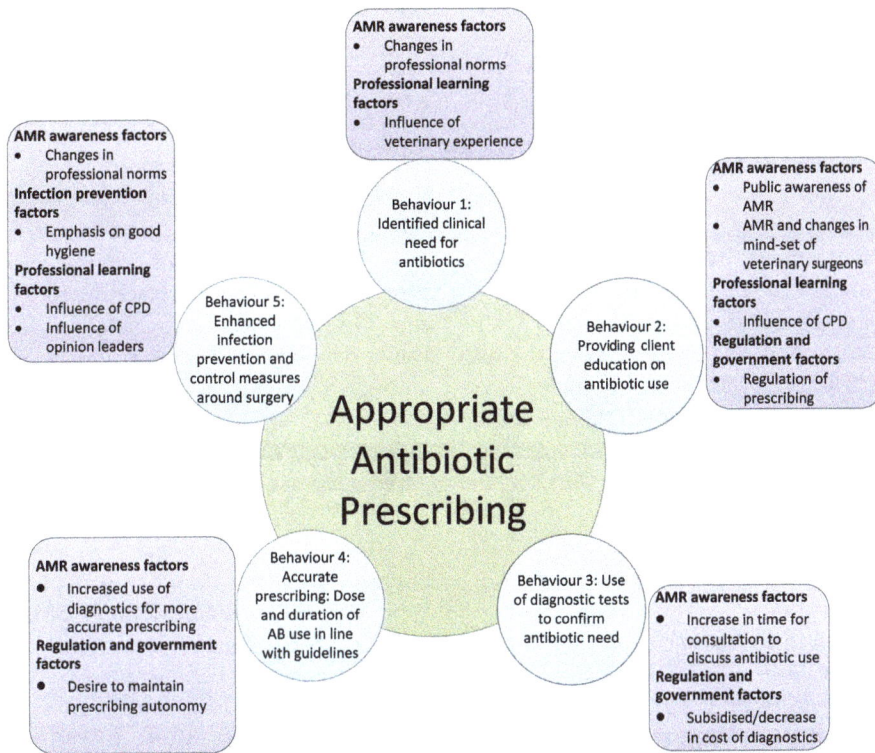

Fig. 2 Facilitators to appropriate antibiotic prescribing

complaint or disciplinary action through their professional bodies:

> ... vets are completely paranoid the Royal Veterinary College [sic Royal College of Veterinary Surgeons] is going to cause them damage or get them struck off (Veterinary surgeon 5)

As such, veterinary surgeons' fears related to outcomes for companion animals and consequences for themselves professionally could act as barriers to appropriate prescribing.

Habitual practice factors

Many of the veterinary surgeons talked about prescribing patterns which had been established over time and which influenced clients' expectations of when their pet would receive an antibiotic. The examples of kennel cough and the treatment of cat abscesses were often used by veterinary surgeons to illustrate this point:

> There is some kind of pattern generated ... this is what I've always treated this with, a jag (Scottish version of the word injection) of penicillin for a cat bite abscess. It's a hard habit to get out of. (Veterinary surgeon 2)

Peer influence was viewed to be a powerful factor in shaping prescribing behaviours within veterinary surgeon practice:

> ... the new grads are initially more prone to not give antibiotics because they were taught, well actually it's bad, and they stand their ground more. But then as they get in to practice and get more experience and maybe they just get worn down or maybe the daily life ... then they start giving antibiotics more loosely. (Veterinary surgeon 4)

Veterinary surgeons also talked about witnessing what they felt to be inappropriate use of antibiotics and the conflict that this caused them:

> ... as I say, I know certain individuals who will happily go and pick up fluoroquinolone before they would touch anything else. (Veterinary surgeon 13)

> So like a skin infection, for example, should ideally have a three-week course ... but in some cases we are discouraged from giving out what I would think would be an appropriate length of course, just because it will keep costs down. (Veterinary surgeon 3)

As such, entrenched prescribing behaviours and the peer processes that could encourage these behaviours to develop, were barriers to appropriate prescribing.

Pharmaceutical factors

Veterinary surgeons also identified that pharmaceutical companies influenced antibiotic prescribing. This opportunity to influence prescribing was created by the marketing of products to address challenges around the administration of antibiotics, such as, difficulties in getting cats to consume tablets. Veterinary surgeons, themselves, were conflicted about whether the use of these antibiotic products was likely to increase or decrease AMR. Irrespective of the nature of the impact on AMR, however, the influence of pharmaceutical companies on prescribing behaviours was articulated:

> ... we do use [antibiotic injections] in cats and we know the problems with it, but we do it when we feel that the owners will not be able to give tablets ... we prescribe it quite often to be honest. ... I am not aware of much evidence that it contributes to specific antimicrobial resistance, but it is a third generation Cephalosporin ... (Veterinary surgeon 11)

As such, prescribing trends were influenced by internal and external factors. These factors included the prescribing norms of veterinary surgeons' practice and the influence of the pharmaceutical companies on prescribing.

Facilitators of appropriate prescribing:

AMR awareness factors

Veterinary surgeons talked about how an increase in public awareness around AMR could help to shape clients' expectations of antibiotic prescribing and use:

> The public are aware ... there are certain things that aren't needing antibiotics that they thought they were generations ago, and that doctors are being a lot more tight with them. ... they know it's an issue. (Veterinary surgeon 2)

Many of the veterinary surgeons interviewed felt that they were often advocating for the appropriate use of antibiotics to colleagues who were less engaged with the issue of AMR. Over time, however, they found that they were able to influence colleagues to be more reflective of their prescribing behaviours:

> I mean we just used antibiotics willy-nilly, so I think it's only since a few of us have got interested in it, that it's actually brought it home to everyone that it's quite important what we do. (Veterinary surgeon 13)

Increased awareness of AMR for both the public and within the veterinary surgeon profession was seen as an important driver of appropriate prescribing.

Infection prevention factors

Emphasis on good hygiene was an important facilitator relating to prophylactic prescribing of antibiotics for surgery. Veterinary surgeons felt that, with good infection prevention practices in place, antibiotics are not necessary. Overall, it was felt by veterinary surgeons that there was a definite trend away from the prophylactic use of antibiotics for surgery:

> Prophylactically after surgery we do it very rarely, it's certainly not a routine thing ... (Veterinary surgeon 12)

Shifts in antibiotic prescribing relating to their prophylactic use were a useful example of how prescribing behaviours had changed over time and in relation to concerns about AMR.

Professional learning factors

Patterns of antibiotic prescribing were established over time and linked closely to clients' expectations around antibiotic use. However, veterinary surgeons talked about how these established behaviours could be mediated or changed with the correct professional education, experience and peer support:

> I say from 30 years ago till now, I think there is a vast improvement in awareness ... younger generations that are coming out [from] the vet schools, it's becoming almost part of just their mind-set. (Veterinary surgeon 15)

Both graduate and post-graduate learning were talked about as important influences, along with the application of new knowledge in practice, peer support and willingness to change practices:

> ... it gets easier as you get older and the clients respect you a bit more and your opinions. ... if you can educate the more established vets in good ways, they're the ones that are teaching the younger vets and they're the ones who are teaching, in inverted commas, the clients what to expect. (Veterinary surgeon 2)

In summary, learning from graduate education, experience of working as a practising veterinary surgeon and learning from peers were working in synergy with one another to create a positive climate of support for AMS, including appropriate prescribing.

Regulation and government factors

Currently, veterinary surgeons in the UK can both prescribe and dispense antibiotics. The decoupling of prescription from the sale of antibiotics within veterinary practice would mean that veterinary surgeons could no longer dispense antibiotics to their clients. The potential for decoupling to happen in the UK was discussed by many of the veterinary surgeons. A lack of agreement about whether decoupling would facilitate AMS was evident. Some veterinary surgeons felt that it would improve AMS and others felt that it would be detrimental to animal welfare and act to limit veterinary surgeons' professional autonomy. Irrespective of veterinary surgeons' personal perspective on decoupling, however, there was agreement that appropriate prescribing was necessary. Improved prescribing could either be enabled by de-coupling or more appropriate prescribing could ward it off, as these two opposing viewpoints illustrate:

I think that [decoupling] would be a good idea, because it would make us think very hard before handing them [antibiotics] out. As I say, they're so accessible for us that it's the easiest thing to do. (Veterinary surgeon 13)

... in the future we may not be able to prescribe them [antibiotics], or the prescription of them may be taken out of our hands, is the other possibility, that we don't have the power to prescribe them and therefore we are completely stuffed then. (Veterinary surgeon 1)

Governments were also seen to have a facilitative role in enabling AMS through the monitoring of antibiotic use and subsidising the cost of diagnostics:

... thinking of government input, if they're going to start subsidising culture and sensitivity in labs, so the clients aren't really having to pay too much for it, that might make it a little bit easier. (Veterinary surgeon 2)

As such, regulation and governmental input, although contested in terms of the form it should take, were talked about by veterinary surgeons as facilitative of appropriate prescribing.

Discussion

The qualitative study reported in this paper takes a behavioural approach, providing new insights and ways of thinking about the contribution to AMR of the prescribing behaviours of companion animal veterinary surgeons. This study identified barriers and facilitators which drive the appropriate and inappropriate prescribing behaviours of companion animal veterinary surgeons.

The antibiotic prescribing behaviours of veterinary surgeons has now been the focus of a number of studies [6, 8, 12, 13], providing an important knowledge base to inform AMR-related behaviour change interventions. These studies use a range of research methodologies and show that antimicrobial prescribing among large-animals in the agricultural sector is influenced by a wide range of social, cultural and political factors [6], provide a pan-European perspective on veterinary surgeon antibiotic prescribing habits and use of sensitivity testing [12], explore the factors influencing prescribing in antibiotic dry cow therapy [13], and document factors influencing decision-making in antimicrobial prescribing in small animal veterinary practice in the UK [8].

With the exception of the work of Mateus and colleagues (2014) [8], the majority of the research to-date focuses primarily on food-producing animals with less attention paid to companion animal prescribing. Mateus et al. (2014) [8] explore influences on antimicrobial prescribing in relation to companion animals and highlight intrinsic factors relating to the veterinary surgeons, and extrinsic factors relating to the workplace and colleagues and to the pet owners and animals and their influence on decision-making. In the present study, we build on this research focusing primarily on the behavioural aspects of prescribing with the intent of developing the evidence-base on the drivers of AMR to inform future behavioural interventions aimed at AMS in the context of companion animal veterinary prescribing. Elsewhere we discuss factors associated with the interactions between veterinary surgeons and their clients [11]. In this paper, we focus on the factors driving the prescribing behaviours of the veterinary surgeons. In what follows, we reflect on our findings in light of the factors identified in Mateus et al.'s (2014) [8] study therefore building the field of knowledge about the promotion of AMS in companion animals.

Our research showed that business factors, including the importance of client retention were barriers to appropriate prescribing. Mateus et al. (2014) [8] report that business factors, although present in the accounts of veterinary surgeons, were not key drivers of decision-making. We found that veterinary surgeons were focused on maintaining good interactions with their clients to ensure the future of their veterinary business. Client expectations rarely related to a direct request for an antibiotic, but rather to veterinary surgeons' perceptions that the costs of diagnostic tests would be too high and take too much time. Other studies have also shown that economic factors play an important role in shaping prescribing behaviours of veterinary surgeons, for example, in relation to veterinary surgeons' awareness of farmers' financial pressures and the intersection between antibiotic use as a short-term measure and more expensive but longer-term solutions to managing infections [6]. The identification of economic factors in studies carried out in different contexts suggests that interventions aimed at changing prescribing behaviours must recognise the economic context which influences veterinary surgeon prescribing.

Diagnostic factors, related to the cost and use of diagnostics, were a key barrier to appropriate prescribing. Mateus et al. (2014) [8] also highlighted factors related to diagnostic use as important influences on decision-making in antibiotic prescribing. Studies have shown that the rate of use of laboratory tests to support prescribing decisions can be very low [14–16]. Eschler and colleagues (2011) [14] found that only 3.7% cases of fluoroquinalone prescriptions for companion animals were supported with laboratory testing; and only around half of the respondents in Hughes and colleagues (2012) [15] survey of antimicrobial prescribing patterns in small animal practice identified laboratory tests to be an important influence on their antimicrobial decision-making. Although veterinary surgeons talk about laboratory tests as being a useful guide for appropriate prescribing, currently financial and time costs appear to be prohibitive factors in their actual use.

Fear factors, in particular in relation to the consequences of untreated infection, were identified as drivers of inappropriate prescribing. This type of cautionary prescribing appears to be context-dependent to companion animal practice. In studies exploring the barriers and facilitators to prescribing in other sectors such as pigs [6] and dairy cows [17], barriers tended to related more to managing the health and welfare of herds and groups of animals and the economic factors of farming and less to ensuring the survival of any one animal.

Habitual practice factors, related to veterinary surgeons' opportunities to develop their knowledge and awareness of AMR and to change their prescribing behaviours, are key barriers to appropriate prescribing. Although trends in antibiotic prescribing are changing, the pace of behaviour change can be slow due to factors such as time pressures in veterinary surgeon practices and lack of access to continuing professional development. In Mateus et al.'s (2014) [8] study veterinary surgeons' past experiences and habits were also found to be major contributors to their prescribing decisions. Behavioural interventions, which aim to change prescribing behaviours, need to acknowledge the importance of these factors.

Pharmaceutical factors were found to have a strong-hold on prescribing behaviours, which has been demonstrated in other studies. In one study of small animal veterinary practices [15], 70% of survey respondents reported that pharmaceutical companies were an important source of prescribing information.

AMR awareness and professional learning factors relating to a change in veterinary surgeons' collective mind-set in relation to antibiotic prescribing was reported to facilitate appropriate prescribing. Although in Mateus et al's (2014) [8] study peer pressure was not deemed to be a direct influence on which antibiotic was prescribed, our study suggests that peer influence may work through subtle and indirect mechanisms which could be beneficial for developing AMS interventions. As awareness of AMR increases, there are also opportunities for the use of techniques such as social comparison. This technique is where veterinary surgeons assess their stewardship performance in relation to that of others. Overall, both this and Mateus et al's study [8] suggest that access to opportunities for continuing professional development and engagement with peers around AMR are likely to be important contributors to countering established habits and norms related to prescribing.

Infection prevention factors identified in this study as facilitative of appropriate prescribing are a useful example of how behaviours can and do change through the availability of alternatives to ensure animal health and welfare.

Regulation and government factors were identified as facilitative to appropriate prescribing, although there was not always agreement among veterinary surgeons about what form regulation should take. The identification of these facilitators suggests that the focus for behavioural change cannot be at the level of individual veterinary surgeons alone. Studies describing prescribing patterns of antimicrobial prescribing in small animal veterinary surgeon practice in the UK [1, 15, 18] and internationally [19] highlight that more antimicrobial prescribing guidelines, which encourage appropriate and more limited use, could be helpful and could act as a more tacit form of regulation.

Limitations of the study

The study sample is limited to a self-selected group of veterinary surgeons with a professional interest in AMR and does not necessarily reflect the diversity of veterinary surgeons' views. As such, it is likely that the veterinary surgeons who were interviewed would have been more progressive both in their ideal and actual behaviours relating to antibiotic prescribing than other veterinary surgeons who are less engaged with the AMR agenda. Although it is not possible to generalise the findings of this study, the authors believe that the value of the research is in describing the components of inappropriate prescribing behaviour, and the barriers and facilitators which drive these behaviours, in depth. Despite the limitation of the self-selected sample, the authors believe that the findings have relevance, for veterinary surgeons, and for all parties interested in a 'One Health' approach to tackling AMR.

Future directions

This study was part of a larger programme of work focused on developing interventions to reduce AMR. It is intended that this data set will be combined with the other data sets of the study and using Theoretical Domains Framework [20, 21], the Behaviour Change Wheel [7] and the Behaviour Change Taxonomy [22] will be used to design AMS evidence-based behaviour change interventions.

Conclusions

By applying a behavioural lens to the qualitative analysis reported in the findings of this paper, we have been able to identify specific antibiotic prescribing behaviours which result in inappropriate antibiotic prescribing practices, which existing evidence suggests are likely to contribute to AMR. The development and implementation of behavioural interventions based on evidence are one way in which the emerging and developing public health problem of AMR can be addressed.

Abbreviations
AMR: Antimicrobial Resistance; AMS: Antimicrobial Stewardship; CARS Advisory Group: Control of Antimicrobial Resistance Scotland Advisory Group; HPS: Health Protection Scotland

Acknowledgements
We would like to acknowledge the contribution of the CARS Advisory Group in supporting the conduct of this study.

Funding
This study was funded by NHS Health Protection Scotland.

Authors' contributions
PF and KC were involved in the initial conception and design of the research. CK, MS, KC, AD, FS, MD and PF were involved in data collection, analysis, and interpretation of data for the paper. All authors contributed to the intellectual ideas within the paper. CK drafted the paper and CK, MS, KC, AD, MD and PF critically revised the paper. All authors have agreed and are accountable for the work presented within the paper. All authors read and approved the final manuscript.

Consent for publication
Not applicable.

Competing interests
The authors declare that they have no competing interests.

Author details
[1]Department of Nursing and Community Health, School of Health and Life Sciences, Glasgow Caledonian University, Cowcaddens Road, Glasgow G4 0BA, Scotland, UK. [2]School of Social Sciences, Monash University, Melbourne, Australia.

References
1. Singleton DA, et al. Patterns of antimicrobial agent prescription in a sentinel population of canine and feline veterinary practices in the United Kingdom. Vet J (London, England: 1997). 2017;224:18–24.
2. PFMA's Pet Data Report 2018. London: Pet Food Manufacturers' Association; 2018.
3. Guardabassi L, Schwarz S, Lloyd DH. Pet animals as reservoirs of antimicrobial-resistant bacteria. J Antimicrob Chemother. 2004;54(2):321–32.
4. Pomba C, et al. Public health risk of antimicrobial resistance transfer from companion animals. J Antimicrob Chemother. 2017;72(4):957–68.
5. Lloyd DH, et al. Antimicrobial selective pressure in pet-owning healthcare workers. Vet Rec. 2012;170(8):211–2.
6. Coyne LA, et al. Understanding the culture of antimicrobial prescribing in agriculture: a qualitative study of UK pig veterinary surgeons. J Antimicrob Chemother. 2016;71(11):3300–12.
7. Michie S, van Stralen M, West R. The behaviour change wheel: a new method for characterising and designing behaviour change interventions. Implement Sci. 2011;6(42).
8. Mateus A, et al. Qualitative study of factors associated with antimicrobial usage in seven small animal veterinary practices in the UK. Prev Vet Med. 2014;117(1):68–78.
9. Smith JA, Flowers P, Larkin M. Interpretative Phenomenological Analysis Theory, Method and Research. United Kingdom: sage; 2009. p. 232.
10. Braun V, Clarke V. Using thematic analysis in psychology. Qual Res Psychol. 2006;3(2):77–101.
11. Smith M, et al. Pet owner and vet interactions: exploring the drivers of AMR. Antimicrob Resist Infect Control. 2018;7(1):46.
12. De Briyne N, et al. Factors influencing antibiotic prescribing habits and use of sensitivity testing amongst veterinarians in Europe. Vet Rec. 2013;173(19):475.
13. Higgins HM, et al. Understanding veterinarians' prescribing decisions on antibiotic dry cow therapy. J Dairy Sci. 2017;100(4):2909–16.
14. Escher M, et al. Use of antimicrobials in companion animal practice: a retrospective study in a veterinary teaching hospital in Italy. J Antimicrob Chemother. 2011;66(4):920–7.
15. Hughes LA, et al. Cross-sectional survey of antimicrobial prescribing patterns in UK small animal veterinary practice. Prev Vet Med. 2012;104(3–4):309–16.
16. Fowler H, et al. A survey of veterinary antimicrobial prescribing practices, Washington state 2015. Vet Rec. 2016;179(25):651.
17. McDougall S, Compton C, Botha N. Factors influencing antimicrobial prescribing by veterinarians and usage by dairy farmers in New Zealand. N Z Vet J. 2017;65(2):84–92.
18. Buckland EL, et al. Characterisation of antimicrobial usage in cats and dogs attending UK primary care companion animal veterinary practices. Vet Rec. 2016;179(19):489.
19. Chipangura JK, et al. An investigation of antimicrobial usage patterns by small animal veterinarians in South Africa. Prev Vet Med. 2017; 136(Supplement C):29–38.
20. Michie S, et al. From theory to intervention: mapping theoretically derived behavioural determinants to behaviour change techniques. Appl Psychol. 2008;57(4):660–80.
21. Cane J, O'Connor D, Michie S. Validation of the theoretical domains framework for use in behaviour change and implementation research. Implement Sci. 2012;7(1):37.
22. Michie S, et al. The behavior change technique taxonomy (v1) of 93 hierarchically clustered techniques: building an international consensus for the reporting of behavior change interventions. Ann Behav Med. 2013;46(1):81–95.

21

Factors contributing to the decision to perform a cesarean section in Labrador retrievers

Gaudenz Dolf[1]* (iD), Claude Gaillard[1], Jane Russenberger[2], Lou Moseley[2] and Claude Schelling[3]

Abstract

Background: In the past 10 years, the frequency of unplanned cesarean sections in the Labrador Retriever breeding colony at Guiding Eyes for the Blind stayed around 10% (range 5% to 28%). To reduce the number of cesarean sections, factors influencing the occurrence of a cesarean section need to be known. The goal of this study was to identify factors that contribute to the decision to perform a cesarean section.

Results: Of the 688 Labrador Retriever litters whelped between 2003 and 2016, 667 litters had sufficient data and remained in the analysis. The target trait was ordinal with the three levels "normal whelping", "assisted whelping" and "cesarean section". A general ordinal logistic regression approach was used to analyze the data. Model selection with possible predictors resulted in a final model including weight of the dam, the weight of the heaviest puppy of a litter, the number of fetuses malpositioned and the quality of uterine contractions. Weight and size of a litter, parity, maternal inbreeding coefficient, whelping season, dam and sire were dropped from the model because they were not significant. The risk of a cesarean section was influenced by the combination of the weight of the dam and the weight of the heaviest puppy in the litter, as well as by the number of malpositioned fetuses and the quality of the contractions. Larger puppies increased the risk of cesarean section especially when the dam had a lighter weight. For dams weighing 23.6 kg and 32.8 kg the predicted probability of a cesarean section was low, with 0.06 and 0.02, respectively, when the heaviest puppy in a litter was light (0.42 kg), contractions were normal and no fetus was malpositioned. However, the probability of a cesarean section was much higher, ranging from 0.24 to 0.08, when the heaviest puppy in a litter was heavy (0.66 kg).

Conclusions: Means to reduce the cesarean section frequency in this Labrador Retriever breeding colony should include genetic selection for ideal puppy weight. In addition, dams with an adult body weight substantially below average should not be selected as breeders in this colony.

Keywords: Cesarean section, Assisted delivery, Labrador retriever, Risk factors

Background

A cesarean section (c-section) is the surgical intervention applied when a dam with dystocia fails to respond to the medical treatment or fetal distress is evident [1]. The term dystocia is used to describe a difficult birth or the failure of a normal vaginal delivery. In dogs, dystocia is a frequently encountered complication during parturition and for roughly 60% of these cases the decision to perform a c-section is taken [2]. Although health surveillance is an important epidemiological tool to improve canine health and welfare, the collection of disease information for dogs is still problematic [3]. Incident rates for dystocia and c-sections have been reported for the general dog population as well as for specific breeds [2, 4], but as they are based on insurance data or questionnaires they may not be representative. Based on the observation in humans that dystocia runs in families a genetic background has been suggested [5, 6]. Knock-out mice implicated several genes to be involved in dystocia [7], but the relevance of these models for dystocia in humans could not be shown [8, 9].

* Correspondence: gaudenz.dolf@vetsuisse.unibe.ch
[1]Institute of Genetics, Vetsuisse Faculty, University of Berne, Bremgartenstrasse 109a, 3001 Berne, Switzerland
Full list of author information is available at the end of the article

Maternal and fetal factors are known to cause dystocia often resulting in a c-section. The most common cause of maternal dystocia is uterine inertia whereas malpositioned fetuses are the most common cause of fetal dystocia [10]. In some dog breeds, particularities of the pelvic anatomy of the dam or the facial skeleton of a puppy may result in a predisposition for obstructive dystocia [4, 11]. Bergström and coworkers [2] identified the breed, age of the dam, and the geographical region as possible risk factors for a dam to be in need of a c-section. In addition, the veterinarian and the owner seem to have a rather high influence on the decision of a surgical intervention.

In the past ten years, the frequency of c-sections in a breeding colony of Labrador Retrievers at Guiding Eyes for the Blind never dropped markedly under 10% and even reached a high of 28% in 2012.

The aim of the present study was to identify factors, other than uterine inertia and malpositioned fetuses that have an influence on the occurrence of a c-section in the Labrador Retriever breeding colony at Guiding Eyes for the Blind and could be improved by breeding and/or adapting management.

Methods

Guiding Eyes for the Blind is a non-for profit organization that breeds and trains mostly Labrador Retrievers (LR) and a few German Shepherd guide dogs to serve people who are blind or have visual impairment. Dams receive a complete physical examination at the start of each estrus cycle and the decision to mate is made based on receiving medical clearance and the need for puppies. The dam is tested for *Brucella canis* using a rapid slide agglutination test at the beginning of each heat where a mating is planned. Males are tested for antibodies against *Brucella canis* every 6 months. On average 65 LR matings are realized per year resulting in 61 whelpings with an average litter size of 7.9 and a litter size at weaning of 7.2. Stillborn puppies and neonatal losses account for 65% and 35% of the puppy losses, respectively.

The timing of matings is based on determining the peak fertile window of the dam through progesterone level testing. The "initial rise" (IR) generally occurs when the serum progesterone level rises to between 1.5 and 2.0 ng/ml (Antech Diagnostics – Fountain Valley, CA 92708 and in-house Tosoh 360 – Tosoh Bioscience – King of Prussia, PA 19406 progesterone assays) and typically coincides with the release of luteinizing hormone. Matings occur most often on days 3 or 4 and 5 or 6 post IR. Estrus is also monitored through vaginoscopy, vaginal cytology and receptivity.

After mating, dams are returned to their foster homes from the start of diestrus until 3 to 5 days prior to their due date which is based on 65 days post IR. An ultrasound to verify pregnancy and approximate the litter size is performed at approximately 33 days post IR.

Dams are admitted to the Guiding Eyes whelping kennel approximately 3 days prior to their due date, which allows sufficient time to acclimate to the kennel environment, and housed in a private, specially equipped whelping suite. Experienced staff monitor for prepartum changes such as nesting, changes in food intake and most notably the drop in rectal temperature below 37.2 degrees Celsius. Individual dam progesterone levels are monitored daily during the 2 to 3 days prior to the anticipated whelp date. If progesterone levels are 2 ng/ml, whelps are typically within 24–36 h; if progesterone levels are 1 ng/ml, whelps are typically within 18–24 h; if progesterone levels are below 1 ng/ml, early stages of whelp have either begun or will begin within 18 h.

Normal parturition is monitored via video monitors by staff in a nearby room with occasional visits to the whelping suite to provide needed elimination walks, food, water or support for the puppies. The decision points for assisted whelping are guided by an established protocol. A c-section will be performed if labor fails to initiate by day 66 from the progesterone IR date measured during estrus or within 24 to 36 h after the progesterone level drops below 2 ng/ml. If the dam has exhibited visible contractions without delivering a puppy the protocols depend on the presence of a fetus in the vaginal canal, strength of contractions and fetal heart rates.

In cases of obstructive dystocia where a fetus is palpated in the vaginal canal and the dam is exhibiting tail arching contractions for 30 min without delivering a puppy a vaginal examination is performed to check for malposition and/or structural maternal abnormalities. Attempts are made to reposition the malpositioned fetus through digital manipulation and/or manually deliver the puppy. The staff veterinarian is called in for a c-section if a puppy is not delivered within 20 min.

If a fetus is palpated upon vaginal examination, however tail arching contractions are very weak or absent, fetal heart rates are measured by ultrasound twice, 10 min apart. If fetal heart rates are 150 beats per minute or slower, the staff veterinarian is called in to provide support which often results in a c-section. If fetal heart rates are above 160 beats per minute, staff will feather the dorsal vagina, often resulting in stronger and/or more consistent contractions which move the fetus within reach to manually deliver the puppy. If a puppy is not delivered, fetal heart rates are monitored and if they are above 160 beats per minute, intermittent periods of allowing the dam to deliver the puppy, feathering the dorsal vagina and monitoring heart rates continue, and the veterinarian is consulted. If heart rates drop below 150 beats per minute, a c-section is performed.

In cases where no tail arching contractions have occurred for a period of two hours since a puppy was delivered and the dam is sleeping or resting the dam is taken for a short exercise walk and fed a small meal. A vaginal examination is performed to check for a fetus in the vaginal canal and fetal heart rates are measured. If fetal heart rates drop below 150 beats per minute, the staff veterinarian is called in and a c-section is performed. If fetal heart rates are at least 170 beats per minute, the vaginal examination is repeated 30 min later along with feathering. If no contractions result, the staff person handling the whelp obtains approval to administer 2 units of oxytocin (Henry Schein Animal Health – Dublin, OH 43017) frequently administered subcutaneously and occasionally by intramuscular injection along with 23% calcium solution (Vedco – Saint Joseph, MO 64507) administered subcutaneously at the dosage of 0.5 ml per 4.5 kg body weight. If within 30 min a puppy is not delivered and/or no contractions resulted from feathering, oxytocin and calcium are repeated provided fetal heart rates are at least 170 beats per minute. If within an additional 30 min a puppy is still not delivered and/or fetal heart rates drop below 150 beats per minute, the staff veterinarian is called in and a c-section is performed.

Statistical analyses were carried out using Stata/SE 14.1 (StataCorp, 4905 Lakeway Drive, College Station, Texas 77,845, USA). The initial data set comprised 688 litters of LR from 2003 to 2016 by 256 different dams and 150 sires. The target trait, ease of whelping (EOW), was ordinal with the three levels "normal whelping", "assisted whelping without c-section" and "c-section with or without prior assistance". Correlation coefficients between possible predictors were calculated to avoid the inclusion of highly correlated predictors. Possible predictors were the parity ranging from 1 to 6, the number of malpositioned fetuses (defined as birth position not either head first and front legs forward or rear first and rear legs extended at time of delivery), ranging from 0 to 3 or more, as well as that number squared, the quality of contractions coded 0 if normal and 1 if poor (poor was coded when medical treatment fails to improve contraction strength sufficiently to deliver the puppy), as an indicator for uterine inertia, the whelping season with 4 levels (January to March, April to June, July to September and October to December), and the inbreeding coefficient of the dam. Dam age was not included as a variable because dams are bred on a regular basis so that the age at a given parity would not differ greatly among dams. Most parities and c-sections are in dams 4 years of age and younger. The identity of the dam and the identity of the sire were evaluated as random effects. In addition, two groups of variables were considered as predictors. The first group comprised variables that describe the body condition of the dam, including the adult weight in kg, the height at withers in cm, the body mass index in kg/m^2, and the weight (kg) to height (cm) ratio. The second group comprised variables describing the litter, including the litter size ranging from 2 to 13, the litter weight in kg, the average puppy weight in kg, the standard deviation of the puppy weights in kg, and the variance of the puppy weights in kg^2, and the weight of the heaviest puppy in kg.

The ordinal target trait EOW was analyzed with ordered logistic regression. The different steps of the model development are described in Additional file 1.

Results

Dropping 13 observations because c-sections were planned, 7 observations because of missing data and a single observation with parity 7 left 667 litters in the analyses. With the body mass index, height at withers or weight to height ratio in the model an additional 203 observations were lost due to missing values for the height of the dams, leaving 464 observations in the analyses. Details of the descriptive statistics of all variables are presented in Additional file 2.

P-values, df, Akaike's information criterion and the Bayesian information criterion for the full and the final model are given in Table 1.

Figures 1, 2, 3, 4, 5 and 6 visualize the probabilities of the three different outcomes of EOW for different representative combinations of the four predictors adult weight of the dam, weight of the heaviest puppy in a litter, number of malpositioned fetuses and quality of contractions. All predictions and their probabilities depicted in Figs. 1, 2, 3, 4, 5 and 6 are listed in Additional file 3.

Table 1 Comparison of the full model and the final model for EOW

Variable	Full model	Final model
Adult weight of the dam	0.001	0.003
Weight of the heaviest puppy in a litter	0.000	0.000
std of the puppy weights in a litter	0.333	
Litter size	0.128	
Parity	0.881	
Season of whelping	0.667	
Number of malpositioned fetuses, linear	0.000	0.000
Number of malpositioned fetuses, quadratic	0.000	0.042
Quality of the contractions	0.000	0.000
Inbreeding coefficient of the dam	0.973	
df	12	8
Akaike's information criterion	896.69	858.23
Bayesian information criterion	950.73	894.25

The full model was calculated with an ordered logit regression. The final model was calculated with a generalized ordered logit regression. P-values are given for each independent variable in the model

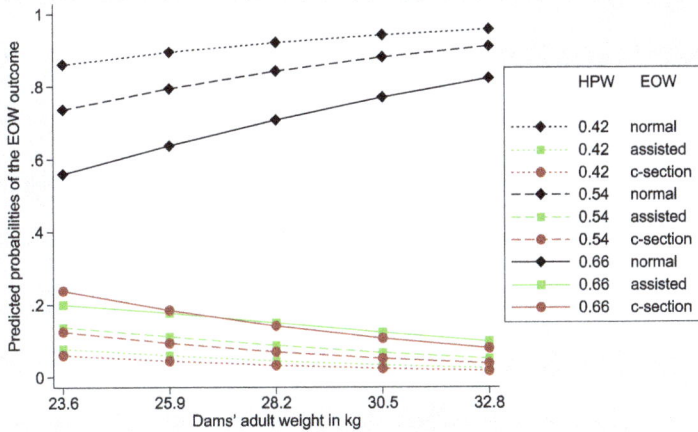

Fig. 1 Predicted probabilities of EOW outcomes if contractions are normal and no malpositioned fetus is present. On the y-axis are the predicted probabilities of the nine outcomes of the target trait EOW for the weight of the dam ranging from the mean − 2sd (23.6 kg) to the mean + 2sd (32.8 kg) on the x-axis. HPW is the weight of the heaviest puppy in a litter in kg. All predicted probabilities are significantly different from zero

Figure 1 shows the implications of an increasing adult weight of the dam for 3 different weights of the heaviest puppy in a litter in the case where the dams have normal contractions and no fetus is malpositioned. Actually, this constellation was observed in 507 litters, which is 76% of the total number of litters. Predicted probabilities for an assisted delivery and a c-section are very similar and low if the weight of the heaviest puppy in a litter is average or below average. If the weight of the heaviest puppy in a litter is high, these probabilities increase for both, but more steeply for a c-section, if the adult weight of the dam is low. The predicted probabilities of c-sections and assisted deliveries decrease slightly with an increasing adult weight of the dam. The differences between the extreme weights range from 0.04 probability points in the case of a c-section with a lightest weight of the heaviest puppy in a litter to 0.16 probability points in the case of a c-section with a heaviest weight of the heaviest puppy in a litter.

Figure 2 shows the huge impact of poor contractions on the probabilities of the c-section outcome in comparison to the situation in Fig. 1. The delivery conditions, poor contraction and no malpositioned fetus in a litter, are not very frequent in our data set (n = 14 or 2%). The risk for a c-section is highest (0.84) when the dam is light (23.6 kg) and the heaviest puppy of a litter

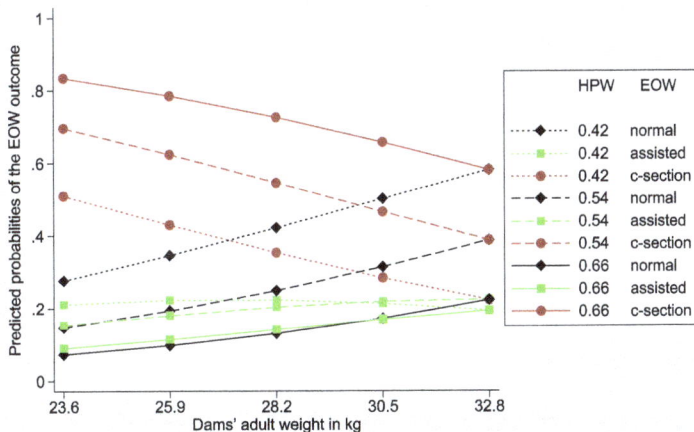

Fig. 2 Predicted probabilities of EOW outcomes if contractions are poor and no malpositioned fetus is present. On the y-axis are the predicted probabilities of the nine outcomes of the target trait EOW for the weight of the dam ranging from the mean − 2sd (23.6 kg) to the mean + 2sd (32.8 kg) on the x-axis. HPW is the weight of the heaviest puppy in a litter in kg. All predicted probabilities are significantly different from zero with the exception of the estimate for a c-section at 32.8 kg in the case of a light heaviest puppy and the estimates at 23.6 kg in the case of a heavy heaviest puppy

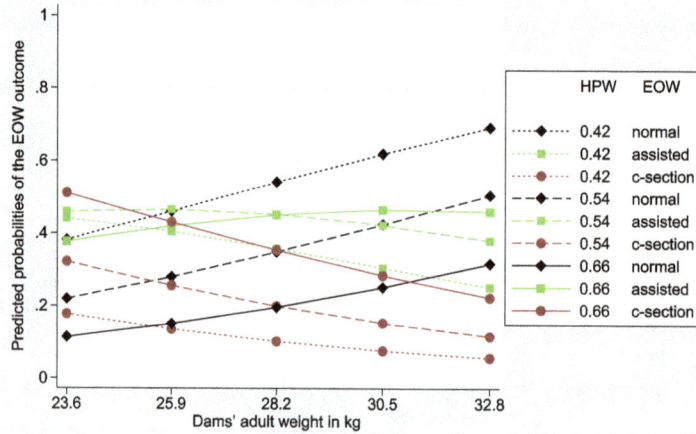

Fig. 3 Predicted probabilities of EOW outcomes if contractions are normal and one fetus is malpositioned. On the y-axis are the predicted probabilities of the nine outcomes of the target trait EOW for the weight of the dam ranging from the mean − 2sd (23.6 kg) to the mean + 2sd (32.8 kg) on the x-axis. HPW is the weight of the heaviest puppy in a litter in kg. All predicted probabilities are significantly different from zero

is heavy (0.66 kg) that is 0.60 probability points higher than in Fig. 1. The decline of the risk of a c-section from light (23.6 kg) to heavy dams (32.8 kg) seems very similar for all 3 levels of the heaviest puppy in a litter (0.29, 0.31, and 0.25 probability points). Differences of probabilities of a c-section between light and heavy weights of the heaviest puppy in a litter are similar and vary over the whole range of the adult weight of the dam from 0.32 to 0.37 probability points. In contrast, the probabilities for an assisted whelping are only slightly higher as in Fig. 1 (0.12 probability points at an adult weight of the dam of 28.2 kg and a weight of the heaviest puppy in a litter of 0.54 kg). As a consequence of the high

probabilities of a c-section, the probabilities of a normal whelping are much lower than in Fig. 1. The differences in the probabilities between light and heavy dams are more pronounced in Fig. 2.

Figure 3 shows that the impact of one malpositioned fetus is not as severe as poor contractions considering the predicted probability of a c-section. In our data, the combination of normal contractions and one malpositioned fetus occurred in 93 litters or 14% of the deliveries. Compared to Figs. 1 and 2 the probabilities for an assisted whelping are much higher (0.36 and 0.25 probability points, respectively) when the adult weight of the dam and the weight of the heaviest puppy in a litter are

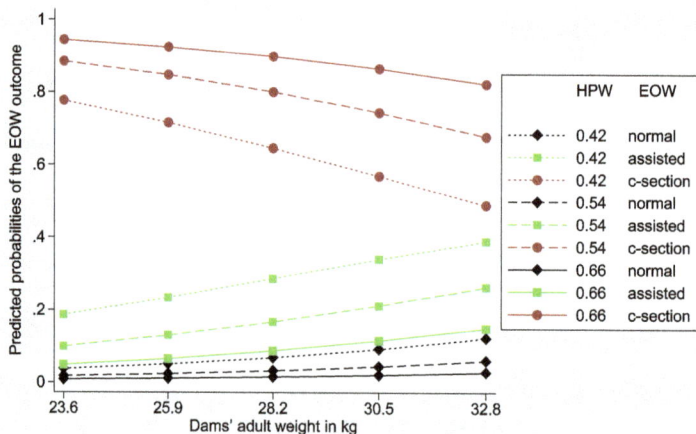

Fig. 4 Predicted probabilities of EOW outcomes if contractions are poor and one fetus is malpositioned. On the y-axis are the predicted probabilities of the nine outcomes of the target trait EOW for the weight of the dam ranging from the mean − 2sd (23.6 kg) to the mean + 2sd (32.8 kg) on the x-axis. HPW is the weight of the heaviest puppy in a litter in kg. All predicted probabilities for a normal delivery, as well as for an assisted delivery of a heavy heaviest puppy, are not significantly different from zero whereas all others are

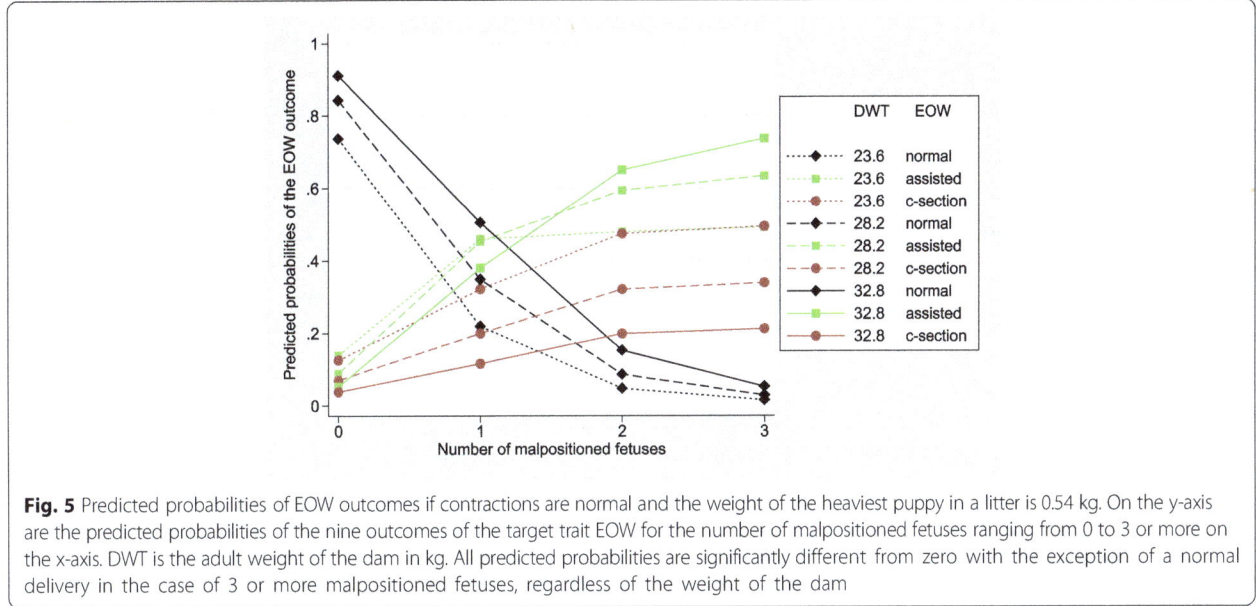

Fig. 5 Predicted probabilities of EOW outcomes if contractions are normal and the weight of the heaviest puppy in a litter is 0.54 kg. On the y-axis are the predicted probabilities of the nine outcomes of the target trait EOW for the number of malpositioned fetuses ranging from 0 to 3 or more on the x-axis. DWT is the adult weight of the dam in kg. All predicted probabilities are significantly different from zero with the exception of a normal delivery in the case of 3 or more malpositioned fetuses, regardless of the weight of the dam

average. The risks for a c-section are higher than the ones in Fig. 1 but clearly lower than in Fig. 2 (0.13 and − 0.35 probability points, respectively) when the adult weight of the dam and the weight of the heaviest puppy in a litter are average. The probabilities of c-sections decrease with an increasing adult weight of the dam about twice as much for a heavy than for a light weight of the heaviest puppy in a litter (0.29 and 0.12 probability points, respectively).

Figure 4 shows an extremely unfavorable scenario where the dam has poor contractions and one fetus is malpositioned. Fortunately there were only 3 cases in our data set which makes about 0.4%. Comparing the curve patterns with those of Fig. 2 and Fig. 3, Fig. 4 is much more similar to Fig. 2 than to Fig. 3. This seems to confirm the impression from the comparison of Fig. 3 with Fig. 2, that poor contractions do affect whelping more than malpositioned fetuses. The probabilities for a normal delivery are all not significantly different from zero that is the weight of the heaviest puppy in a litter has no influence. If the weight of the heaviest puppy in a litter is heavy and the adult weight of

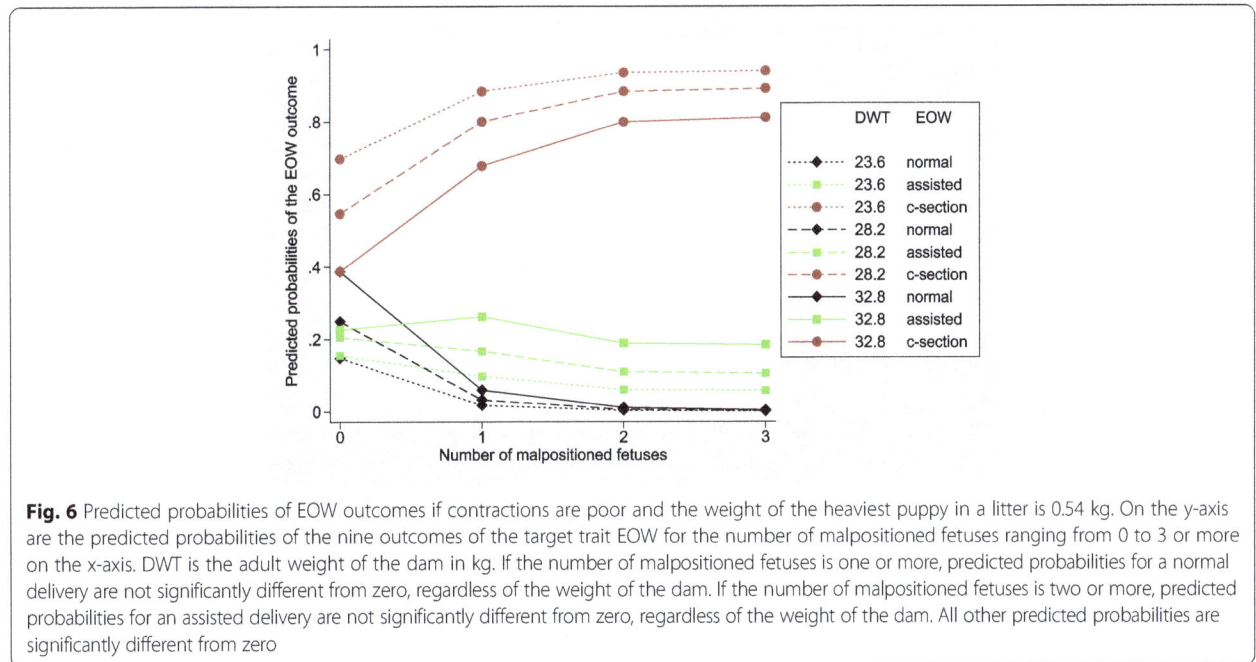

Fig. 6 Predicted probabilities of EOW outcomes if contractions are poor and the weight of the heaviest puppy in a litter is 0.54 kg. On the y-axis are the predicted probabilities of the nine outcomes of the target trait EOW for the number of malpositioned fetuses ranging from 0 to 3 or more on the x-axis. DWT is the adult weight of the dam in kg. If the number of malpositioned fetuses is one or more, predicted probabilities for a normal delivery are not significantly different from zero, regardless of the weight of the dam. If the number of malpositioned fetuses is two or more, predicted probabilities for an assisted delivery are not significantly different from zero, regardless of the weight of the dam. All other predicted probabilities are significantly different from zero

the dam below average a c-section is practically unavoidable.

Figures 5 and 6 show the influence of the number of malpositioned fetuses for 3 different adult weights of the dam on the outcome of EOW in the case where the weight of the heaviest puppy in a litter is average (0.54 kg).

Figure 5 shows the situation for dams with normal contractions which was observed in 97% of our data. Probabilities for a normal delivery drop to or close to zero if there is more than one malpositioned fetus. In the case of 3 or more malpositioned fetuses the predicted probabilities for a normal delivery for all three levels of the adult weight of the dam are not significantly different from zero. In the case of one malpositioned fetus, the probability for a normal delivery is much higher in the case of a heavy adult weight of the dam (0.51) in comparison to a light adult weight of the dam (0.22). The increase of the risk for a c-section from 0 to 2 malpositioned fetuses is linear but much greater for a light than for a heavy adult weight of the dam (0.35 and 0.16 probability points, respectively). The increase of that risk between 2 and 3 malpositioned fetuses is much smaller (0.02 and 0.01 probability points, respectively). The increase of the risk of assisted deliveries from 0 to 2 malpositioned fetuses is similar for a heavy and average adult weight of the dam (0.60 and 0.51 probability points, respectively), whereas the increase from 2 to 3 is clearly smaller (0.09 and 0.04 probability points, respectively). For a light adult weight of the dam the risk of assisted delivery increased by 0.32 probability points when the number of malpositioned fetuses increased from zero to one, with no real increase thereafter (0.03 probability points), when the number of malpositioned fetuses increased from one to three or more.

Figure 6 shows the situation where the dam has poor contractions. This situation was observed only 22 times in our data set or in 3% of all cases. It is apparent that the 3 c-section curves are positioned at much higher predicted probabilities in comparison to Fig. 5, e.g. the increase at 0 malpositioned fetuses for an average adult weight of the dam (28.2 kg) amount to 0.48 probability points and at 1 malpositioned fetus to 0.60 probability points. A c-section practically is unavoidable in the case of a light dam and 2 or more malpositioned fetuses. The probabilities of assisted deliveries decrease marginally from 0 to 3 or more malpositioned fetuses but the range between a light and heavy adult weight of the dam are smallest at 0 with 0.07 probability points and about double at the other malposition levels with 0.13 to 0.17 probability points.

Discussion

Dystocia is a common emergency in dogs and criteria for the decision to perform a timely c-section have been proposed [10]. Most of the dystocia cases in dogs are of maternal origin [1]. In a multicenter study in the USA and Canada the LR was among the top five breeds for emergency and elective c-sections during 1994 to 1997 [12]. In a multi-breed study c-sections were performed in 20% of the parturitions in LR [4]. c-sections bring a health risk for both the dam and the puppies. Therefore, the reduction of emergency c-sections is desirable in dog breeding to enhance animal welfare.

The comprehensive and large data set for parturitions recorded by the Guiding Eyes for the Blind (Additional file 4) allows for the analysis of possible predictors for c-sections. In the present data set there was one heaviest puppy weight, 0.11 kg (weight of the dam 25.40 kg) that could be considered an extreme value. Plotting the leverage against the normalized residual squared clearly showed that it did have a large residual but no leverage meaning that it had no great impact on the estimates of the regression coefficients (Additional file 1). The weight of the dams showed no extreme values. Neither the dam nor the sire could significantly explain part of the total variance in our data. It is not surprising that the body mass index of the dams did not affect the probability of the occurrence of a c-section as the body mass index in dogs probably does not reflect the condition of the body as it does it in humans. The Guiding Eyes breeding stock are also closely monitored and managed to maintain their established target weight within ±1.5 kg. We hypothesized that the weight to height ratio characterizes the body condition of a dog much better than the body mass index. Also we considered the weight to height ratio a better metric than the weight as the weighting with the height at withers will bring extreme values of the weight nearer to the mean. The fact that the weight to height ratio did not stay in the model probably is due to missing measurements of the height that led to a loss of about one third of the observations in comparison to weight. The inbreeding coefficient of the dam had no impact on the probability of the occurrence of a c-section, which may be due to the relatively low inbreeding rates with two thirds of the dams having an inbreeding coefficient below 10%. There was no influence of the whelping season. The seasonal occurrence of c-sections ranged from 11% (fall) over 14% (spring) and 15% (summer) to 16% (winter). Also the parity had no influence. Looking at the 6 parities, the percentage of c-sections is more or less evenly distributed over parities, ranging from 14% in parity 3 to 18% in parity 4 with the exception of parities 2 and 6 with only 9% c-sections. Of the litter characteristics, the weight of the heaviest puppy had an impact on the probability of the occurrence of a c-section. It is plausible that a heavier puppy is a greater physical challenge to the whelping dam than a lighter puppy, due to feto-maternal disproportion. The influence of the observer, here the whelpers, on the observations as described in other studies [13, 14] was not taken into account because whelpers were assigned to whelpings according to a schedule and had to follow a clear protocol. Therefore, the occurrence of c-sections does not reflect the presence of specific whelpers but rather is the consequence of the procedure in the protocol. The duration of a whelping was not considered in the analyses because it rather seems to be a consequence of whelping problems than its source. Also the number of stillborn puppies was not considered as a predictor because the death of a puppy could also be caused by factors leading to a c-section, e.g. suffocation during a prolonged whelping.

Our data confirms that poor contractions of a dam, as an indicator for uterine inertia, as well as malpositioned fetuses increase the probability that a whelping has to be assisted or that a c-section cannot be avoided. These factors can be related because contracting against a malpositioned fetus can lead to uterine inertia from exhaustion of uterine muscles. Malpositioned fetuses are likely the result of a feto-maternal disproportion or maternal characteristics resulting in the vaginal vault being too small for the fetus to reposition itself. Our study allowed for the examination of two additional factors leading to c-sections, the weight of the dam and the weight of the heaviest puppy in a litter. Although not significant, dams at first parity are with an average weight of 28.07 kg lighter than dams at later parities with an average weight of 28.31 kg. Dams at second or higher parity with a normal delivery on average were 0.60 kg heavier than dams with a c-section that weigh on average 27.91 kg. In the case of the first parity they are on average 1.46 kg heavier. The weight of the dams certainly has a genetic background. In another colony of LR at The Seeing Eye in New Jersey, heritabilities were estimated to be 0.44 for adult weight and 0.46 for adult height [15]. The influence of the birthweight on the probability of requiring assistance at delivery or a c-section was expected as this phenomenon is known in cattle (e.g. [16, 17]). Besides direct genetic effects, paternal and especially maternal genetic effects could, as in cattle, also play a role in dog. The genetic correlation between pelvic opening and the maternal genetic effect of dystocia scores in cattle is high with − 0.62 in heifers and − 0.77 in cows [18]. Heritabilities of direct and maternal effects were 0.25 and 0.08 respectively while heritability of cow pelvic opening was 0.21. Other authors obtained even larger heritabilities for pelvic opening with $h^2 = 0.42$ [19].

Conclusions

The four predictors, poor contractions, number of malpositioned fetuses, weight of the dam and the weight of the heaviest puppy in a litter, had an impact on the probability of the occurrence of a c-section in LR.

Therefore, the consideration of the adult weight of the dam may reduce the risk of c-sections in this colony. Dams with an adult body weight substantially below average should not be selected as breeders in this colony. The problem of the weight of the heaviest puppy in a litter must be tackled on the genetic track resorting to the estimation of breeding values that allow for maternal and paternal effects.

Our findings apply to this colony of LR and are not necessarily, but could be, also meaningful for breeds of similar stature at large. To evaluate the impact of our results on the general LR population data on the weights of the puppies at birth and the weight and possibly the height of the dam at mating are needed. Whether our findings help to improve the situation with respect to c-sections in guide dogs depends heavily on how they can be implemented in a breeding strategy that is focused on the guiding abilities of the dogs.

Additional files

Additional file 1: Presenting the model development for the analysis of EOW.

Additional file 2: Presenting descriptive statistics for all variables in the analyses.

Additional file 3: Displaying for Figs. 1, 2, 3, 4, 5 and 6 the predicted probabilities for the EOW outcomes, together with the P-values for the tests of predicted probabilities being different from zero.

Additional file 4: Displaying the data analyzed.

Abbreviations
EOW: Ease of whelping; IR: Initial Rise; LR: Labrador Retriever

Acknowledgements
The authors want to thank Barbara Havlena, Guiding Eyes for the Blind, for data editing and the two reviewers for their suggestions to improve the manuscript.

Funding
Not applicable.

Authors' contributions
JR and LM provided the data files. GD, CG and CS did the data analyses. All authors contributed to the writing and review of the manuscript and approved of its submission.

Consent for publication
Not applicable.

Competing interests
The authors declare that they have no competing interests.

Author details

[1]Institute of Genetics, Vetsuisse Faculty, University of Berne, Bremgartenstrasse 109a, 3001 Berne, Switzerland. [2]Guiding Eyes for the Blind, 611 Granite Springs Road, Yorktown Heights, NY 10598, USA. [3]Clinic of Reproductive Medicine, Vetsuisse Faculty, University of Zurich, Winterthurerstrasse 260, 8057 Zurich, Switzerland.

References

1. Davidson A. Problems during and after parturition. In: England GCW, von Heimendahl A, editors. BSAVA manual of canine and feline reproduction and neonatology. Gloucester: BSAVA; 2010. p. 121–34.
2. Bergström A, Nødtvedt A, Lagerstedt AS, Egenvall A. Incidence and breed predilection for dystocia and risk factors for cesarean section in a Swedish population of insured dogs. Vet Surg. 2006;35:786–91.
3. O'Neill DG, Church DB, McGreevy PD, Thomson PC, Brodbelt DC. Approaches to canine health surveillance. Canine Genet Epidemiol. 2014; https://doi.org/10.1186/2052-6687-1-2.
4. Evans KM, Adams VJ. Proportion of litters of purebred dogs born by cesarean section. JSAP. 2010;51:113–8.
5. Berg-Lekås ML, Högberg U, Winkvist A. Familial occurrence of dystocia. Am J Obstet Gynecol. 1998;179:117–21.
6. Algovik M, Nilsson E, Cnattingius S, Lichtenstein P, Nordenskjöld A, Westgren M. Genetic influence on dystocia. Acta Obstet Gynecol Scand. 2004;83:832–7.
7. Ratajczak CK, Muglia LJ. Insights into parturition biology from genetically altered mice. Pediatr Res. 2008;64:581–9.
8. Algovik M, Lagercrantz J, Westgren M, Nordenskjöld A. No mutations found in candidate genes for dystocia. Hum Reprod. 1999;14:2451–4.
9. Algovik M, Kivinen K, Peterson H, Westgren M, Kere J. Genetic evidence of multiple loci in dystocia – difficult labour. BMC Med Genet. 2010;11:105.
10. Gendler A, Brourman JD, Graf KE. Canine dystocia: medical and surgical treatment. Compendium. 2007;29:551–63.
11. Eneroth A, Linde-Forsberg C, Uhlhorn M, Hall M. Radiographic pelvimetry for assessment or dystocia in bitches: a clinical study in two terrier breeds. JSAP. 1999;40:257–64.
12. Moon PF, Erb HN, Ludders JW, Gleed RD, Pascoe PJ. Perioperative management and mortality rates of dogs undergoing cesarean section in the United States and Canada. JAVMA. 1998;213:365–9.
13. Meyer F, Schawalder P, Gaillard C, Dolf G. Estimation of genetic parameters for behavior based on results of German shepherd dogs in Switzerland. Appl Anim Behav Sci. 2012;140:53–61.
14. Lauper M, Gerber V, Ramseyer A, Burger D, Lüth A, Koch C, Dolf G. Heritabilities of health traits in Swiss warmblood horses. Equine Vet J. 2017;49:15–8.
15. Helmink SK, Rodriguez-Zas SL, Shanks RD, Leighton EA. Estimated genetic parameters for growth traits of German shepherd dog and Labrador retriever dog guides. J Anim Sci. 2001;79:1450–6.
16. Bellows RA, Lammoglia MA. Effects of severity of dystocia on cold tolerance and serum concentrations of glucose and cortisol in neonatal beef calves. Theriogenology. 2000;53:803–13.
17. Hickson RE, Morris ST, Kenyon PR, Lopez-Villalobos N. Dystocia in beef heifers: a review of genetic and nutritional influences. New Zealand Vet J. 2006;54:256–64.
18. Renand G, Vinet A, Krauss D, Saintilan R. Genetic relationship between pelvic opening and calving ease in the Charolais cattle breed. Renc Rech Ruminants. 2010;17:451–4.
19. Upton WH, Bunter KL. Pelvic measurement as an aid to selection in beef cattle. Proc Aust Assoc Anim Breed Genet. 1995;11:615–9.

22

Postoperative pain and short-term complications after two elective sterilization techniques: ovariohysterectomy or ovariectomy in cats

Marco Aurélio A. Pereira[1], Lucas A. Gonçalves[1], Marina C. Evangelista[2], Rosana S. Thurler[1], Karina D. Campos[1], Maira R. Formenton[1], Geni C. F. Patricio[1], Julia M. Matera[1], Aline M. Ambrósio[1] and Denise T. Fantoni[1*]

Abstract

Background: Surgical sterilization of cats is one of the most commonly performed procedures in veterinary practice and it can be accomplished by two different techniques: ovariohysterectomy (OVH) or ovariectomy (OVE). Although there is an apparent preference for OVH in United States and Canada, OVE seems to be the standard of care in many European countries due to its advantages, such as a smaller surgical incision and potentially less complications associated with surgical manipulation of the uterus. The aim of this randomized, blind, prospective study was to compare postoperative pain and short-term complications in cats undergoing ovariohysterectomy or ovariectomy.

Methods: Twenty female cats were randomly assigned into two groups (OVH, $n = 10$ and OVE, n = 10). Pain was assessed prior to surgery (baseline) and 1, 2, 4, 8 12 and 24 h after the procedure using pain and sedation scales, physiologic parameters and blood glucose levels. Short-term complications were evaluated in the early postoperative period and reassessed at day 7 and day 10.

Results: Changes in cardiovascular parameters were not clinically relevant, however cats in OVH group had higher heart rates at T1 h compared with baseline ($p = 0.0184$). Blood glucose levels in OVH group were also higher at T1 h compared with baseline ($p = 0.0135$) and with OVE group ($p = 0.0218$). Surgical time was higher in OVH group ($p = 0.0115$). Even though no significant differences in pain scores were observed between groups or time points, cats in OVH group had greater need for rescue analgesia compared with OVE (2/10 and 0/10, respectively). Complications were not observed in any cat during surgery, at days 7 and 10 postoperatively or at discharge.

Conclusions: Both surgical techniques promoted similar intensity of postoperative pain in cats and there were no short-term complications throughout the study's evaluation period. Therefore, both techniques may be indicated for surgical sterilization of cats, according to the surgeon's preference and expertise. Cats that underwent ovariectomy did not require rescue analgesia and surgical time was shorter in that group.

Keywords: Analgesia, Reproductive sterilization, Ovariohysterectomy, Ovariectomy, Cats, Pain

* Correspondence: dfantoni@usp.br
[1]Faculty of Veterinary Medicine and Animal Sciences, Department of Surgery, University of Sao Paulo, 87, Av Professor Doutor Orlando Marques de Paiva, Sao Paulo 05508-270, Brazil
Full list of author information is available at the end of the article

Background

Elective surgical sterilization of female dogs and cats is one of the most commonly performed procedures in veterinary practice due to its potential benefits, such as population control, prevention of reproductive tract diseases, attenuation of undesirable behaviors associated with hormonal activity and reduction of stray and feral populations of dogs and cats [1].

Sterilization of female cats can be accomplished by surgically removing the ovaries and the uterus (ovariohysterectomy - OVH) or by removing the ovaries only (ovariectomy - OVE). OVH is the most frequently performed technique in some countries like the United States and Canada [1]. Meanwhile, in the Netherlands and some other European countries, OVE is usually performed instead of OVH as the standard of care for sterilization [2]. Furthermore, with the development of minimally invasive surgical techniques, laparoscopic ovariectomy in cats has gained popularity [3–5].

Potential development of uterine diseases and post-surgical complications are important factors to consider in the choice of the sterilization technique. The risk of post-surgical hemorrhage is lower in OVE, partially because this complication is often related to removal of the uterus [6]. Moreover, ovariectomy has several advantages over OVH: it is technically less complicated, it allows shorter surgical and anesthetic time, there is less morbidity due to a smaller incision, less trauma in the abdomen and the broad ligaments are not torn [1, 6, 7]. Regarding postoperative pain in bitches, no significant difference between the two techniques was found [6, 8], however, there are no known studies in cats.

The aim of this study was to assess postoperative pain and short-term complications in cats undergoing either OVH or OVE.

Methods

Experimental design

This prospective, randomized, blinded, controlled study was performed at the Veterinary Hospital of the School of Veterinary Medicine and Animal Science, University of Sao Paulo, Brazil.

Animals

Twenty healthy female domestic cats undergoing OVH or OVE. All animals were deemed healthy (ASA status I) based on physical examination, medical history and laboratory tests (complete blood count, serum chemistry profile and blood glucose). Exclusion criteria included aggressiveness, signs of pre-existing pain or inflammation, underlying diseases and use of analgesic or anti-inflammatory drugs prior to the study. Animals with history of excessive fear when handled were also excluded. Written informed consent was obtained from the owners before inclusion of the animals and the study protocol (8,461,060,715/2016) was approved by the institutional Animal Ethics Committee (AEC).

Anesthetic procedure

Cats were randomly assigned to two groups (OVH or OVE; $n = 10$ each) with the help of an online random sequence generator (http://www.randomization.com). All cats received acepromazine maleate[1] (0.1 mg/kg) intramuscularly as premedication. Fifteen minutes after, a 22-gauge catheter was placed in the cephalic vein for fluids (Lactated Ringer's solution[2] at 3 mL/kg/h) and drugs administration, then anesthesia was induced with propofol[3] (5–8 mg/kg). Orotracheal intubation was performed and anesthesia was maintained with isoflurane[4] diluted in 70% of oxygen in a circular anesthesia circuit. Pressure-controlled mechanical ventilation[5] was performed (peak inspiratory pressure: 8–10 mmHg, tidal volume: 8 mL/kg and positive end-tidal expiratory pressure: 1 cm H_2O) and the respiratory rate was adjusted to maintain normocapnia (end tidal carbon dioxide, $ETCO_2$: 30–40 mmHg). Remifentanil[6] constant rate infusion (0.2–0.4 µg/kg/min) was performed to ensure intraoperative analgesia. A single anesthesiologist (LAG) and a single surgeon (JMM) performed all procedures in different dates. Animals were placed on a heating pad with caution to avoid thermal trauma. At the end of the procedure, cats in both groups received meloxicam[7] (0.1 mg/kg) intravenously at skin closure and 24 h later before hospital discharge.

Heart rate (HR), electrocardiogram (lead II), respiratory rate (RR), oxyhemoglobin saturation, and ventilatory parameters were monitored with a multiparameter bedside monitor[8]; $ETCO_2$ and end tidal isoflurane concentration (ET_{iso}) were measured by a gas analyzer[9] and non-invasive systolic blood pressure was measured with the ultrasonic Doppler method.[10]

An increase greater than 15% of baseline values of HR or systolic blood pressure was interpreted as nociception and led to an increase of 0.1 µg/kg/min in remifentanil constant rate infusion.

Surgical procedures

All surgeries were performed by a single surgeon with more than 25 years of experience (JMM) and one assistant. Standardized surgical protocols were used and the duration of all procedures was recorded, which consisted of the time from the beginning of the skin incision up to its complete closure.

Hair was clipped at the surgical site and skin was aseptically prepared. A ventral midline celiotomy was performed, with its incision starting at the caudal border of the umbilicus. The initial length of the incision was estimated by the surgeon and extended during surgery if necessary. Skin and subcutaneous tissues incision was achieved with an electrosurgical equipment,[11] which was also used for hemostasis. A small incision was made in the *linea alba* and extended in either direction with scissors to access the abdominal cavity. The left uterine horn was located and the ovary was retracted from the abdomen. Three-clamp technique was used. After section of the ovarian pedicle, an encircling ligature with 4–0 nylon[12] is placed distal to the two forceps; the ovarian artery and vein were doubly ligated.

In ovariectomy procedures, the ovaries were dissected and excised; the ovarian arteries and veins were ligated with 4–0 nylon[12] and the uterine horns were returned to their anatomic position. In ovariohysterectomy procedures, after the mesovarium was cut, the broad ligaments were torn parallel to the uterine vessels toward the cervix. The round ligaments were cut with scissors and small vessels were cauterized in case of bleeding. The uterus was removed, and the uterine pedicle was repositioned in its normal anatomic position. All ligated vessels were inspected (in their normal anatomic positions) for bleeding, and used surgical sponges were counted before the abdominal incision was closed.

The abdominal and skin closure were performed with size 4–0 nylon[12] suture material in a simple interrupted pattern.

Pain assessment

Prior to the beginning of the study, cats were clinically examined and acclimatized to the observers, cages and sedation and pain assessment tools. Pain was assessed through objective and subjective analysis before premedication (baseline, TBL) and up to 24 h after the end of the surgery, at the following time points: T1 h, T2 h, T4 h, T8 h, T12 h and T24 h.

The objective pain assessment included physiological parameters (HR, RR and rectal temperature – RT) and blood glucose levels.[13] Subjective pain scores consisted of four pain scales, the Visual Analogue Scales – VAS and three other scales described for the feline species (The Colorado State University Feline Acute Pain Scale - Colorado, The UNESP-Botucatu multidimensional composite pain scale for assessing postoperative pain in cats – UNESP, The Glasgow Feline Composite Measure Pain Scale – Glasgow) [9–12]. Sedation was assessed with a scale adapted from Valverde et al. (2004) [13]. Rescue analgesia (tramadol hydrochloride,[14] 2 mg/kg intravenously) was administered if the cat reached a score greater than or equal to the cut-off value for rescue in any scale (VAS ≥ 4, Colorado ≥2, UNESP ≥7, Glasgow ≥5). The person responsible for pain assessment (MAAP) was unaware of the surgical technique performed.

Meloxicam 0.1 mg/kg (PO, q 24 h for 1 day) and tramadol 2 mg/kg (PO, q 12 h for 3 days) were prescribed at hospital discharge.

Postoperative complications

The occurrence of adverse effects such as intra-abdominal hemorrhage during and after surgery, erythema, swelling, vaginal discharge, urinary incontinence, suture dehiscence and signs of infections, was investigated in the early postoperative period (up to 24 h after surgery) and reassessed at day 7 (follow up for complete blood count and serum chemistry) and day 10 (suture removal) of the postoperative period. The owners were contacted daily (by telephone) and asked about the cats' general condition (appetite, comfort), presence of abnormal behaviors and general appearance of the surgical wound.

Statistical analysis

Statistical analysis was performed using a statistical software.[15] Significance was defined as $p < 0.05$ (two-tailed). Results are presented as mean ± standard deviation (SD). Weight and surgical time were compared between groups by unpaired t-tests. For physiological parameters and blood glucose levels, two way-ANOVA and Sidak's post-test were performed to compare groups and time points. Differences between baseline and other time points' values in each group were assessed by Dunnett's post-test. For nonparametric data, such as pain and sedation scores, Krukal-Wallis test and Dunn post-test were used to compare groups throughout time, and the Friedman test followed by Dunn post-test was used to identify differences within a group. Fisher's exact test was used to analyze the number of rescue analgesia interventions.

Results

Twenty-two cats were initially selected, however two had to be excluded due to early pregnancy ($n = 1$) and mesenteric lymphadenitis (n = 1). Finally, 20 healthy female cats, without gross reproductive abnormalities were included in this study; OVH group ($n = 10$) and OVE group (n = 10).

Body weight (mean ± SD – OHE: 2.71 ± 0.49 kg, OVE: 2.88 ± 0.58 kg; $p = 0.5032$) and age (OHE - 15 ± 13 months, OVE – 11 ± 6 months; $p = 0.4327$) were not different between groups.

Surgical time differed significantly between groups. The OVH technique was longer than OVE (30 ± 4 min and 25 ± 5 min, respectively, $p = 0.0115$).

Physiological parameters

Baseline parameters were similar between groups. Respiratory rate did not differ between groups, or among time points observed. Heart rate was higher in OVH than in OVE group at 1 h ($p = 0,0184$). Rectal temperature decreased in both groups at T1 h, compared to baseline. Blood glucose levels were higher in OVH compared to OVE ($p = 0.0218$) and to baseline values ($p = 0,0135$) at 1 h. (Table 1).

Pain assessment

Sedation scores both in OVH and OVE groups were higher than baseline at 1 h ($p < 0.0001$ and $p = 0,0014$, respectively).

Although no significant difference was observed between groups or among time points, OVH group had higher pain scores and greater overall need for rescue analgesia. (Fig. 1).

In the OVH group, 2/10 cats required rescue analgesia. One cat received tramadol at T2 h (Scores: VAS = 4, Colorado = 2, UNESP = 11 and Glasgow = 12) and the other received it at T4 h (Scores: VAS = 4.5, Colorado = 2, UNESP = 10 and Glasgow = 6). No cats required additional analgesia in OVE group.

Short-term complications

Owners did not notice any changes in the cats' behavior or in the general appearance of the surgical wound. No complications were observed during the follow-up consultations at day 7 and day 10.

Discussion

Both surgical sterilization techniques produced similar postoperative pain levels and there were no short-term complications throughout the study's period of evaluation. This clinical study mimics the setting of veterinary practice, where young, healthy female cats are commonly spayed. A standardized anesthetic protocol and a single surgeon were chosen to reduce potential bias in the intraoperative period and postoperative pain assessments. Anesthetic and surgical complications were not observed.

Corroborating the results of previous studies performed in bitches [2, 8], surgical time differed between groups. Duration of the procedures was significantly longer in OVH than in OVE. This result confirms ovariectomy's potential advantage.

The choice of remifentanil as part of the anesthetic protocol was based on its short half-life and minimal residual analgesic effect, so that it does not interfere in postoperative sedation and analgesia [14]. Acepromazine was administered as premedication in all animals. Its antinociceptive effect was studied previously in cats and increased pressure nociceptive thresholds were observed up to 2 h [15]. In the present study, 90% of the animals showed sedation scores of 0 at T2 h, including those who needed rescue analgesia at this time point.

Changes in physiologic parameters, despite significantly different, were not clinically relevant. These changes may have been influenced by several factors other than pain, such as environmental conditions, stress associated with manipulation and behavior of the animal [16, 17]. Consequently, HR alone is a poor indicator of pain in cats [16–21]. Nevertheless, one of the cats showed increased HR and blood glucose levels in the moment it required rescue analgesia, which could be associated with pain.

Rectal temperature decreased in all groups at T1 h when compared with TBL. This is justified by the central nervous system depression caused by the inhalation anesthetic (isoflurane), which decreases the sensitivity of the thermoregulatory center of the hypothalamus, and also by the fact that small animals (under 5 kg) have higher risk of developing hypothermia due to their larger surface area to volume ratio [22]. Moreover, acepromazine is known to cause mild hypotension due to vasodilation, which contributes to decreasing body temperature [15]. An attempt to attenuate hypothermia was performed by placing the animals on a heating pad during surgery.

Table 1 Physiological parameters and blood glucose of cats undergoing ovariohysterectomy (OVH) or ovariectomy (OVE) at baseline and up to 24 h postoperatively

		Baseline	T_{1h}	T_{2h}	T_{4h}	T_{8h}	T_{12h}	T_{24h}
HR (bpm)	OVH	208 ± 28	241 ± 22*	215 ± 26	207 ± 17	206 ± 26	202 ± 20	205 ± 29
	OVE	214 ± 42	238 ± 23	215 ± 20	210 ± 28	205 ± 28	200 ± 13	196 ± 15
RR (mpm)	OVH	56 ± 19	52 ± 26	48 ± 13	52 ± 20	54 ± 12	52 ± 14	56 ± 12
	OVE	56 ± 13	53 ± 12	47 ± 12	48 ± 12	51 ± 11	47 ± 11	46 ± 11
RT (°C)	OVH	38,5 ± 0	36,6 ± 1*	37,8 ± 1	38,6 ± 1	38,3 ± 1	37,9 ± 0	37,8 ± 0
	OVE	38,3 ± 0	36,5 ± 1*	37,7 ± 1	38,2 ± 1	38,3 ± 1	38,3 ± 1	38,2 ± 1
Blood glucose (mg/dL)	OVH	78 ± 16	103 ± 34* [b]	95 ± 22	92 ± 14	84 ± 7	81 ± 9	79 ± 12
	OVE	77 ± 9	79 ± 21 [a]	85 ± 24	98 ± 17	76 ± 8	73 ± 14	73 ± 10

Data are expressed as mean ± SD. *HR* Heart rate expressed in beats per minute; *RR* Respiratory rate expressed in movements per minute; *RT* Rectal temperature in Celsius; *Value significantly different ($p < 0.05$) from TBL for that group. Letters means values significantly different among the groups in each time point, as b > a

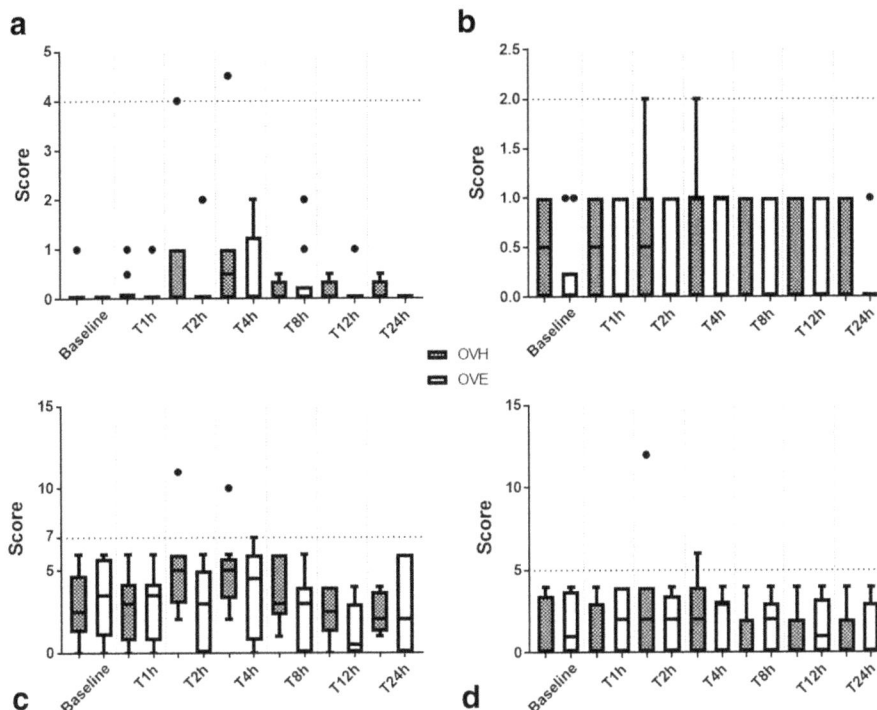

Fig. 1 Box plot showing median, interquartile range, minimum and maximum pain scores according to the subjective pain scales during the study. Differences between groups or time points compared with baseline were not observed in the Visual Analogue Scale (**a**), Colorado state university feline acute pain scale (**b**), UNESP-Botucatu multidimensional composite pain scale for assessing postoperative pain in cats (**c**) and Glasgow feline composite measure pain scale (**d**)

In the first postoperative assessment time point (T1 h), blood glucose levels were significantly higher in the OVH group compared both with its baseline values and with OVE group. That could have been caused by the substantial increase observed in one cat that required analgesic rescue (T2 h). This cat's blood glucose levels at baseline, T1 h and T2 h were 73, 164 and 130 mg/dL, respectively. Pain, as a stress factor, may be associated with increases in blood glucose concentration. Changes in blood glucose levels were previously described as part of analgesic efficacy assessment [23, 24].

Pain scores were not significantly different between groups or compared with baseline values. Similar findings have been previously observed in bitches undergoing OVH or OVE [6, 8]. In the present study, four subjective pain measurement tools [9–12] were used to further quantify differences after surgery, however no statistical differences between groups was found. This may be explained by the fact that the analgesic regimen used during and after surgery was satisfactory for both surgical techniques, thus the pain experienced by the cats was only mild.

The subjective nature of pain assessment and the difficulty in recognizing behavioral signs that may be indicative of painful states, especially in a hospital environment, are some of the inherent limitations of pain scales. A study that investigated the correlation between the UNESP-Botucatu and the CMPS-Feline pain scales have shown strong association between the tools, however outcome for rescue analgesia would differ when using each of scales [25]. In the present study, all cats showed scores above the cut-off values of all scales in the moments when they required rescue analgesia.

The Portuguese version (native language of the evaluators) of the UNESP-Botucatu scale was used. The Colorado and Glasgow pain scales were used in their original language of publication (English). The observer's level of experience and cultural and language differences are other factors that might influence pain assessment using scales [26]. Due to the difficulty in measuring blood pressure in non-anesthetized or sedated cats in a reliable way [12, 27] we did not use this part of the UNESP-Botucatu scale (subscale 3 - physiological variables). This scale has been previously validated to be used not only in its full version, but also considering each of the subscales, so that they could be independently evaluated and even omitted if necessary. Considering the descriptive and ROC curve analysis, rescue analgesia should be performed if scores reach at least 26.6% of the scale's maximum score and is strongly recommended if it reaches at least 33.3% [12]. Therefore, 7/27 in the UNESP-Botucatu pain scale was defined as the cut-off value for the administration of rescue analgesia.

The anesthetic and analgesic protocols provided adequate analgesia in the postoperative period in most of the cats. Two cats in OVH group required rescue analgesia, while there was no need for additional analgesia in the OVE group. This could be related to the greater degree of trauma in the abdomen and to the rupture of the broad ligaments that occur during ovariohysterectomy, which may correspond to a higher level of nociception [8, 28] and might have contributed to the need for rescue analgesia in OVH group. The administration of tramadol as rescue analgesia controlled pain adequately.

One of the limitations of the present study is that abdominal echography was not performed in the perioperative period. We could only evaluate the complications based on expected clinical signs or behavioral changes based on owners' report.

Conclusions

Both OVH and OVE promoted similar intensity of postoperative pain and absence of surgical complications in cats. Either technique may be indicated for surgical sterilization, according to the surgeon's preference and expertise. Although no significant differences were observed in pain scores between groups, two cats in OVH group required rescue analgesia, whereas none required it in OVE group, and surgical time was shorter in OVE procedure. No short-term complications were observed throughout the study's evaluation period.

Endnotes

[1]Acepran 0,2%, Vetnil, SP, Brazil.

[2]Ringer Lactato, Baxter Hospitalar Ltda., SP, Brazil

[3]Propovan, Cristália, SP, Brazil

[4]Isoflorane, Cristália, SP, Brazil

[5]Anesthetic Machine Inter Linea A, Intermed, SP, Brazil

[6]Ultiva 2 mg, GlaxoSmithKline, RJ, Brazil

[7]Maxicam 0,2%, Ourofino Saúde Animal, SP - licensed for IV use in Brazil

[8]Multi-parameter Patient Monitor DX 2020, Dixtal Biomédica Ind. Com. Ltda., SP, Brazil

[9]Anesthetic Gas Monitor The Poet IQ2, Critcare Systems, Inc., North Kingstown, U.S

[10]Ultrasonic Doppler Flow Detector Model 812, Parks Medical Eletronics, Inc., Oregon, U.S

[11]Aspen Excalibur Plus PC Electrosurgical Unit, CONMED, New Jersey, U.S

[12]Mononylon Ethilon 4.0, Ethicon US, LLC, U.S

[13]Glycosimeter Optium Xceed™, Abbott Laboratories, Philippines

[14]Cronidor 2%, Agener União Saúde Animal, SP, Brazil

[15]GraphPad Prism 7.03 Software Inc., La Jolla, U.S

Abbreviations

HR: Heart rate; OVE: Ovariectomy; OVH: Ovariohysterectomy; RR: Respiratory rate; RT: Rectal temperature

Acknowledgements
Not applicable.

Funding
This research had no funding sources.

Authors' contributions

MAAP collected and analyzed data, and drafted the manuscript. LAG, MCE, RST, KDC and GPF participated in sample collection and technical assistance. JMM performed the surgeries. MCE, MRF, JMM and DTF participated in statistical analysis and manuscript writing. MAAP, JMM, AMA and DTF participated in the conceptualization and study design. All authors read and approved the final manuscript.

Ethics approval

This study which involved the use of animals belonging to the phylum Chordata, subphylum Vertebrata (except human beings), for scientific research purpose is in accordance with Law 11.794 of October 8, 2008, Decree 6899 of July 15, 2009, as well as with the rules issued by the National Council for Control of Animal Experimentation (CONCEA), and was approved by the Ethic Committee on Animal Use of the School of Veterinary Medicine and Animal Science (University of São Paulo) (CEUA/FMVZ) (protocol number 8461060715/2016). The cat owners were informed about the methods and purpose of the study and gave their written informed consent.

Consent for publication

Not applicable.

Competing interests

The authors declare that they have no competing interests.

Author details

[1]Faculty of Veterinary Medicine and Animal Sciences, Department of Surgery, University of Sao Paulo, 87, Av Professor Doutor Orlando Marques de Paiva, Sao Paulo 05508-270, Brazil. [2]Faculty of Veterinary Medicine, Department of Clinical Sciences, Université de Montréal, Saint-Hyacinthe, Quebec, Canada.

References

1. Detora M, Mccarthy RJ. Commentary ovariohysterectomy versus ovariectomy for elective sterilization of female dogs and cats: is removal of the uterus necessary? J Am Vet Med Assoc. 2011;11:1409–12.
2. Van Goethem B, Schaefers-Okkens A, Kirpensteijn J. Making a rational choice between ovariectomy and ovariohysterectomy in the dog: a discussion of the benefits of either technique. Vet Surg. 2006;35:136–43.
3. Coisman JG, Case JB, Shih A, Harrison K, Isaza N, Ellison G. Comparison of surgical variables in cats undergoing single-incision laparoscopic ovariectomy using a LigaSure or extracorporeal suture versus open ovariectomy. Vet Surg. 2014;43:38–44.
4. van Nimwegen SA, Kirpensteijn J. Laparoscopic ovariectomy in cats: comparison of laser and bipolar electrocoagulation. J Feline Med Surg. 2007;9:397–403.
5. Shih AC, CASE JB, Coisman JG, Isaza NM, Junior DA, III Maisenbacher HW. Cardiopulmonary effects of laparoscopic Ovariectomy of variable duration in cats. Vet Surg. 2015;44:2–6.

Postoperative pain and short-term complications after two elective sterilization techniques: ovariohysterectomy...

189

6. Peeters ME, Kirpensteijn J. Comparison of surgical variables and short-term postoperative complications in healthy dogs undergoing ovariohysterectomy or ovariectomy. J Am Vet Med Assoc. 2011;238:189–94.

7. Okkens AC, Kooistra HS, Nickel RF. Comparison of long-term effects of ovariectomy versus ovariohysterectomy in bitches. J Reprod Fertil. 1997;51:227–31.

8. Tallant A, Ambros B, Freire C, Sakals S. Comparison of intraoperative and postoperative pain during canine ovariohysterectomy and ovariectomy. Can Vet J. 2016;57:741–6.

9. Jensen MP, Chen C, Brugger AM. Interpretation of visual analog scale ratings and change scores: a reanalysis of two clinical trials of postoperative pain. J Pain. 2003;4:407–14.

10. Hellyer PW, Uhrig SR, Robinson NG. Feline Acute Pain Scale. Fort Collins: State University Veterinary Medical Center; 2006. http://csu-cvmbs.colostate.edu/Documents/anesthesia-pain-management-pain-score-feline.pdf>. Accessed 10 May 2015

11. Reid J, Scott EM, Calvo G, Nolan AM. Definitive Glasgow acute pain scale for cats: validation and intervention level. Vet Rec. 2017;180:449.

12. Brondani JT, Luna SPL, Minto BW, Santos BPR, Beier SL, Matsubara LM, Padovani CR. Validade e responsividade de uma escala multidimensional para avaliação de dor pós-operatória em gatos. Arq Bras Med Vet Zootec. 2012;6:1529–38.

13. Valverde A, Cantwell S, Hernández J, Brotherson C. Effects of acepromazine on the incidence of vomiting associated with opioid administration in dogs. Vet Anaesth Analg. 2004;31:40–5.

14. Pypendop BH, Brosnan RJ, Siao KT, Stanley SD. Pharmacokinetics of remifentanil in conscious cats and cats anesthetized with isoflurane. Am J Vet Res. 2008;69:531–6.

15. Steagall PV, Taylor PM, Brondani JT, Luna SP, Dixon MJ. Antinociceptive effects of tramadol and acepromazine in cats. J Feline Med Surg. 2008;10:24–31.

16. Hellyer P, Rodan I, Brunt J, Downing R, Hagedorn JE, Robertson SA. AAHA/AAFP pain management guidelines for dogs and cats. J Feline Med Surg. 2007;6:466–80.

17. Brondani JT, Luna SP, Beier SL, et al. Analgesic efficacy of perioperative use of vedaprofen, tramadol or their combination in cats undergoing ovariohysterectomy. J Feline Med Surg. 2009;11:420–9.

18. Mollenhoff A, Nolte I, Kramer S. Anti-nociceptive efficacy of carprofen, levomethadone and buprenorphine for pain relief in cats following major orthopaedic surgery. J Vet Med A Physiol Pathol Clin Med. 2005;52:186–98.

19. Smith JD, Allen SW, Quandt JE, Tackett RL. Indicators of postoperative pain in cats and correlation with clinical criteria. Am J Vet Res. 1996;57:1674–8.

20. Cambridge AJ, Tobias KM, Newberry RC, et al. Subjective and objective measurements of postoperative pain in cats. J Am Vet Med Assoc. 2000;217:685–90.

21. Epstein M, Rodan I, Griffenhagen G, Kadrlik J, Petty M, Robertson S, Simpson W. 2015 AAHA/AAFP pain management guidelines for dogs and cats. J Am Anim Hosp Assoc. 2015;2:67–84.

22. Murison P. Prevention and treatment of perioperative hypothermia in animals under 5 kg bodyweight. Pract. 2001;23:412–8.

23. Smith JD, Allen SW, Quandt JE. Changes in cortisol concentration in response to stress and postoperative pain in client-owned cats and correlation with objective clinical variables. Am J Vet Res. 1999;60:432–6.

24. Carroll GL, Howe LB, Peterson KD. Analgesic efficacy of preoperative administration of meloxicam or butorphanol in onychectomized cats. J Am Vet Med Assoc. 2005;226:913–9.

25. Steagall PV, Benito J, Monteiro BP, Doodnaught GM, Beauchamp G, Evangelista MC. Analgesic effects of gabapentin and buprenorphine in cats undergoing ovariohysterectomy using two pain-scoring systems: a randomized clinical trial. J Feline Med Surg. 2017. https://doi.org/10.1177/1098612X17730173.

26. Doodnaught GM, Benito J, Monteiro BP, Beauchamp G, Grasso SC, Steagall PV. Agreement among undergraduate and graduate veterinary students and veterinary anesthesiologists on pain assessment in cats and dogs: a preliminary study. Can Vet J. 2017;58:805–8.

27. Brondani JT, Luna S, Padovani CR. Refinement and initial validation of a multidimensional composite scale for use in assessing acute postoperative pain in cats. Am J Vet Res. 2011;2:174–83.

28. Höglund OV, Olsson K, Hagman R, Öhlund M, Olsson U, Lagerstedt AS. Comparison of haemodynamic changes during two surgical methods for neutering female dogs. Res Vet Sci. 2011;91:159–63.

Treatment of calvarial defects by resorbable and non-resorbable sonic activated polymer pins and mouldable titanium mesh in two dogs

Pierre Langer[*] ⓘ, Cameron Black, Padraig Egan and Noel Fitzpatrick

Abstract

Background: To date, calvarial defects in dogs have traditionally been addressed with different types of implants including bone allograft, polymethylmethacrylate and titanium mesh secured with conventional metallic fixation methods. This report describes the use of an absorbable and non absorbable novel polymer fixation method, Bonewelding® technology, in combination with titanium mesh for the repair of calvarial defects in two dogs. The clinical outcomes and comparative complication using resorbable and non-resorbable thermoplastic pins were compared.

Case presentation: This report of two cases documents the repair of a traumatic calvarial fracture in an adult male Greyhound and a cranioplasty following frontal bone tumor resection in an adult female Cavalier King Charles Spaniel with the use of a commercially available titanium mesh secured with an innovative thermoplastic polymer screw system (Bonewelding®). The treatment combination aimed to restore cranial structure, sinus integrity and cosmetic appearance. A mouldable titanium mesh was cut to fit the bone defect of the frontal bone and secured with either resorbable or non-resorbable polymer pins using Bonewelding® technology. Gentamycin-impregnated collagen sponge was used intraoperatively to assist with sealing of the frontal sinuses. Calvarial fracture and post-operative implant positioning were advised using computed tomography. A satisfactory restoration of skull integrity and cosmetic result was achieved, and long term clinical outcome was deemed clinically adequate with good patient quality of life. Postoperative complications including rostral mesh uplift with minor associated clinical signs were encountered when resorbable pins were used. No postoperative complications were experienced in non-resorbable pins at 7 months follow-up, by contrast mesh uplift was noted 3 weeks post-procedure in the case treated using absorbable pins.

Conclusions: The report demonstrates the innovative use of sonic-activated polymer pins (Bonewelding® technology) alongside titanium mesh is a suitable alternative technique for skull defect repair in dogs. The use of Bonewelding® may offer advantages in reduction of surgical time. Further, ultrasonic pin application may be less invasive than alternative metallic fixation and potentially reduces bone trauma. Polymer systems may offer enhanced mesh-bone integration when compared to traditional metallic implants. The use of polymer pins demonstrates initial potential as a fixation method in cranioplasty. Initial findings in a single case comparison indicate a possible advantage in the use of non-absorbable over the absorbable systems to circumvent complications associated with variable polymer degradation, further long term studies with higher patient numbers are required before reliable conclusions can be made.

Keywords: Titanium mesh, Bonewelding®, Calvarial defect, Polymer pins, Bioresorbable, Non-resorbable

* Correspondence: pierre.langer@hotmail.com
Fitzpatrick Referrals, Orthopaedic and Neurology Hospital, Halfway Lane, Eashing, Godalming GU7 2QQ, UK

Background

Calvarial defects are an unavoidable consequence following resection of primary bone tumors of the skull [1–6] and less frequently following traumatic calvarial fracture [7]. A range of cranioplasty techniques including bone allograft, polymethylmethacrylate (PMMA) and titanium (Ti) mesh have been used to repair skull defects following tumour resection in dogs [1–3, 5]. Calvarial defects of traumatic origin in humans have been treated using customisable mouldable materials including Ti mesh, polyetheretherketone, PMMA and bioceramic hydroxyapatite (HA) [8, 9].

Cranial fractures experience complication due to paucity of available bone stock and limited soft tissue coverage, further complications may arise due to sinus involvement and in such cases care must be given to restore sinusal architecture with internal fixation [10]. Establishing an adequate air-tight seal is of paramount importance in sinus fracture repair [10]. The challenge of repairing irregular bone defects with associated bone-stock loss restricts the use of conventional metal implants in maxillofacial surgery [11]. As an alternative to metallic screws, polymer pins have been used clinically in human craniomaxillary surgery [12]. BoneWelding® technology (WW Technology AG, Schlieren, Switzerland) utilises thermoplastic polymer screws melted by ultrasonic activation, the melted polymer infiltrates surrounding bone geometry, subsequent rapid cooling and hardening providing a comprehensive bone-implant interface [13]. BoneWelding® technology can be applied rapidly with minimal bone trauma and may offer an effective alternative to metallic fixation in calvarial repair.

This case report documents the repair of a traumatic calvarial fracture in a Greyhound and a cranioplasty following frontal bone tumor resection in a Cavalier King Charles Spaniel with the use of a commercially available Ti mesh secured with an innovative thermoplastic polymer screw system. The treatment combination aimed to restore cranial structure, sinus integrity and cosmetic appearance. The clinical application, outcomes and complications are reported and contrasted when using resorbable (case 1) and non-resorbable (case 2) thermoplastic pins. The authors acknowledge that only one case of each system is represented therefore definitive recommendations cannot be made on the suitability of one system versus the other, however the authors do propose that findings described may contribute to clinical decision making in future scenarios.

Case presentation
Case 1

A nine-year-old entire male greyhound presented with head trauma resulting from a collision with a park bench. The dog had no previous significant clinical history. On examination, cardiovascular parameters were stable overt distress in the animal not apparent. The dog was ambulatory with normal gait and posture devoid of proprioceptive deficits.

Thorough head inspection revealed subcutaneous emphysema between the eyes and a superficial cut to the right dorso-orbital region. Mild right unilateral epistaxis was noted. The dog resented palpation of the right frontal bone and a communication with the sinonasal cavity was inferred by the presence of a flail segment movement of the bone synchronous with respiration. Cranial nerve examination demonstrated bilateral delayed pupillary light reflex (PLR) and normal pupil size, the remainder of the neurological examination was within normal limits.

A right-sided frontal bone depression fracture was suspected founded on clinical findings. Radiographs and Computer Tomography (CT) imaging with a three-dimensional reconstruction of the skull were performed under general anaesthesia (see Fig. 1a-c). Radiographs of the cervical spine were unremarkable.

CT imaging revealed a comminuted, depressed fracture of the frontal bone that extended from the level of the maxillary recesses up to the caudal aspect of the frontal sinuses at the level of the dorsal aspect of the right maxillary, nasal and frontal bones. Surgical repair of the defect was warranted to reestablish sinus architecture and mechanical stability [10]. Further, fracture comminution is associated with soft tissue contracture leading to cavitation with connective tissue scarring and sequestrum formation [14], fracture repair addresses soft tissue injury and may minimize long-term risks of complication [15]. Surgery was carried out three days after admission.

A standard dorsal approach to the frontal bone was taken (Fig. 2-a). A malleable highly porous Ti mesh (0.2 mm thickness with 1.4 mm by 0.6 mm elongated pores) was contoured to the patient's skull (Fig. 2-b).

The Ti mesh was firmly seated against the skull and a 1.6 mm drill bit, with a 6 mm stop, was used to drill pilot holes through the mesh into the skull. A 2.1 mm diameter resorbable poly-L, D-lactic acid (PLDLA) thermoplastic pin was placed into the pilot hole and the ultrasonic trode applied to the proximal end of the pin (Fig. 2-c). The ultrasonic device was activated melting the outer surface of the pin and allowing it to be advanced into the pilot hole. Further pilot holes were drilled around the periphery of the Ti mesh at 20-25 mm intervals and thermoplastic pins inserted until the Ti mesh was adequately secured.

The surgical site was flushed with copious volumes of sterile saline and a sheet of gentamycin-impregnated collagen (Collatamp®, EusaPharma) was overlaid on the implant to prevent infection and assist in achieving a pneumatic seal. Prophylactic intravenous antibiotic cover

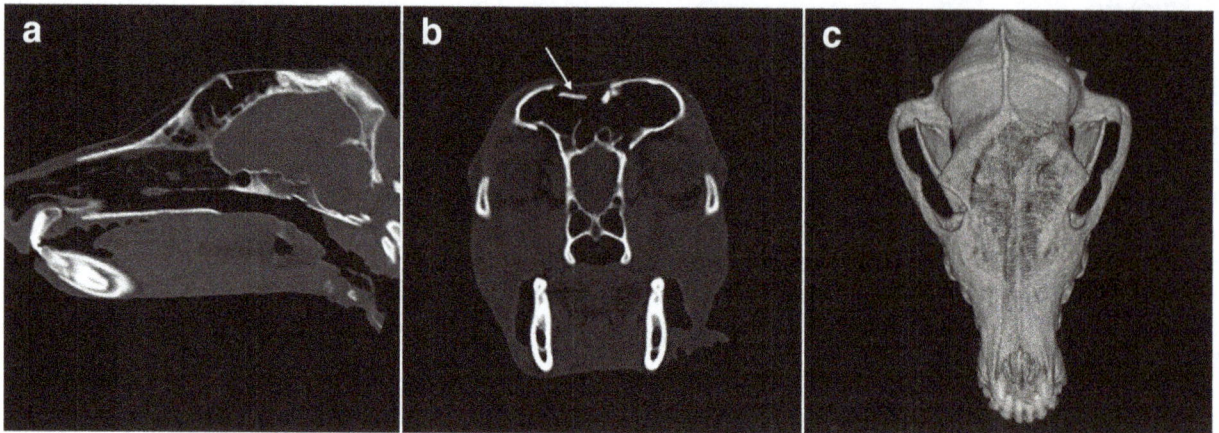

Fig. 1 a Parasagittal reconstruction of the skull showing the calvarial fracture at the level of the frontal bone. **b** Transverse image at the level of the frontal sinuses showing two calvarial fragments were displaced with the main one being depressed into the lumen of the left frontal sinus (white arrow). **c** Three-dimensional reconstructed volume rendering of the skull showing a right frontal depressed bone fracture

was provided by clavulanated amoxicillin (20 mg/kg; Augmentin, GSK) given 30 min pre-operatively and every 90 min thereafter for surgery duration. Recovery from anaesthesia was uneventful. Post-operative analgesia was provided with intravenous methadone (0.2 mg/kg q4hours; Comfortan, Dechra). Postoperative radiographs and CT images showed satisfactory positioning of the Ti mesh and adequate coverage of the calvarial defect (Fig. 3-a, b, c).

The dog was discharged two days after surgery with a 10 day course of oral carprofen (2 mg/kg q24hours; Rimadyl, Zoetis) and oral clavulanic acid-amoxicillin (20 mg/kg q12h; Synulox, Zoetis).

The dog re-presented two weeks after discharge, with hyperthermia and swelling around the surgical site. Subcutaneous oedema was present in the absence of emphysema. Sampling for culture and sensitivity was prevented by the absence of nasal and surgical

site discharge, exposure of the wound to obtain a swab sample was deemed inappropriate. Antibiotic therapy effective against common nasal pathogens [16] was introduced with oral cefalexin (20 mg/kg q 12 hours; Therios, Ceva) for ten days. Clinical signs had resolved at 1 week post treatment.

At the six weeks recheck, the physical examination was within normal limits. No pain was elicited upon palpation of the surgical site and no indications of infection recurrence was found. Radiographs and CT of the skull revealed a slight uplift of the mesh at its most rostral aspect from the frontal bone. Mesh uplift was not a clinical concern at this stage. Radiographs and CT scan at 6 months revealed soft tissue swelling between the rostral mesh portion and the skull (see Fig. 4-a). Decision was made to trim and re-contour the uplifted mesh. The procedure and recovery were uneventful and no further complications were experienced.

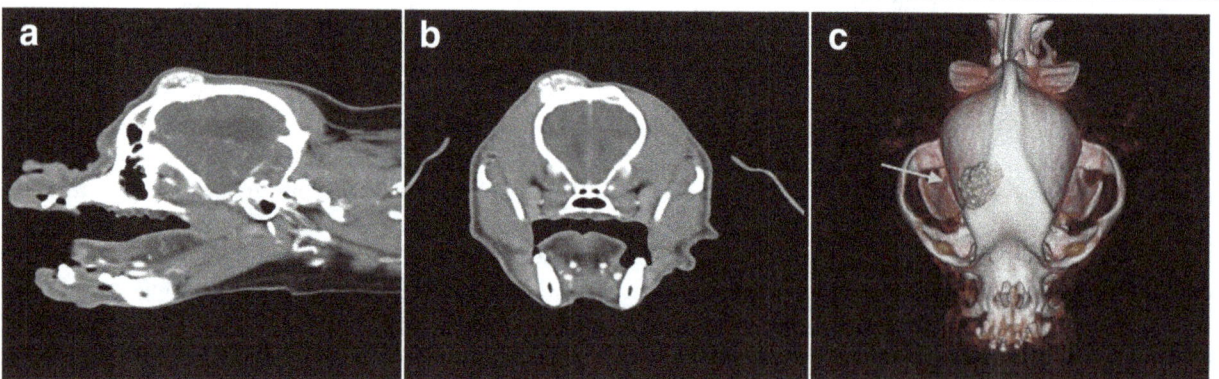

Fig. 2 a Parasagittal CT scan reconstruction showing a 25mm height x 20mm diameter ovoid mass arising from the right frontal bone above the right orbital globe. **b** Transverse CT scan image of the skull showing the mass arising from the right frontal bone. **c** Three-dimensional reconstructed volume rendering of the skull showing the mass arising from the right frontal bone (white arrow).

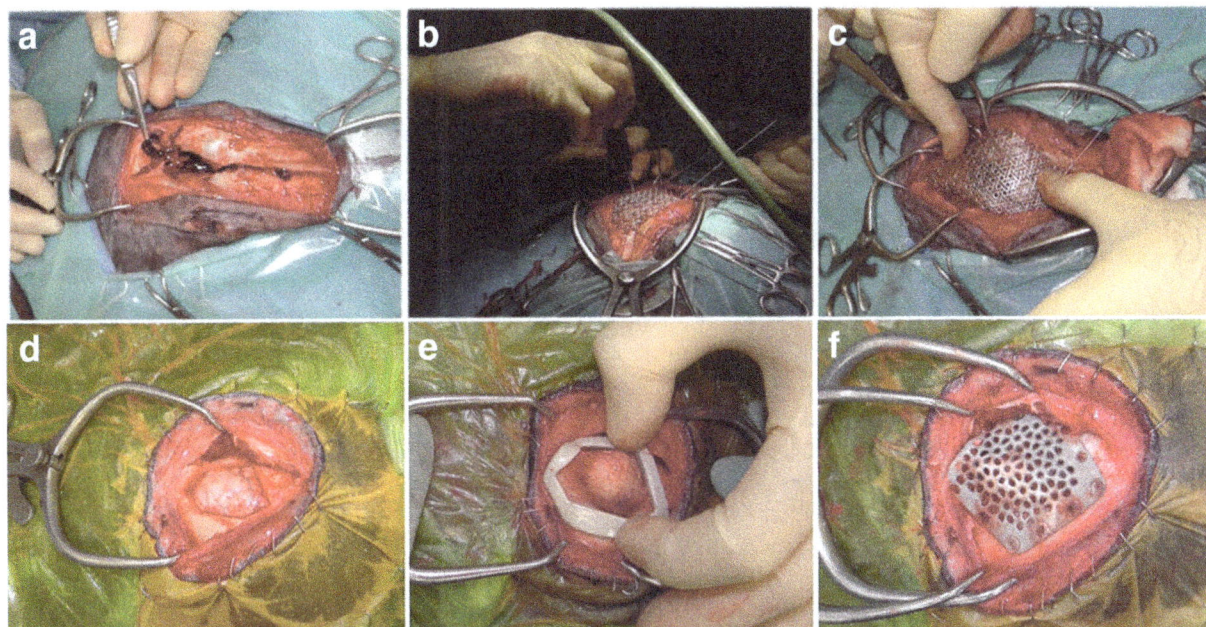

Fig. 3 a Surgical exposure of the calvarial fracture site. **b** Intraoperative use of the ultrasonic device and **c** Intraoperative contouring of the titanium mesh (Case 1). **d** Surgical exposure of the calvarial resection site. E) Custom template designed for border demarcation and (F) Titanium mesh secured with nonresorbable polymer pins covering the defect (Case 2)

At 2 years assessment, radiographs and CT scan confirmed adequate contouring and positioning of the Ti mesh. Radiographs revealed a bone-dense opacity between the rostral part of the mesh and the skull potentially associated with mesh micromotion stimulating periosteal reaction (Fig. 4-b). The degree of new bone formation around the mesh periphery was difficult to ascertain radiographically, however, clinical examination was unremarkable and cosmetic result was satisfactory. The owners did not raise any further concerns regarding the patients ability to participate in normal lifestyle and activity.

Case 2

A ten-year-old neutered female Cavalier King Charles Spaniel presented for a gradually enlarging mass on the right frontal bone with no associated clinical signs. The mass was bone-like and non-painful upon palpation. The remainder of clinical examination was within normal limits. Fine needle aspirates of the mass revealed evidence of bone remodeling compatible with a neoplastic process yet were not diagnostic, further investigation was declined and mass excision by surgery was planned. Radiography and CT imaging of the

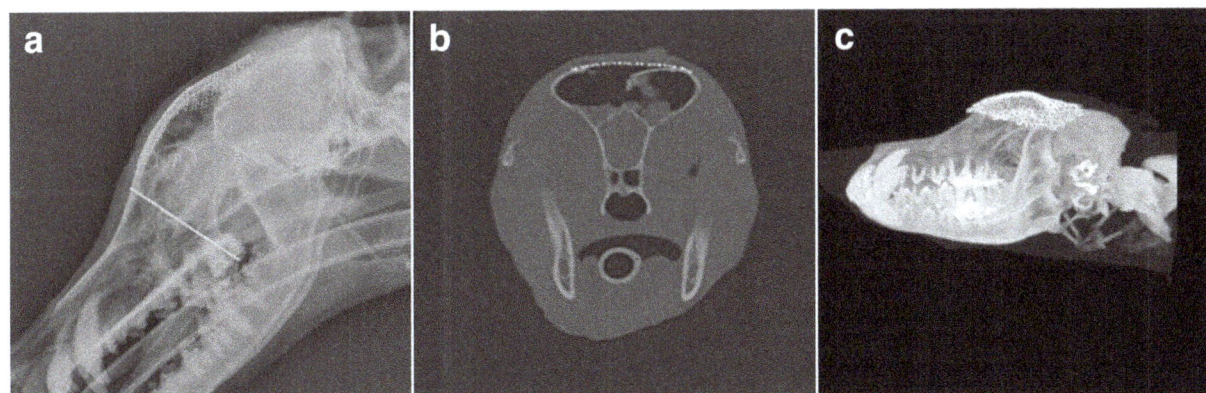

Fig. 4 a Lateral immediate postoperative radiographic view of the skull showing titanium mesh spanning from the level of the third premolar maxillary tooth (grey line) until the level of the parietal bones. **b** Immediate postoperative transverse CT reconstruction at the level of the frontal sinuses showing a titanium mesh repair spanning the right frontal bone fracture. **c** Three-dimensional reconstruction of the skull showing the titanium mesh covering the caudal aspect of the maxillary bones and rostral frontal bone

skull were performed under general anaesthesia to advise surgical planning and custom 3D Ti mesh design for use in reconstruction following tumour resection. Thoracic and abdominal CT scan were also taken for staging and were negative for metastatic disease. CT imaging of the skull revealed a 25 mm (h) × 20 mm (diam.) ovoid mass arising from the right frontal bone above the right orbital globe (see Fig. 5a-c). Surgery was implemented a week later.

The same surgical approach was performed (Fig. 2-d). A craniotomy with resection margins guided by the use of customised template was performed (Fig. 2-e). The resection guide was computer modelled from CT imaging and printed using a sterolithographic system. A pre-contoured Ti mesh aided by computer modeling and computed manufacture was firmly seated to the patient's skull covering the defect (see Fig. 2-f). The protocol for thermoplastic pin placement and application of gentamycin-impregnated collagen sheet was as described for patient 1. Non-resorbable methacrylate-butadiene-styrol (MBS) pins were used in case 2 for fixation in contrast to resorbable PLDLA described in case 1.

Prophylactic intravenous antibiotic cover was provided by cefuroxime (20 mg/kg; Zinacef, GSK) given 30 min pre-operatively and every 90 min thereafter for surgery duration. Recovery from anaesthesia was uneventful. Post-operative analgesia was provided with intravenous methadone (0.2 mg/kg q 4 h) and in travenous paracetamol (10 mg/kg q12hours; Perfalgan, BristolMyers squibb). Postoperative radiographs and CT images showed satisfactory positioning of the Ti mesh and adequate coverage of the calvarial defect (Fig. 6-a, b, c). The dog was discharged six days after surgery after uneventful hospitalisation.

The dog re-presented two weeks after discharge for suture removal. Surgical wound has healed and physical examination was within normal limits. At the ten weeks recheck, physical examination was within normal limits and the owner reporting no restrictions on the patient's activity. There was no pain elicited upon surgical site palpation. Radiographs and CT of the skull revealed satisfactory positioning of the mesh. A histological diagnosis of multilobular osteochondrosarcoma was made with potential of local recurrence advised.

At 7 months assessment, owners reported a small bone-like mass near the resection site. This clinical finding was consistent with either local recurrence or reactive osseus proliferation. CT scan identified the region of proliferation as dorsal and to the right side of the Ti mesh. The mesh remained well localised and confluent with the skull. The remaining clinical examination was unremarkable and cosmetic result was satisfactory. Owners did not raise concerns regarding overall quality of life and further investigation of the mass was declined. A request to examine the patient at 1 year follow up was again declined by the owner due to long travel distance.

Discussion

Three main goals should be achieved when reconstructive maxillofacial surgery is performed: biomechanical stability, cerebral protection and cosmetic restoration [17, 18]. In case 1, medical management was not deemed appropriate as the scale of damage and exposure of nasal sinus was considered significant enough to undermine mechanical integrity of the facial and skull bones. Referenced surgical treatment modalities of maxillofacial fractures in humans advocates sinus reconstruction and restoration of mechanical stability for the protection of sensitive intracranial structures and limitation of infection risk [10]. Although specific guidelines pertaining to canine surgery could not be found it was the authors' clinical decision that guidelines for humans be consistent with the clinical need in case 1, relating to similarity of intracranial structure and

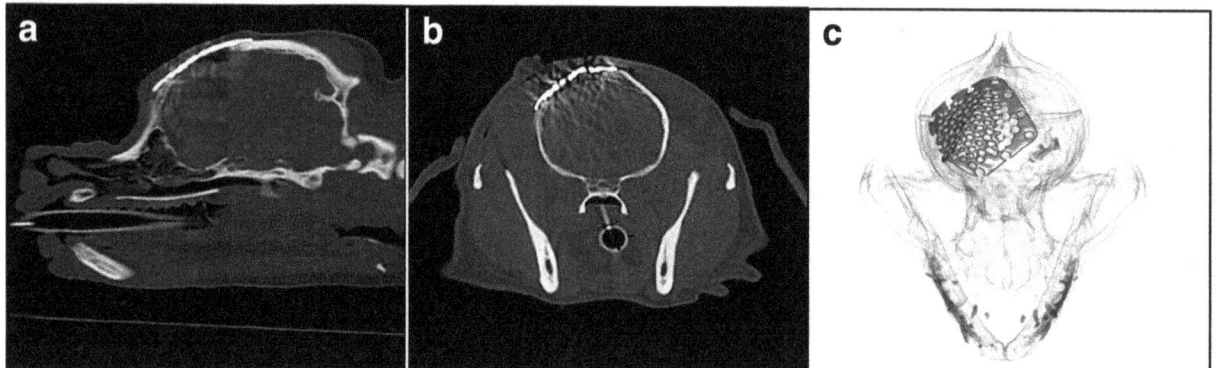

Fig. 5 a Immediate postoperative sagittal CT scan reconstruction of the skull showing adequate covering of the surgical defect in the right frontal bone by titanium mesh. **b** Immediate postoperative transverse CT scan reconstruction. **c** Three-dimensional volume rendering reconstruction of the skull with mesh in situ

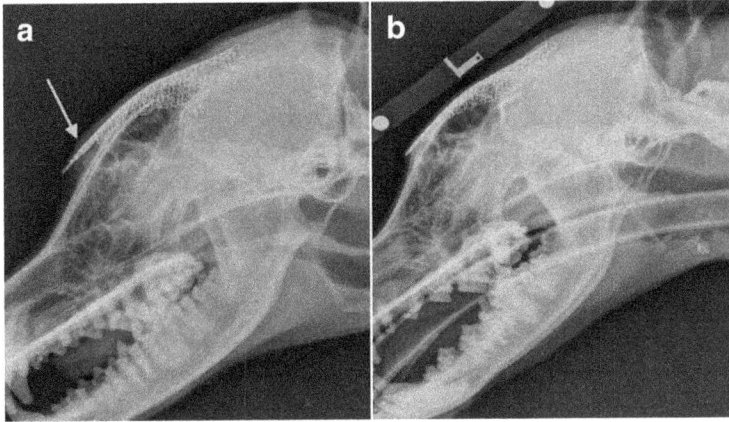

Fig. 6 a 6 months postoperative lateral radiographic view of the skull showing rostral uplift of the mesh (white arrow). **b** 2 years postoperative lateral radiographic view of the skull showing adequate positioning of the mesh

infection risk. Of importance was the possibility for infection originating from sinus flora, advanced sequencing of nasal canine flora highlights a number of potentially pathogenic bacteria present in healthy dogs [19], hence the potential for infection as a consequence of a compromised sinus architecture supports the require of surgical management in this scenario.

Materials used for skull defect reconstruction can include autologous bone, allogenic and alloplastic materials, synthetic and organic biomaterials, or biocompatible metals and their alloys. Titanium mesh is used in human surgery for its strength, malleability, ability for easy intraoperative handling, biocompatibility and low infection rate [20–23]. These systems are routinely used for defect reconstruction in maxillofacial surgery for the treatment of depressed skull fractures and reconstruction of paranasal sinuses. Application of Ti mesh within veterinary medicine is less widespread but is documented in skull reconstruction following primary bone tumour removal [2, 5].

In case 2, the Ti mesh was placed over an intact dura after tumor resection. In the event of compromise to the dura, augmentation of the dural layer facility is indicated as previously described [5]. Dural repair materials should be biocompatible, non-toxic and may include autologous substances (pericranium, temporalis fascia and fascia lata) or biological substitute materials such as Small Intestinal Submucosa [20].

Titanium mesh provides long-term biomechanical stability [23] and may be used as a framework for soft tissue reconstruction over the damaged sinus. In the current cases, a complete air-tight sealing of the sinuses was obtained with the combination of Ti mesh, gentamycin-collagen sponge and soft tissue closure after accurate reconstruction and remained unchanged in the long-term follow-up (up to two years).

The innovative use of polymeric pins with Bonewelding® technology may carry several advantages compared to traditional metallic screws and plates. Biocompatibility of the polymer screw technology was demonstrated in an ovine spine fusion model. The system demonstrated bone-screw integration, high bonding strength when assessed by screw pull-out and clear new bone growth surrounding the implant [24, 25]. Application of Bonewelding® is considered less traumatic than traditional metallic screw fixation [26] and is advantageous in cases where the skull defect originated from trauma, minimising further inflammation whilst achieving surgical repair and implant integration. In case 1, the calvarial defect originated from trauma precipitating severe localised tissue inflammation, the decision to use Bonewelding® technology was in part based on an intention to minimise further damage to traumatised tissue.

In an advantage, pins are not constrained to pre-determined trajectory as defined by implant design and threading; the angle of application can be varied without undue application of torque forces [25]. This ease of use improves the procedural flexibility lending itself to use in the repair of irregular bone defects and in clinical scenarios involving areas of complex morphology. In the reported two cases, the location and complex geometry of bone defects benefitted from the procedural flexibility afforded by employing Bonewelding® technology. The unusual nature of the reported cases negates the possibility of comparing surgical time to standard fixation and comparable reported procedures do not document surgical duration [5]. Application of the polymer pin system was perceived as being faster compared to conventional screws, as it has been reported by Pilling et al. [25] and Eckelt et al. [12]. However, categorical demonstration of this fact in this instance was not possible.

Polymer pins are radiolucent and therefore have an advantage for postoperative CT studies compared to metal implants generating fewer artefacts allowing more accurate assessment of the operated site [13, 27]. Quantification of postoperative bone formation and mesh-skull integration was complicated although satisfactory mesh positioning at long-term follow up may be interpreted as an adequate clinical indicator of tissue incorporation. The authors thought it warranted to use both radiographic and CT scan modalities as diagnostic tools thoroughly reflect of the postoperative appearance of this novel polymeric fixation material. Although CT scan is the technique of choice to assess such an implant, radiography remains the most widely available and easy to perform modality in first opinion practice and as such the accurate description of the radiographic presentation of the material carries direct clinical relevance.

Complications associated with the use Ti mesh for skull defect reconstruction in humans include infection, haemorrhage, seizures and postoperative pain [27, 28]. In previous veterinary reports, postoperative complications after Ti mesh cranioplasty have not been described [2, 5, 29].

In case 1, the mesh uplift in its rostral aspect six weeks postoperatively was an incidental finding on imaging. It is the authors' opinion that the irregular rostral border of the mesh implant may have required further fixation to the rostral frontal and caudal maxillary bones. It was intended that accurate contouring of the mesh in combination with pin placement would have secured the mesh sufficiently. Melting and fusion of the polymer pins in the host bone by ultrasound increase the mechanical resistance to shearing forces compared to a conventional screw-plate construct [30] and provide sufficient mesh fixation. Increased pin number and density may circumvent complications of inadequate implant constraint although conjecture remains regarding the suitability of a resorbable system in the reported case. In case 2, non-resorbable pins made of an acryl-based multipolymer compound, MBS, were used and despite the presence of an osseous response which could not be investigated, mesh positioning remained well seated to the defect and no implant related complications were experienced.

Use of polymeric pins poses challenges to the new user. Attention must be given to the angle of pin placement and degree of ultrasonic exposure received. Incomplete insertion can occur if ultrasound application is removed too early [31]. Similarly, if the process of pin introduction during ultrasound application is excessively delayed, it can impair proper fusion and result in inadequate linkage of the pin-bone interface [32]. Resorbable polymers may be contraindicated where high mechanical load or movement occur as their degradation may occur before new bone formation, leading to implant loosening [31]. Bonewelding® resorbable pins were made of PLDLA and resorb within approximately 10–12 weeks. The degradation profile of

PLDLA pins was designed to facilitate tissue in-growth consistent with rate of polymer absorption [33].

Ideally, the breakdown, resorption and excretion of a resorbable system should coincide with new tissue growth and ease transition from synthetic fixation to bony integration with the implant. The breakdown of PLDLA in vivo occurs by hydrolysis, subsequent phagocytosis and cyclic breakdown into lactic acid. Initial hydrolysis reduces polymer molecular weight without affecting the total bulk (and by extension strength). As the PLDLA is further cleaved, the number of polymer chains exposed for hydrolytic and enzymatic degradation increases, accelerating the rate of degradation. Polymer breakdown is influenced by implant shape, size, molecular weight, pH and the water content of the surrounding tissue (contributing to hydrolysis) [34]. Polymer breakdown products can influence implant microenvironment stimulating an inflammatory response and, although documented in humans, reaction to PLDLA is uncommon in animal models [35]. In a clinical setting, factors influencing tissue repair and new bone growth may result in a disconnect between polymer breakdown and the intended transition towards biological fixation. In this scenario the implant would no longer be adequately secured and migration related complications would be expected. Mesh stabilization was better maintained in the patient wherein non-degradable pins were used for fixation. The authors would propose that the uplift of mesh in case 1, which appears concurrent with the expected timing of pin degradation, and the degradable poly-pin can be causally linked. In case 2, the absence of mesh uplift may be linked to the use of non-resorbable pins although no further consensus is possible with larger and extensive case series.

A gentamycin-collagen sponge was used to deliver high-concentration perioperative antibiotics to reduce risks of infection [36]. Collagen has been used as a natural polymer scaffold for applied growth factors, cytokines and transplanted cells which may enhance osseointegration and bone repair [37].

Osseointegration at the mesh-bone interface could have been achieved through traditional autograft or allograft or synthetic materials. The use of octacalcium phosphate combined with collagen disks enhanced bone regeneration up to six months after application in a canine calvarial defect suggesting a potential role as a bone substitute graft material [38]. The application of exogenous Bone Morphogenic Protein 2 by a polymer delivery system significantly increased bone formation compared to collagen implant alone in calvarial defect model in rats [39]. Pro-osteogenic material coatings such as HA enhance osteoblastic activity and increase mesh osteoconductivity [40].

Conclusions

We report the successful repair of a traumatic calvarial fracture in a greyhound and calvarioplasty in a Cavalier King Charles Spaniel using a Ti mesh secured with thermoresponsive polymer pins. It is in the authors' opinion that Bonewelding ® technology may be a suitable adjunct technique for fixation of calvarial defects as it yields easy application with minor bone trauma. The short-term postoperative mesh uplift encountered in case 1 with the use of resorbable pins was a potential consequence of their variable degree of degradation and incomplete biological integration, comparatively no complications relating to implant movement were reported with the use of the non-resorbable system in case 2, post-operatively and at 7 month follow up. The varying outcome using absorbable and non-absorbable systems may suggest a clinical advantage to the non- absorbable pins, however a multiple patient case series with long term follow up would be required to demonstrate this proposal.

Abbreviations

CT: Computer tomography; HA: Hydroxyapatite; MBS: Methacrylate-butadiene-styrol; PMMA: Polymethylmethacrylate; Ti: Titanium

Authors' contributions

PL made substantial contributions to conception, design, analysis and interpretation of data, writing process of the paper and revising the manuscript. CB made significant contribution to drafting, editing the manuscript and revising it critically for important intellectual content. PE and NF executed both surgeries and performed clinical follow-up and data acquisition and contribution to editing of manuscript. Each author have participated sufficiently in the work to take public responsibility for appropriate portions of the content and agreed to be accountable for all aspects of the work in ensuring that questions related to the accuracy or integrity of any part of the work are appropriately investigated and resolved. All authors gave final approval of the version to be published.

Consent for publication

Not applicable

Competing interests

The authors declare that they have no competing interests.

References

1. Bryant KJ, Steinberg H, McAnulty JF. Cranioplasty by means of molded polymethylmethacrylate prosthetic reconstruction after radical excision of neoplasms of the skull in two dogs. J Am Vet Med Assoc. 2003;223:67–72.
2. Bordelon JT, Rochat MC. Use of titanium mesh for cranioplasty following radical rostrotentorial craniectomy to remove an ossifying fibroma in a dog. J Am Vet Med Assoc. 2007;231:1692–5.
3. Moissonnier P, Devauchell P, Delisle F. Cranioplasty after en bloc resection of calvarial chondroma rodens in two dogs. J Small Anim Pract. 1997;38:358–63.
4. Gordon PN, Kornegay JN, Lattimer JC, et al. Use of a rivet-like titanium clamp closure system to replace an external frontal bone flap after transfrontal craniotomy in a dog. J Am Vet Med Assoc. 2005;226:752–5.
5. Rosselli DD, Platt SR, Freeman C, et al. Cranioplasty using titanium mesh after skull tumor resection in five dogs. Vet Surg. 2016;0:1–7.
6. Mouatt JG. Acrylic and axial pattern flap following calvarial and cerebral mass excision in a dog. Aust Vet J. 2002;80(4):211–5.
7. Philipps IR. A survey of bone fractures in the dog and cat. J Small Anim Pract. 1979;20:661–74.
8. Stefini R, Esposito G, Zanotti B, et al. Use of "custom made" porous hydroxyapatite implants for cranioplasty: postoperative analysis of complications in 1549 patients. Surg Neurol Int. 2013;4:12.
9. Park EY, Lim JY, Yun IS, et al. Cranioplasty enhanced by three-dimensional printing: custom-made three-dimensional-printed titanium implants for skull defects. J Craniofac Surg. 2016;27(4):943–9.
10. Metzinger SE, Guerra AB, Garcia RE. Frontal sinus fractures : management guidelines. Facial Plast Surg. 2005;21(3):199–206.
11. Boudrieau RJ. Miniplate reconstruction of severely comminuted maxillary fractures in two dogs. Vet Surg. 2004;33:154–63.
12. Eckelt U, Nitsche M, Muller A, et al. Ultrasound aided pin fixation of biodegradable osteosynthetic materials in cranioplasty for infants with craniosysnostosis. J Cranio-Maxillofac Surg. 2007;35:218–21.
13. Langhoff JD, Kuemmerle JM, Mayer J, et al. An ultrasound assisted anchoring technique (Bonewelding® technology) for fixation of implants to bone – a histological pilot study in sheep. Open Orthop J 2009; 3: 40–47.
14. Rohrich RJ, Hollier LH. Management of frontal sinus fractures. Changing concepts. Clin Plast Surg. 1992;19:219–32.
15. Boudrieau RJ, Verstraete JM. Principles of maxillofacial trauma repair. In: FJM V, Lommer MJ, editors. Oral and maxillofacial surgeryin dogs and cats. 1st ed. Edinburgh: Saunders Elsevier; 2012. p. 233–42.
16. Clapper WE, Meade GH. Normal flora of the nose, throat and lower intestine of dogs. J Bacteriol. 1963;85(3):643–8.
17. Boudrieau RJ. Maxillofacial fracture repair using miniplates and screws. In: FJM V, Lommer MJ, editors. Oral and maxillofacial surgeryin dogs and cats. 1st ed. Edinburgh: Saunders Elsevier; 2012. p. 293–308.
18. Arzi B, Verstraete FJM. Internal fixation of severe maxillofacial fractures in dogs. Vet Surg. 2015;44:437–42.
19. Tress B, Dorn ES, Suchodolski JS, et al. Bacterial microbiome of the nose of healthy dogs and dogs with nasal disease. PLoS One. 2017;12(5):1–18.
20. He SK, Guo JH, Wang ZL, et al. Efficacy and safety of small intestinal submucosa in dural defect repair in a canine model. Mat Sci Engi. 2017;73:267–74.
21. Blake GB, MacFarlane MR, Hinton JW. Titanium in reconstruction of the skull and face. Br J Plast Surg. 1990;43:528–35.
22. Spetzger U, Vougioukas V, Schipper J. Materials and techniques for osseous skull reconstruction. Min Inv Ther. 2010;19:110–21.
23. Ducic Y. Titanium mesh and hydroxyapatite cement cranioplasty: a report of 20 cases. J Oral Maxillofac Surg. 2002;60:272–6.
24. Heidenreich D, Langhoff JD, Nuss K, et al. The use of BoneWelding technology in spinal surgery: an experimental study in sheep. Eur Spine J. 2011;20:1821–36.
25. Pilling E, Mai R, Theissig F, et al. An experimental in vivo analysis of the resorption to ultrasound activated pins (Sonic weld®) and standard biodegradable screws (ResorbX®) in sheep. Br J Oral Maxillofac Surg. 2007; 45:447–50.
26. Ferguson SJ, Weber U, Mayer J. BoneWelding® technology: micro-scale finite element analysis of load transfer at the implant-bone interface. Oral Presentations J Biomech. 2006;39(1):S10.
27. Hill CS, Luoma AM, Wilson SR, et al. Titanium cranioplasty and the prediction of complications. Br J Neurosurg. 2012;26:832–7.
28. Janecka IP. New reconstructive technologies in skull base surgery: role of titanium mesh and porous polyethylene. Arch Otolaryngol Head Neck Surg. 2000;126:396–401.
29. Dewey CW, Marino DM, Bailey KS, et al. Foramen magnum decompression with cranioplasty for treatment of caudal occipital malformation syndrome in dogs. Vet Surg. 2007;3:406–15.
30. Meissner H, Pilling E, Richter G, et al. Experimental investigations for mechanical joint strength following ultrasonically welded pin osteosynthesis. J Mater Sci Mater Med. 2008;19:2255–9.
31. Kuttenberger JJ, Hardt N. Long-term results following reconstruction of craniofacial defects with titanium micro-mesh systems. J Craniomaxillofac Surg. 2001;29:75–81.

32. Chia CLK, Shelat VG, Low W, et al. The use of Collatamp G, local gentamicin-collagen sponge, in reducing wound infection. Int Surg. 2014;99:565–70.

33. Agarwal R, Garcia AJ. Biomaterial strategies for engineering implants for enhanced osseointegration and bone repair. Adv Drug Deliv Rev. 2015; 94:53–62.

34. Landes CA, Ballon A, Roth C. In-patient versus in vitro degradation of P(L/DL)LA and PLGA. J Biomed Mater Res B Appl Biomater. 2006;76((2):403–11.

35. Woodruff MA, Hutmacher DW. The return of a forgotten polymer - Polycaprolactone in the 21st century. Prog Polym Sci. 2010;35(10):1217–56.

36. Kawai T, Matsui K, Iibuchi S, et al. Reconstruction of critical-sized bone defect on dog skull by octacalcium phosphate combined with collagen. Clin Implant Dent Relat Res. 2011;13(2):112–23.

37. Mariner PD, Wudel JM, Miller DE, et al. Synthetic hydrogel scaffold is an effective vehicle for delivery of INFUSE (rhBMP2) to critical-sized calvaria bone defects in rats. J Orthop Res. 2013;31:401–6.

38. Hirota M, Hayakawa T, Yoshinari M, et al. Hydroxyapatite coating for titanium fibre mesh scaffold enhances osteoblast activity and bone tissue formation. Int J Oral Maxillofac Surg. 2012;41:1304–9.

39. Ferguson SJ, Weber U, Von Rechenberg B, et al. Enhancing the mechanical integrity of the implant-bone interface with Bonewelding® technology: determination of quasi-static interfacial strength and fatigue resistance. J Biomed Mater Res B Appl Biomater 2005; 77: 13–20.

40. Augat P, Robioneck PB, Abdulazim A, et al. Fixation performance of an ultrasonically fused, bioresorbable osteosynthesis implant: a biomechanical and biocompatibility study. J Biomed Mater Res B Appl Biomater. 2016;(1):170–9.

Evaluation of P16 expression in canine appendicular osteosarcoma

B. G. Murphy[1]*, M. Y. Mok[1], D. York[2], R. Rebhun[2], K. D. Woolard[1], C. Hillman[1], P. Dickinson[2] and K. Skorupski[2]

Abstract

Background: Osteosarcoma (OSA) is a common malignant bone tumor of large breed dogs that occurs at predictable anatomic sites. At the time of initial diagnosis, most affected dogs have occult pulmonary metastases. Even with aggressive surgical treatment combined with chemotherapy, the majority of dogs diagnosed with OSA live less than 1 year from the time of diagnosis. The ability to identify canine OSA cases most responsive to treatment is needed. In humans, OSA is also an aggressive tumor that is histologically and molecularly similar to canine OSA. The expression of the tumor suppressor gene product P16 by human OSA tissue has been linked to a favorable response to chemotherapy.

Results: We identified an antibody that binds canine P16 and developed a canine OSA tissue microarray in order to test the hypothesis that P16 expression by canine OSA tissue is predictive of clinical outcome following amputation and chemotherapy. Although statistical significance was not reached, a trend was identified between the lack of canine OSA P16 expression and a shorter disease free interval.

Conclusions: The identification of a molecular marker for canine OSA is an important goal and the results reported here justify a larger study.

Keywords: Canine, Osteosarcoma, P16, Immunohistochemistry, Tissue microarray

Background

Canine osteosarcoma (OSA) is an aggressive and highly metastatic tumor of bone and although it can occur at any age and in any dog breed, it is most often diagnosed in adult to older large to giant breed dogs. OSA is the most common canine skeletal tumor, accounting for approximately 80–85% of all bone tumors in dogs [1–3] and tends to occur at the most active metaphyseal regions of the appendicular skeleton. Relative to other skeletal sarcomas, canine osteosarcoma pursues a more rapid clinical course with earlier lung metastasis than either chondrosarcoma or fibrosarcoma of bone [4]. Early metastatic spread to the lungs contributes to the poor overall prognosis for canine OSA. Human OSA is histologically and molecularly similar to canine OSA [5–7] and both can be difficult to manage clinically [8, 9].

The current treatment of choice for canine OSA is surgical excision (involving limb amputation or limb-salvage surgery) followed by adjuvant platinum-based chemotherapy. Stereotactic radiation therapy has been reported as an alternative means to achieve local control [10, 11]. The survival time of canine appendicular OSA with adequate local control and without adjuvant chemotherapy is 119–175 days with a 12 month survival rate of only 11–21% [12]. In addition to surgery, platinum-based chemotherapy alone or in combination with doxorubicin has been shown to improve survival time [13]. A large study involving 470 dogs identified no difference in outcome between dogs with appendicular osteosarcoma treated with carboplatin vs. alternating carboplatin and doxorubicin [14]. Radiation therapy, bisphosphonates, and analgesics such as non-steroidal anti-inflammatory drugs and opioids can be utilized for palliative therapies. Reflecting owner choices, the use of palliative therapies alone generally result in relatively short survival times [12].

In an attempt to predict biological behavior, canine OSA has been categorized into a number of different histologic subtypes. Some studies have indicated that canine OSA histologic subtyping is not predictive of biological outcome [15] while others have indicated

* Correspondence: bmurphy@ucdavis.edu
[1]Department Pathology, University of California, Davis, School of Veterinary Medicine, Microbiology and Immunology, Davis, CA 95618, USA
Full list of author information is available at the end of the article

that specific OSA subtypes, such as telangiectatic or fibroblastic, may have negative or positive prognostic implications, respectively [2, 16]. Histological classifications have been frequently shown to be less informative than molecular phenotypes when applied to therapeutic outcome across a wide range of cancer types. A molecular biomarker that is predictive of canine OSA disease progression may assist prognostic determinations and treatment decisions.

Expression of the tumor suppressor gene product P16 by tumor tissue has recently been shown to significantly correlate with chemotherapeutic response in human osteosarcoma [9] and loss of P16 expression by OSA cells has been associated with decreased survival time in human patients with OSA [17–20]. Inactivation of tumor suppressor gene products like P16 is an important event in oncogenesis that may contribute to the development of canine OSA. Therefore, P16 expression has the potential to be a predictive signature of canine OSA tumor biology.

The tumor suppressor gene product P16 belongs to a family of cyclin-dependent kinase inhibitors. When bound to their respective cyclin dependent kinase, these proteins increase the inhibitory effects of the retinoblastoma tumor suppressor gene at the G1-S checkpoint, a 'point of no return' for cell division [21, 22]. In a normally regulated cell, growth-inhibiting signals result in P16 expression, blocking DNA synthesis and cell cycle progression [23]. Deletion or mutational inactivation of P16 can defeat the protective effect of the G1-S checkpoint, potentially leading to unregulated cellular division in a genetically damaged cell. Four of 6 previously reported canine OSA cell lines have been shown to have undetectable P16 protein or mRNA expression [23] and numerous human cancers are associated with P16 gene mutations, including osteosarcoma [21, 23].

We hypothesized that the presence or absence of P16 expression by canine OSA tissue is predictive of clinical outcome. In order to test this hypothesis, the identification of a P16 antibody that reliably binds canine P16 protein in immunoblot and immunohistochemistry (IHC) assays was needed. Utilizing a set of control human and canine tissues with known P16 expression patterns [24], we identified an anti-P16 antibody with appropriate binding affinity in both immunoblot and IHC assays. In addition, we developed a set of canine tissue microarrays comprised of retrospective case material from 33 dogs with appendicular OSA with known treatment regimens and long-term outcomes.

Methods
Pathology and clinical features
In this retrospective study, 33 excisional biopsies (amputations) diagnosed as canine appendicular OSA were utilized

from patients enrolled in a randomized prospective study comparing the adjuvant use of single-agent carboplatin or alternating carboplatin and doxorubicin [13]. The inclusion criteria for the current study were the availability of sufficient high quality, formalin fixed, paraffin embedded tumor tissue and known treatment and clinical outcome data. Representative bone and soft tissue biopsy samples had been previously sectioned and fixed in 10% buffered formalin for a minimum of 48 h. Mineralized tissue was thinly sectioned and decalcified in 15% formic acid for 2–4 days, as needed. Tissue samples were routinely processed, cut into 4 μm thick sections, placed on positively charged glass slides and stained with hematoxylin and eosin according to routine protocols. All specimens were confirmed to be consistent with the diagnosis of osteosarcoma by a single pathologist (MYM) based upon published criteria [2]. Canine OSA tumors were subclassified as osteoblastic, chondroblastic, fibroblastic or mixed subtypes based upon published criteria [2].

Tissue microarray
For each paraffin embedded tumor, optimal sites of the formalin-fixed paraffin embedded blocks for core sampling were identified. Characteristics of optimal sites included the following features: high cellularity, minimal necrosis, minimal hemorrhage and minimal matrix or bone deposition. The construction of the tissue microarray (TMA) was based upon a 2009 review by Parsons and Grabsh [25]. An Advanced Tissue Arrayer (model ATA-100, Chemicon International) was used to cut and insert canine OSA tissue core samples, in triplicate, into pre-cast paraffin blocks (Paraplast Plus, Sigma Aldrich). For the 33 canine cases, four canine OSA TMAs were constructed using a 9 × 6 grid pattern. Three, 2 mm diameter core biopsies from each donor tissue block, along with 2 positive control core biopsies (canine glioblastoma tissue) were semi-randomly arranged in the paraffin block while the outer circumferential border was generally comprised of negative control tissue (normal canine cerebrum or renal cortical tissue). To generate unstained paraffin sections, each assembled TMA was cut into 4 μm thick sections with a microtome and placed on positively charged glass slides. TMA sections were stained with either hematoxylin and eosin stains according to standard protocols or were further processed for P16 immunohistochemistry.

Immunohistochemistry for P16
Immunohistochemistry (IHC) assays were performed on whole sections of the positive control tissue (canine glioblastoma), negative control tissue (normal canine brain tissue and canine renal cortical tissue) and the constructed tissue microarrays. IHC assays were performed

on 4 μm thick, formalin-fixed, paraffin-embedded tissue sections, mounted on charged slides, and air-dried overnight at 37° C. In order to ensure reproducible and homogeneous results between the IHC assays, a consistent development time and protocol was utilized.

Sections were deparaffinized through xylene to reagent alcohol, and treated with 0.3% hydrogen peroxide in methanol for 30 min. Sections were then rehydrated to water through graded reagent alcohols, and stabilized in 0.1 M Phosphate Buffered Saline, pH 7.4 (PBS). Antigen retrieval required exposure of sections to Dako Target Retrieval Solution, pH 9 (Dako, S2368) at 95° C for 30 min, followed by a 20 min cool down at room temperature. Sections were blocked for 20 min in 10% normal horse serum in PBS. The primary antibody, a rabbit anti-P16 (SC-373695, F-8, Santa Cruz Biotechnology) diluted 1:100 in PBS-Tween 20 (0.02%) was applied for 1 h. All reagent incubations were at room temperature, and PBS-Tween 20 rinses occurred twice between reagent applications for 3 min each change. Envision + System-HRP (Dako, K4003) was applied for 30 min to label bound rabbit anti-P16 antibodies. The label was visualized with NovaRed for peroxidase (Vector, SK-4800). Sections were counterstained in Mayer's Hematoxylin, air-dried and coverslipped. Non-specific background was evaluated with a duplicate section receiving diluent in place of the primary antibody.

The sub-cellular location of the P16 antigen was determined microscopically as nuclear, cytoplasmic or membranous. To determine the level of P16 expression, a semiquantitative scoring system was used based upon the percent of neoplastic cells expressing P16 in a 100× field of magnification: negative (0%), 1+ (<25%), 2+ (26–79%), 3+ (80–100%) (at 100× magnification the entire TMA biopsy section filled the field of view). The intensity of P16 staining was not scored. The semiquantitative ordinal scoring system was developed in accordance with recommended histopathologic principles [26]. For each canine OSA lesion on the TMA, one, two or three tissue biopsies were examined and scored for P16 expression, as described above (Table 1). For each case, a consensus P16 staining pattern was determined (1 of 1, 2 of 2, 2 of 3, or 3 of 3 sections). Discordant cases (1 of 2 sections) were re-reviewed by two anatomic pathologists (MYM and BGM) until a consensus could be reached. All IHC sections were examined in a blinded fashion where the pathologists were not aware of case signalment, diagnosis or outcome.

Immunoblot

Control human and canine tissues were obtained from cell culture, surgical biopsy or necropsy as previously described [24]. Tissues know to express P16 (positive controls) included the SAOS2 human osteosarcoma cell line, a canine high grade oligodendroglioma (O8) and a

canine grade IV astrocytoma/glioblastoma (GBM, G2); canine tissues previously demonstrated to not express P16 (negative controls) included a different canine GBM (G4), a high grade oligodendroglioma (O5) and normal canine cerebrum (NB) [24].

Briefly, cells and tumor samples were lysed in radioimmunoprecipitation assay buffer (RIPA) lysis buffer (Boston BioProducts, Worcester, MA, USA) with 1X Halt protease and phosphatase inhibitors (Thermo Fisher Scientific, Rockford, IL, USA) and kept on ice or stored at –80 C if not used immediately. Cell lysates were electrophoresed in 4–20% SDS Precast Polyacrylamide Gels (Expedeon) at 150 V for 45 min. The lysates were transferred overnight onto a PVDF membrane (BioRad) at 50 V in a 5 C cold room (PAGEgel Dual Run & Blot Vertical Mini-Gel System). The PVDF membrane was washed three times in tris-buffered saline with 0.1% Tween-20 (TBST), blocked for 1 h with 5% nonfat milk/TBST (blocking buffer), and subsequently washed 3 more times with TBST. The PVDF membrane was then incubated overnight at 5C with mouse monoclonal anti-P16 (1:500, SC-373695, F-8, Santa Cruz Biotechnology) diluted in blocking buffer. Membranes were then washed 3× and incubated with HRP conjugated-goat anti-mouse IgG antibody (Santa Cruz Biotechnology, IgG-HRP sc-2005) for 1 h at room temperature. Finally, membranes were washed 3×, incubated for 1 min with Pierce ECL reagent (Thermo Fisher Scientific, Catalog number 32106) and imaged using a FluorChem E digital imaging system (ProteinSimple).

Analysis and statistics

Disease free interval (DFI) and survival were defined as described in Skorupski et al. [13]. The Kaplan-Meier method was used to estimate DFI and survival and the log-rank test was used to compare DFI and survival times between P16 expression groups. Statistical analyses were performed using commercial software (GraphPad Prism version 6.0f) and a p-value of <0.05 was considered significant. To determine if the decalcification process interfered with P16 detection, the putative correlation between P16 expression and decalcification was determined using Fisher's exact test.

Results
Pathology and clinical features
The anatomic locations of the canine OSA tumors, in general, followed a predictable pattern reflecting the most active growth plates of the appendicular skeleton. There were two exceptions to this rule, in case 2, the OSA lesion was identified in the proximal radius while in case 6, the tumor was identified in the ulnar diaphysis (Table 1). Consistent with the tendency of OSA to occur in larger dogs, most of the dogs were large to giant breeds. Approximately equal numbers of patients

Table 1 Clinical and pathologic data for canine appendicular osteosarcomas

case	De/NDe	tx	sex	breed	tumor location	subtype	# sct	p16 exp
1	De	C/D	MC	Mix	Proximal tibia	C	2	1+
2	De	C/D	FS	GSD	Proximal radius	O	3	3+
3	NDe	C	MC	Lab	Proximal humerus	O	3	3+
4	NDe	C	FS	Grt Dane	Distal radius	C	3	2+
5	NDe	C	FS	Rott	Proximal tibia	O	3	neg
6	NDe	C	MC	Gold	Ulnar diaphysis	O	3	1+
7	De	C/D	MC	Mix	Distal radius	O	3	3+
8	De	C/D	FS	St. Bern	Distal tibia	O	3	3+
9	Nde	C	FS	Gold	Distal femur	O	3	2+
10	De	C	FS	Rott	Distal femur	O	3	3+
11	De	C	MC	Rott	Distal tibia	O	3	neg
12	NDe	C/D	FS	G Pyr	Distal tibia	O	3	2+
13	De	C/D	MC	Bernese MD	Distal radius	O	2	neg
14	NDe	C	FS	Rott	Distal radius	O	3	neg
15	De	C	FS	Mix	Distal femur	O	3	3+
16	NDe	C	FS	OESD	Distal radius	O	1	3+
17	NDe	C/D	FS	Curly C Ret	Proximal humerus	O	3	3+
18	De	C/D	FS	Rott	Proximal tibia	O	1	1+
19	De	C/D	FS	Mix	Distal radius	O	3	3+
20	NDe	C	FS	Lab	Proximal humerus	O	3	3+
21	NDe	C/D	MC	Grey	Prox humerus	O	1	2+
22	NDe	C/D	MC	Mix	Distal radius	F	3	2+
23	Nde	C/D	FS	GSD	Distal tibia	O	3	3+
24	Nde	C/D	FS	Malam	Distal radius	O	3	3+
25	De	C/D	FS	Rott	Distal femur	O	3	neg
26	De	C	MC	Mix	Proximal humerus	O	3	3+
27	NDe	C/D	FS	Mix	Distal tibia	O	3	neg
28	De	C/D	MC	Bernese MD	Distal femur	C	3	1+
29	De	C	FS	Leonberger	Distal radius	O	3	1+
30	De	C/D	MC	Ana Shep	Distal radius	O	2	2+
31	De	C	FS	Lab	Distal femur	O	3	2+
32	De	C	MC	GS Pointer	Proximal humerus	C	3	2+
33	De	C	M	Rhod Rback	Distal radius	M	3	1+

Abbreviations: De- decalcified section, NDe- non-decalcified section, tx- treatment, C- carboplatin, D- doxorubicin, MC- male castrated, FS- female spayed, GSD- German Shepherd dog, Lab- Labrador Retriever, Grt Dane- Great Dane, Rott- Rottweiler, Gold- Golden Retriever, St. Bern- Saint Bernard, G Pyr- Great Pyrenees, Bernese MD- Bernese Mountain dog, OESD- Old English Sheep dog, Curly C Ret- Curly Coat Retriever, Grey- Greyhound, Malam- Malamute, Ana Shep- Anatolian Shepherd, GS Pointer- German Shorthair Pointer, Rod Rback- Rhodesian Ridgeback, C- chondroblastic OSA, O- osteoblastic OSA, F- fibroblastic OSA, M- Mixed type OSA, # sct- number of P16 IHC sections examined

received each chemotherapeutic protocol. The majority of the tumors were of the osteoblastic subtype (n = 27), with fewer numbers of chondroblastic (n = 4) and one case each of fibroblastic and mixed subtypes. Sections of the tissue microarrays stained with hematoxylin and eosin demonstrated histologically recognizable canine positive control (GBM), canine negative control (normal renal cortical or brain tissue) and canine osteosarcoma tissues (Figs. 2 and 3).

Immunoblot

Immunoblot assay with the primary anti-P16 antibody (F-8) revealed the presence of a 15-16 kDa band representing the P16 protein in the SAOS-2 human cell line (lane 1), a canine high grade oligodendroglioma (O8, lane 2) and a canine GBM (G2, lane 3) (Fig. 1). No evidence of P16 protein expression was observed in negative control lanes 4–6 representing a different canine GBM (G4), a canine high grade oligodendroglioma (O5), and normal canine cerebrum

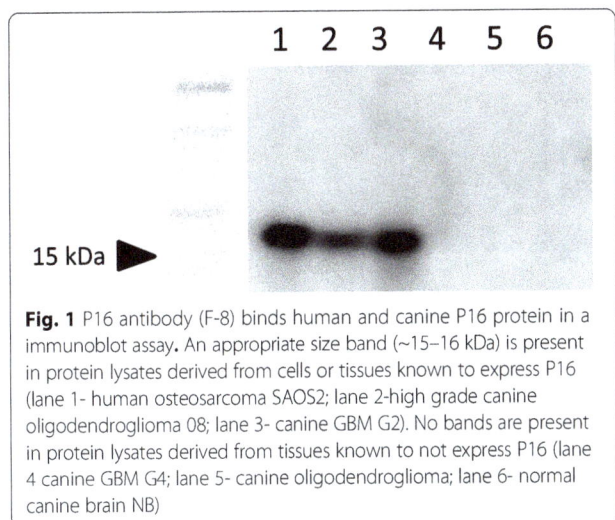

Fig. 1 P16 antibody (F-8) binds human and canine P16 protein in a immunoblot assay. An appropriate size band (~15–16 kDa) is present in protein lysates derived from cells or tissues known to express P16 (lane 1- human osteosarcoma SAOS2; lane 2-high grade canine oligodendroglioma 08; lane 3- canine GBM G2). No bands are present in protein lysates derived from tissues known to not express P16 (lane 4 canine GBM G4; lane 5- canine oligodendroglioma; lane 6- normal canine brain NB)

(NB). These results were consistent with previous results using a different P16 antibody [24].

Immunohistochemistry

Using the same P16 antibody (F-8) as used in the immunoblot assay, P16 immunoreactivity was noted within the cytoplasm and nuclei of the neoplastic cells comprising the canine GBM (G2, positive expression control) but was absent in normal canine cerebrum and canine renal cortical tissue (negative expression controls) (Figs. 2 and 3).

Hence, an antibody capable of identifying the expression of P16 in IHC assays was identified.

OSA biopsy tissues in the TMA were assigned an ordinal value based upon the percent of neoplastic cells expressing P16 in a 100× magnification field: negative (0% cells), 1+ (<25% cells), 2+ (26–79% cells), 3+ (80–100% cells). In the majority of cases, three biopsy cores were examined and scored ($n = 26$ cases). In the remaining 6 cases, less than 3 biopsy cores were available for scoring as a result of loss during sectioning of the TMA blocks. In 3 cases, two biopsy cores were examined, and in 3 cases, a single core was examined and scored (Table 1). Although decalcification had no significant effect on the immunohistochemical scoring for P16 expression ($p = 1.0$) (Table 1), the effect of treatment or lack of treatment with decalcifying agents was not assessed within the same sample.

Survival

Dogs with negative P16 immunoreactivity had a median disease free interval (DFI) of 125 days compared to 201 days for dogs with *any* evidence of P16 immunoreactivity (1+, 2+ or 3+ P16 immunoreactivity, Fig. 4). This difference approached statistical significance with a *p* value 0.055. Dogs with negative P16 immunoreactivity had a median survival time of 179 days compared to 353 days for dogs with any

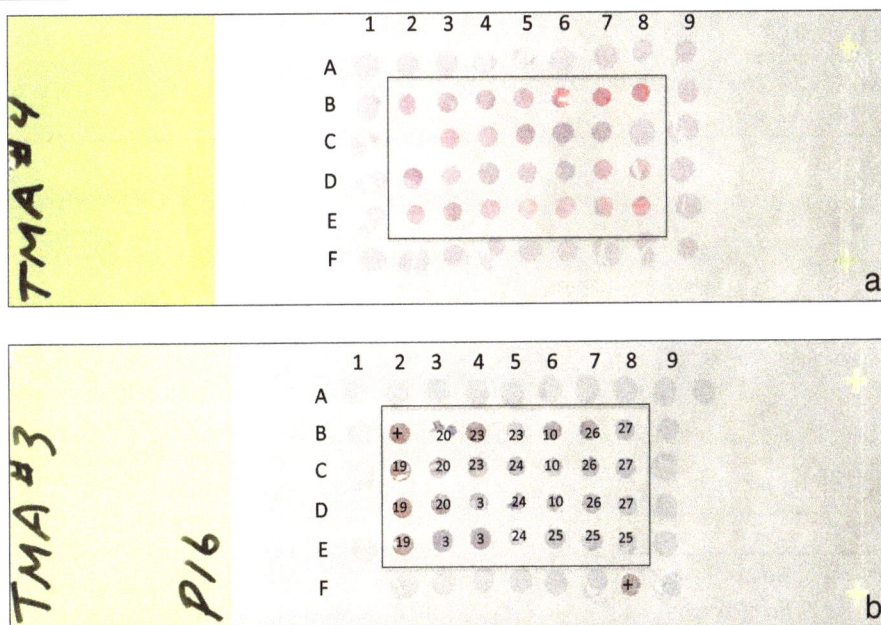

Fig. 2 The organization and appearance of slides derived from canine OSA TMA stained with H&E stains or anti-P16 antibody (IHC). The TMA are arranged in 9 columns (1–9) by 6 rows (A-F) comprising a 9 × 6 grid. The majority of 2 mm diameter biopsy cores are present in hematoxylin & eosin-stained slides (TMA4) (**a**) and anti-P16 IHC (TMA3) (**b**). The outer row (columns 1 and 9, rows A and F) are generally comprised of negative control tissue (canine renal cortical or brain tissue). Triplicate canine OSA biopsy (test) samples are located within the boxed regions and are identified by case numbers (**b**). The location of positive control samples (GBM) are indicated (+) (**b**)

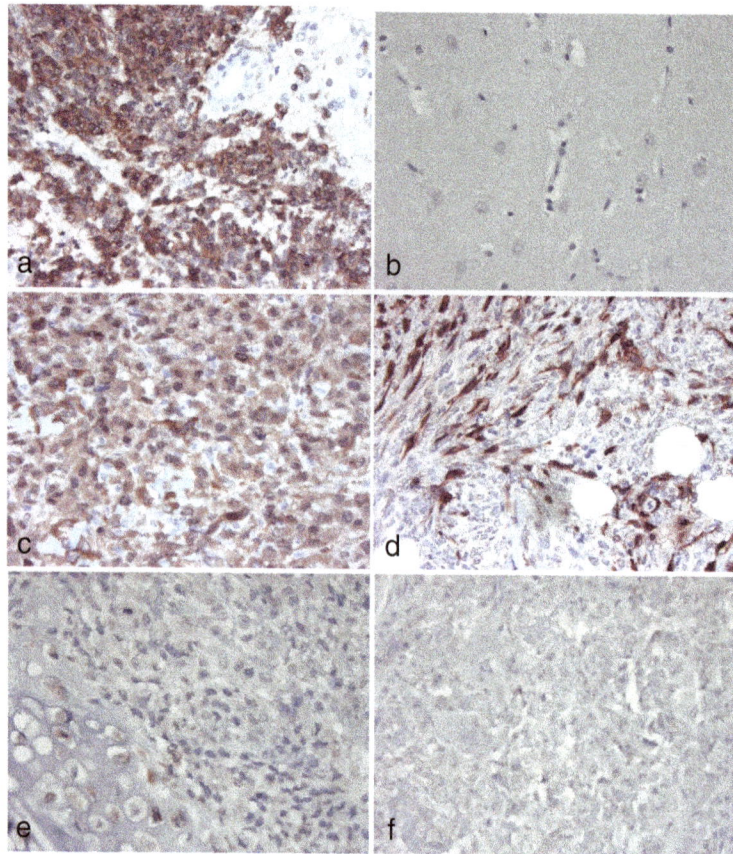

Fig. 3 Immunohistochemistry assays reveal the proportion of neoplastic cells expressing P16. Canine glioblastoma cells demonstrate abundant *red-brown* staining in both the cytoplasm and nucleus (GBM, + control P16 IHC) (**a**). Normal canine brain tissue demonstrates an absence of *red-brown* stained cells (NB, negative control P16 IHC) (**b**). In a canine OSA, a majority of the neoplastic cells demonstrate red-brown cytoplasmic staining (3+ staining, case 19) (**c**). In a canine OSA, approximately 50% of the neoplastic cells demonstrate red-brown cytoplasmic staining (2+ staining, case 9) (**d**). In canine OSA, less than 25% of the neoplastic cells demonstrate red-brown cytoplasmic staining (1+ staining, case 4) (**e**). In canine OSA, none of the neoplastic cells demonstrate red-brown cytoplasmic staining (0+ staining, case 13). P16 immunohistochemistry, original magnification 400×

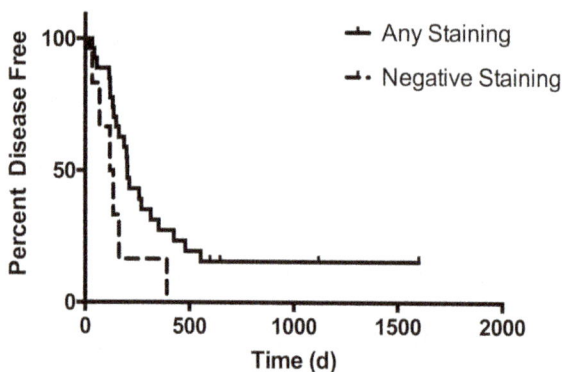

Fig. 4 For dogs with OSA, the disease free interval (DFI) is shorter for tumors expressing P16 relative to tumors without P16 expression. The percent survival of dogs with OSA that exhibit *any* P16 staining (+1, +2 or +3, dashed line) and dogs with OSA that lack P16 staining (*solid line*) are plotted in this survival plot

P16 immunoreactivity. This difference was not significant (p = 0.2). A comparison of samples with strong p16 immunoreactivity (+2 or +3) versus negative immunoreactivity was performed and found to be not significant (p = 0.09 for DFI and 0.3 for survival, respectively; data not shown).

Fourteen dogs treated with a combined chemotherapy regimen (carboplatin and doxorubicin) demonstrated at least some P16 expression while 3 dogs treated with a combined therapy lacked P16 expression. 13 dogs treated with carboplatin alone had P16 expression while 3 dogs treated with carboplatin alone lacked P16 expression (Table 1). As a result, P16 expression did not correlate with chemotherapy protocol (p = 1.00).

Discussion

In this study, we identified an anti-P16 antibody that specifically labeled canine and human cells/tissues previously shown to express P16 protein in immunoblots and immunohistochemistry assays (positive controls); and failed to label cells and tissues known to not express P16 protein (negative controls). The Santa Cruz F-8 antibody is directed towards an epitope mapping between amino acids 4–31 at the N-terminus of human P16. Within this region, there are 4 amino acid mismatches between the human and canine P16 protein sequence (data not shown). This difference between the human and canine P16 sequences is apparently insufficient to abrogate antibody binding.

Using this antibody in IHC assays with a set of 4 canine OSA tissue microarrays demonstrated P16 expression varying from no expression (0% of the neoplastic cells express P16), up to 3+ expression (80–100% of the neoplastic cells express P16). Although statistical significance was not reached, a trend was identified between the lack of P16 expression (negative staining) and a shorter DFI. This finding in canine OSA is intriguing as inactivation of P16 expression by mutation, deletion, or promoter hypermethylation has been associated with continuous cell proliferation in human OSA [9] and loss of P16 expression has been correlated with decreased survival time in human OSA [17].

In all of the examined canine OSA biopsy sections, P16 protein expression, when present, was determined to be cytoplasmic. In the positive control tissue (canine GBM), P16 expression was identified in both the nucleus and cytoplasm of the neoplastic cells. Although the specificity and validity of cytoplasmic localization of P16 observed in some tumors has been questioned, P16 has been shown to be expressed in the cytoplasm of a wide variety of cell types [27–29]. Studies have reported the localization of P16 protein in both the nucleus and the cytoplasm in multiple neoplasms.

Interestingly, four of the six dogs with no P16 expression were Rottweilers, while only two of the 27 dogs with some P16 expression were Rottweilers (Table 1). This finding is intriguing as Rottweilers, along with Greyhounds and Great Danes, have been shown to have an increased risk of developing OSA [30]. McNeill and co-workers found that relative to other dog breeds, Rottweilers are more likely to have an aggressive form of OSA with a higher likelihood of brain metastasis [31]. However, the McNeil study did not confirm that these differences were associated with a worse outcome. Studies have demonstrated an association between specific dog breeds, like Rottweillers, and the distribution of genomic copy number imbalances in canine appendicular osteosarcoma [32]. Such results indicate that individual genetic backgrounds, as defined by dog breed, influence tumor karyotypes in cancers like OSA with extensive genomic instability. Reconciling the findings reported here with these previous studies will require a larger population of animals.

This pilot study had several limitations. Due to sporadic sectional loss in the TMA, three biopsy cores were not available for examination for every case. The concordance for IHC staining between tissue arrays with triplicate cores per tumor and full sections has been shown to be 96–98% [33]. In the study described here, the majority of cases ($n = 26$) had three examined biopsy cores. However, as a result of tissue loss in some of the TMA sections, only two biopsy cores were examined for 3 cases, and a single core was examined and scored for 3 cases. The percent mismatch (nonconcordance) between the immunohistochemical scoring of biopsy cores and the full section has been determined to be 3.7, 4.4 and 9.4% for 3, 2 and 1 core, respectively [33]. Although the examination and scoring of less than 3 sections is considered suboptimal, a nonconcordance rate of <10% was considered to be acceptable for this pilot study.

Overall case numbers were low ($n = 33$), and the number of cases completely lacking P16 expression ($n = 6$) was particularly low. This limitation might have resulted in a type II error ("false negative") in results comparing P16 staining to overall outcome (DFI). This possibility is suggested by the close p-value for DFI and large difference in median survival despite a non-significant p-value. In addition, dogs included in the study received 2 different adjuvant chemotherapy protocols and the study from which the cases were collected showed a significant difference between DFI in these protocols. Although we found no association between P16 staining and chemotherapy protocol, larger studies with uniform treatment would be more ideal.

Conclusions

This study, demonstrating a trend between the lack of P16 expression in canine appendicular OSA lesions and a shorter DFI, provides preliminary data justifying a larger study. The identification of a molecular marker reliably indicating prognosis for canine appendicular OSA is needed.

Abbreviations
DFI: Disease free interval; GBM: Glioblastoma; IHC: Immunohistochemistry; NB: Normal canine cerebrum; OSA: Osteosarcoma; PBS: Phosphate buffered saline; TMA: Tissue microarray

Acknowledgements
The authors would like to thank the histology technicians of the University of California, Davis School of Veterinary Medicine. We are also grateful to Mike Manzer for performing the IHC assays and Stefan Keller for performing the P16 epitope alignment (human vs. canine). Santa Cruz Biotechnology provided the anti-P16 antibody used in this study.

Funding

This work was funded by a resident training grant (MYM) provided by the UC Davis Center for Companion Animal Health.

Authors' contributions

BGM and MYM originally conceived of this study, wrote the training grant proposal and interpreted the histopathology. BGM assisted in the data interpretation, wrote all of the manuscript drafts and created the figures. MYM made all of the tissue microarrays, assisted in performing immunoblots, data interpretation, figure design and manuscript editing. DY performed immunoblot assays, data interpretation and manuscript editing. RR assisted in the experimental design, data interpretation and manuscript editing. KDW assisted in experimental design, data interpretation and manuscript editing. CH performed immuno blot assays, assisted in data interpretation and manuscript editing. PD assisted with the experimental design, data interpretation and manuscript editing. KS assisted with the experimental design, provided the case series database, assisted in data interpretation, performed the statistical analyses, draft editing and created Fig. 4. All of the authors read and approved the final manuscript.

Competing interests

The authors declare that they have no competing interests.

Consent for publication

Not applicable.

Author details

[1]Department Pathology, University of California, Davis, School of Veterinary Medicine, Microbiology and Immunology, Davis, CA 95618, USA. [2]Department of Surgical and Radiological Sciences, Davis, CA 95618, USA.

References

1. Kirpensteijn J, Kik M, Rutteman GR, Teske E. Prognostic significance of a new histologic grading system for canine osteosarcoma. Vet Pathol. 2002;39(2):240-6.
2. Maxie MG. Jubb, Kennedy, and Palmer's pathology of domestic animals, sixth edition. Edn. St. Louis: Elsevier; 2016.
3. Boerman I, Selvarajah GT, Nielen M, Kirpensteijn J. Prognostic factors in canine appendicular osteosarcoma - a meta-analysis. BMC Vet Res. 2012;8:56.
4. Meuten DJ. Tumors in domestic animals. 4th ed. Ames, Iowa: Iowa State University Press; 2002.
5. Scott MC, Sarver AL, Gavin KJ, Thayanithy V, Getzy DM, Newman RA, et al. Molecular subtypes of osteosarcoma identified by reducing tumor heterogeneity through an interspecies comparative approach. Bone. 2011; 49(3):356-67.
6. Fenger JM, London CA, Kisseberth WC. Canine osteosarcoma: a naturally occurring disease to inform pediatric oncology. ILAR J. 2014;55(1):69-85.
7. Fowles JS, Brown KC, Hess AM, Duval DL, Gustafson DL. Intra- and interspecies gene expression models for predicting drug response in canine osteosarcoma. BMC bioinformatics. 2016;17:93.
8. Mertens WC, Bramwell V. Osteosarcoma and other tumors of bone. Curr Opin Oncol. 1994;6(4):384-90.
9. Borys D, Canter RJ, Hoch B, Martinez SR, Tamurian RM, Murphy B, et al. P16 expression predicts necrotic response among patients with osteosarcoma receiving neoadjuvant chemotherapy. Hum Pathol. 2012;43(11):1948-54.
10. Coomer A, Farese J, Milner R, Liptak J, Bacon N, Lurie D. Radiation therapy for canine appendicular osteosarcoma. Vet Comp Oncol. 2009;7(1):15-27.
11. Farese JP, Milner R, Thompson MS, Lester N, Cooke K, Fox L, et al. Stereotactic radiosurgery for treatment of osteosarcomas involving the distal portions of the limbs in dogs. J Am Vet Med Assoc. 2004;225(10):1567 72. 1548
12. North SM, Banks TA. Small animal oncology : an introduction. Edinburgh. New York: Saunders/Elsevier; 2009.
13. Skorupski KA, Uhl JM, Szivek A, Allstadt Frazier SD, Rebhun RB, Rodriguez CO Jr. Carboplatin versus alternating carboplatin and doxorubicin for the adjuvant treatment of canine appendicular osteosarcoma: a randomized, phase III trial. Vet Comp Oncol. 2016;14(1):81-7.
14. Selmic LE, Burton JH, Thamm DH, Withrow SJ, Lana SE. Comparison of carboplatin and doxorubicin-based chemotherapy protocols in 470 dogs after amputation for treatment of appendicular osteosarcoma. J Vet Intern Med. 2014;28(2):554-63.
15. Straw RC, Powers BE, Klausner J, Henderson RA, Morrison WB, McCaw DL, et al. Canine mandibular osteosarcoma: 51 cases (1980-1992). J Am Anim Hosp Assoc. 1996;32(3):257-62.
16. Sivacolundhu RK, Runge JJ, Donovan TA, Barber LG, Saba CF, Clifford CA, et al. Ulnar osteosarcoma in dogs: 30 cases (1992-2008). J Am Vet Med Assoc. 2013;243(1):96-101.
17. Benassi MS, Molendini L, Gamberi G, Ragazzini P, Sollazzo MR, Merli M, et al. Alteration of pRb/p16/cdk4 regulation in human osteosarcoma. Int J Cancer. 1999;84(5):489-93.
18. Maitra A, Roberts H, Weinberg AG, Geradts J. Loss of p16(INK4a) expression correlates with decreased survival in pediatric osteosarcomas. Int J Cancer. 2001;95(1):34-8.
19. Mohseny AB, Tieken C, van der Velden PA, Szuhai K, de Andrea C, Hogendoorn PC, et al. Small deletions but not methylation underlie CDKN2A/p16 loss of expression in conventional osteosarcoma. Genes Chromosom Cancer. 2010;49(12):1095-103.
20. Righi A, Gambarotti M, Sbaraglia M, Sisto A, Ferrari S, Dei Tos AP, et al. p16 expression as a prognostic and predictive marker in high-grade localized osteosarcoma of the extremities: an analysis of 357 cases. Hum Pathol. 2016;58:15-23.
21. Robbins SL, Kumar V, Cotran RS. Robbins and Cotran pathologic basis of disease. 8th ed. Philadelphia: Saunders/Elsevier; 2010.
22. Scott MC, Sarver AL, Tomiyasu H, Cornax I, Van Etten J, Varshney J, et al. Aberrant retinoblastoma (RB)-E2F transcriptional regulation defines molecular phenotypes of Osteosarcoma. J Biol Chem. 2015;290(47):28070-83.
23. Levine RA, Fleischli MA. Inactivation of p53 and retinoblastoma family pathways in canine osteosarcoma cell lines. Vet Pathol. 2000;37(1):54-61.
24. Boudreau CE, York D, Higgins RJ, LeCouteur RA, Dickinson PJ. Molecular signalling pathways in canine gliomas. Vet Comp Oncol. 2015;15(1):133-50.
25. M. Parson HG. How to make tissue microarrays. Diagnostic Histpathology. 2009;15(3):142-50.
26. Gibson-Corley KN, Olivier AK, Meyerholz DK. Principles for valid histopathologic scoring in research. Vet Pathol. 2013;50(6):1007-15.
27. Nilsson K, Landberg G. Subcellular localization, modification and protein complex formation of the cdk-inhibitor p16 in Rb-functional and Rb-inactivated tumor cells. Int J Cancer. 2006;118(5):1120-5.
28. Lai S, Wenaas AE, Sandulache VC, Hartman C, Chiao E, Kramer J, et al. Prognostic significance of p16 cellular localization in Oropharyngeal Squamous cell carcinoma. Ann Clin Lab Sci. 2016;46(2):132-9.
29. Zhao N, Ang MK, Yin XY, Patel MR, Fritchie K, Thorne L, et al. Different cellular p16(INK4a) localisation may signal different survival outcomes in head and neck cancer. Br J Cancer. 2012;107(3):482-90.
30. Rosenberger JA, Pablo NV, Crawford PC. Prevalence of and intrinsic risk factors for appendicular osteosarcoma in dogs: 179 cases (1996-2005). J Am Vet Med Assoc. 2007;231(7):1076-80.
31. McNeill CJ, Overley B, Shofer FS, Kent MS, Clifford CA, Samluk M, et al. Characterization of the biological behaviour of appendicular osteosarcoma in Rottweilers and a comparison with other breeds: a review of 258 dogs. Vet Comp Oncol. 2007;5(2):90-8.
32. Thomas R, Wang HJ, Tsai PC, Langford CF, Fosmire SP, Jubala CM, et al. Influence of genetic background on tumor karyotypes: evidence for breed-associated cytogenetic aberrations in canine appendicular osteosarcoma. Chromosom Res. 2009;17(3):365-77.
33. Hoos A, Urist MJ, Stojadinovic A, Mastorides S, Dudas ME, Leung DH, et al. Validation of tissue microarrays for immunohistochemical profiling of cancer specimens using the example of human fibroblastic tumors. Am J Pathol. 2001;158(4):1245-51.

Permissions

List of Contributors

Verena von Babo, Nina Eberle, Daniela Betz, Ingo Nolte and Patrick Wefstaedt
Small Animal Hospital, University of Veterinary Medicine Hannover, Foundation, Bünteweg 9, D-30559 Hannover, Germany

Vladimir Galindo-Zamora
Small Animal Hospital, University of Veterinary Medicine Hannover, Foundation, Bünteweg 9, D-30559 Hannover, Germany
Small Animal Clinic, Faculty of Veterinary Medicine, National University of Colombia, Carrera 30 # 45-03 (Ciudad Universitaria), Bogotá, Colombia

Noriyuki Nakashima
Department of Physiology, Graduate School of Medicine, Kyoto University, Yoshida-Konoe, Sakyo-ku, Kyoto 606-8501, Japan
Department of Physiology, School of Medicine, Kurume University, 67, Asahi-machi, Kurume-shi, Fukuoka 830-0011, Japan

Claire Legallet and Kelley Thieman Mankin
Department of Small Animal Clinical Sciences (Thieman Mankin, Legallet), College of Veterinary Medicine, Texas A&M University, College Station, TX 77843-4474, USA

Laura E. Selmic
The Department of Veterinary Clinical Medicine (Selmic), College of Veterinary Medicine, University of Illinois at Urbana-Champaign, Urbana, IL 61802, USA

Eva Haltmayer
Department of Small Animals and Horses, Clinic for Horses, Equine Surgery, University of Veterinary Medicine Vienna, Veterinärplatz 1, A-1210 Vienna, Austria

Theresia F. Licka
Department of Small Animals and Horses, Clinic for Horses, Equine Surgery, University of Veterinary Medicine Vienna, Veterinärplatz 1, A-1210 Vienna, Austria
Department of Veterinary Clinical Studies, Royal (Dick) School of Veterinary Studies, University of Edinburgh, Easter Bush Campus, Midlothian EH25 9RG, Scotland

Ilse Schwendenwein
Department of Pathobiology, Clinical Pathology, University of Veterinary Medicine Vienna, Veterinärplatz 1, A-1210 Vienna, Austria

Fuxin Wei, Le Wang, Shaoyu Liu, Rui Zhong, Xizhe Liu, Shangbin Cui and Manman Gao
Department of Spine Surgery, the First Affiliated Hospital and Orthopedic Research, Institute of Sun Yat-sen University, Guangzhou, China

Zhiyu Zhou
Department of Spine Surgery, the First Affiliated Hospital and Orthopedic Research, Institute of Sun Yat-sen University, Guangzhou, China
The medical school of Shenzhen University, Shenzhen, China

Ximin Pan
Department of Radiology, the First Affiliated Hospital of Sun Yat-sen University, Guangzhou, China

Yajing Zhao
The medical school of Sun Yat-sen University, Guangzhou, China

Xin-Wei Li, Qiu-Shi Xu, Ren-He Zhang, Yu-Ming Zhang, Yu Tian, Min Zhang, Zhe Wang, Guo-wen Liu and Xiao-Bing Li
Key Laboratory of Zoonosis, Ministry of Education, College of Veterinary Medicine, Jilin University, 5333 Xi'an Road, Changchun, Jilin 130062, China

Cheng Xia and Wei Yan
College of animal science and veterinary medicine, Heilongjiang Bayi Agricultural University, Daqing 163319, Heilongjiang, China

Yu Li
College of Animal Science and Technology, Anhui Agricultural University, 130 West Changjiang Road, Hefei 230036, Anhui, China

K. Lucas, I. Nolte and P. Wefstaedt
Small Animal Hospital, University of Veterinary Medicine Hannover, Foundation, Bünteweg 9, D-30559 Hannover, Germany

V. Galindo-Zamora
Small Animal Clinic, Faculty of Veterinary Medicine, National University of Colombia, Bogotá, Colombia

M. Lerch and C. Stukenborg-Colsman
Department of Orthopaedic Surgery, Hannover Medical School, Hanover, Germany

B. A. Behrens, A. Bouguecha, S. Betancur and A. Almohallami
Institute of Forming Technology and Machines, Leibniz University Hannover, Hannover, Germany

Luís Belo, Isa Serrano, Eva Cunha, Carla Carneiro, Luis Tavares, L. Miguel Carreira and Manuela Oliveira
Centre for Interdisciplinary Research in Animal Health (CIISA) / Faculty of Veterinary Medicine, University of Lisbon, Avenida da Universidade Técnica, 1300-477 Lisbon, Portugal

Lucia Bel
Department of Surgery, University of Agricultural Sciences and Veterinary Medicine, 3-5 Mănăştur Street, Cluj-Napoca 400372, Romania

Marco Tecilla
Department of Veterinary Sciences and Public Health, University of Milan, Milan, Italy

Gabriel Borza and Marian Taulescu
Department of Veterinary Pathology, University of Agricultural Sciences and Veterinary Medicine, 3-5 Mănăştur Street, Cluj-Napoca 400372, Romania

Cosmin Pestean
Department of Anesthesiology and Intensive Care, University of AgriculturalSciences and Veterinary Medicine, 3-5 Mănăştur Street, Cluj-Napoca 400372, Romania

Robert Purdoiu
Department of Radiology, University of Agricultural Sciences and Veterinary Medicine, 3-5 Mănăştur Street, Cluj-Napoca 400372, Romania

Ciprian Ober and Liviu Oana
Department of Surgical Techniques, University of Agricultural Sciences and Veterinary Medicine, 3-5 Mănăştur Street, Cluj-Napoca 400372, Romania

Ahmed Ibrahim and Magda M. Ali
Department of Surgery, Anesthesiology and Radiology, Faculty of veterinary medicine, Assuit University, Assuit 70155, Egypt

Nasser S. Abou-Khalil
Department of Medical physiology, Faculty of medicine, Assuit University, Assuit, Egypt

Marwa F. Ali
Department of Pathology and clinical pathology, Faculty of veterinary medicine, Assuit University, Assuit, Egypt

Luca Bellini and Matteo Candaten
Veterinary Teaching Hospital, University of Padua, Viale dell'Università 16, 35020 Legnaro, PD, Italy

Irene A. Veladiano, Magdalena Schrank and Antonio Mollo
Department of Animal Medicine, Production and Health, University of Padua, Viale dell'Università 16, 35020 Legnaro, PD, Italy

Stephanie Lindley, Harry W. Boothe and Ralph A. Henderson
Department of Clinical Sciences, Auburn University College of Veterinary Medicine, Auburn University, Auburn, AL, USA

Janet A. Grimes
Department of Clinical Sciences, Auburn University College of Veterinary Medicine, Auburn University, Auburn, AL, USA
Department of Small Animal Medicine and Surgery, College of Veterinary Medicine, University of Georgia, 2200 College Station Road, Athens, GA 30602, USA

Nripesh Prasad and Shawn Levy
Genomics Services Laboratory, HudsonAlpha Institute for Biotechnology, Huntsville, AL, USA

Russell Cattley
Department of Pathobiology, Auburn University College of Veterinary Medicine, Auburn University, Auburn, AL, USA

Bruce F. Smith
Scott Ritchey Research Center, Auburn University College of Veterinary Medicine, Auburn University, Auburn, AL, USA

Carla Faria Orlandini, Denis Steiner, André Giarola Boscarato, Gabriel Coelho Gimenes and Luiz Romulo Alberton
Department of Veterinary Medicine and Graduate Program in Animal Science, Universidade Paranaense, Praça Mascarenhas de Moraes 4282, Zona III, 87502-210 Umuarama, Paraná, Brazil

Yumiko Yamazaki
Advanced Research Centres, Keio University, 35 Shinanomachi, Shinjuku-ku, Tokyo 160-8582, Japan
Laboratory for Symbolic Cognitive Development, RIKEN BSI, 2-1 Hirosawa, Wako-shi, Saitama 351-0198, Japan

Shinpei Kawarai
Laboratory of Small Animal Clinics, Veterinary Teaching Hospital, Azabu University, 1-17-71 Fuchinobe, Chuo-ku, Sagamihara-shi, Kanagawa 252-5201, Japan

Atsushi Iriki
Laboratory of Small Animal Clinics, Veterinary Teaching Hospital, Azabu University, 1-17-71 Fuchinobe, Chuo-ku, Sagamihara-shi, Kanagawa 252-5201, Japan
RIKEN-NTU Research Centre for Human Biology, Nanyang Technological University, Singapore 639798, Singapore

Hidetoshi Morita
Graduate School of Environmental and Life Science, Okayama University, 1-1-1 Tsushimanaka, Kita-ku, Okayama-shi, Okayama 700-8530, Japan

Takefumi Kikusui
Companion Animal Research, School of Veterinary Medicine, Azabu University, 1-17-71 Fuchinobe, Chuo-ku, Sagamihara-shi, Kanagawa 252-5201, Japan

M. E. Olson
Alberta Veterinary Laboratories, 411 19th Street SE, Calgary, Alberta T2E 6J7, Canada

Brenda Ralston and Les Burwash
Alberta Agriculture and Forestry, 97 East Lake Ramp NE, Airdrie, Alberta T4A 0C3, Canada

Heather Matheson-Bird
Alberta Horse Industry Association, 97 East Lake Ramp NE, Airdrie, Alberta T4A 0C3, Canada

Nick D. Allan
4Chinook Contract Research, 97 East Lake Ramp NE, Airdrie, Alberta T4A 0C3, Canada

I. Airikkala-Otter and L. Gamble
Worldwide Veterinary Service, 4 Castle Street, Cranborne, Dorset BH21 5PZ, UK

S. Mazeri, I. G. Handel, B. M. de C. Bronsvoort and N. V. Meunier
The Epidemiology, Economics and Risk Assessment (EERA) Group, The Roslin Institute and the Royal (Dick) School of Veterinary Studies (R(D)SVS), Easter Bush, Midlothian EH25 9RG, UK

R. J. Mellanby
The Royal (Dick) School of Veterinary Studies (R(D) SVS) and the Roslin Institute, Hospital for Small Animals, Easter Bush Veterinary Centre, Midlothian EH25 9RG, UK

James C. Ferguson, Veronika Hruschka, Heinz Redl and Thomas Nau
Ludwig Boltzmann Institute for Experimental and Clinical Traumatology in AUVA research center, Vienna, Austria
Austrian Cluster for Tissue Regeneration, Vienna, Austria

Patrick Heimel
Ludwig Boltzmann Institute for Experimental and Clinical Traumatology in AUVA research center, Vienna, Austria
Austrian Cluster for Tissue Regeneration, Vienna, Austria
Karl Donath Laboratory for Hard Tissue and Biomaterial Research, Department of Oral Surgery, School of Dentistry, Medical University of Vienna, Vienna, Austria

Stefan Tangl
Department of Evolutionar Anthropology, Faculty of Life Sciences, University of Vienna, Vienna, Austria
Karl Donath Laboratory for Hard Tissue and Biomaterial Research, Department of Oral Surgery, School of Dentistry, Medical University of Vienna, Vienna, Austria

Dirk Barnewitz and Antje Genzel
Research Centre of Medical Technology and Biotechnology, fzmb GmbH, Bad Langensalza, Germany

Heather A. Richbourg
Department of Orthopaedic Surgery, University of California San Francisco, San Francisco, CA, USA
Department of Comparative Biomedical Sciences, Louisiana State University School of Veterinary Medicine, Baton Rouge, LA, USA

Ashley N. Gillett
Department of Comparative Biomedical Sciences, Louisiana State University School of Veterinary Medicine, Baton Rouge, LA, USA

Margaret A. McNulty
Department of Comparative Biomedical Sciences, Louisiana State University School of Veterinary Medicine, Baton Rouge, LA, USA
Department of Anatomy and Cell Biology, Indiana University School of Medicine, Indianapolis, IN, USA

Colin F. Mitchell
Department of Veterinary Clinical Sciences, Louisiana State University School of Veterinary Medicine, Baton Rouge, LA 70803, USA

Matthew D. Winter and Daniel D. Lewis
Department of Small Animal Clinical Sciences, College of Veterinary Medicine, University of Florida, Gainesville, FL 32610-0126, USA

Marije Risselada
Department of Small Animal Clinical Sciences, College of Veterinary Medicine, University of Florida, Gainesville, FL 32610-0126, USA
Department of Veterinary Clinical Sciences, College of Veterinary Medicine, Purdue University, Lynn Hall, 625 Harrison Street, West Lafayette, IN47907, USA

Antonio Pozzi
Department of Small Animal Clinical Sciences, College of Veterinary Medicine, University of Florida, Gainesville, FL 32610-0126, USA
Department for Small Animals, Vetsuisse University of Zurich, Winterthurerstrasse 258c, 8057 Zurich, Switzerland

Emily Griffith3
Department of Statistics, College of Agriculture and Life Sciences, North Carolina State University, Raleigh, NC, USA

C. King, M. Smith, K. Currie, A. Dickson, F. Smith and P. Flowers
Department of Nursing and Community Health, School of Health and Life Sciences, Glasgow Caledonian University, Cowcaddens Road, Glasgow G4 0BA, Scotland, UK

M. Davis
School of Social Sciences, Monash University, Melbourne, Australia

Gaudenz Dolf and Claude Gaillard
Institute of Genetics, Vetsuisse Faculty, University of Berne, Bremgartenstrasse 109a, 3001 Berne, Switzerland

Jane Russenberger and Lou Moseley
Guiding Eyes for the Blind, 611 Granite Springs Road, Yorktown Heights, NY 10598, USA

Claude Schelling
Clinic of Reproductive Medicine, Vetsuisse Faculty, University of Zurich, Winterthurerstrasse 260, 8057 Zurich, Switzerland

Marco Aurélio A. Pereira, Lucas A. Gonçalves, Rosana S. Thurler, Karina D. Campos, Maira R. Formenton, Geni C. F. Patricio, Julia M. Matera, Aline M. Ambrósio and Denise T. Fantoni
Faculty of Veterinary Medicine and Animal Sciences, Department of Surgery, University of Sao Paulo, 87, Av Professor Doutor Orlando Marques de Paiva, Sao Paulo 05508-270, Brazil

Marina C. Evangelista
Faculty of Veterinary Medicine, Department of Clinical Sciences, Université de Montréal, Saint Hyacinthe, Quebec, Canada

Pierre Langer, Cameron Black, Padraig Egan and Noel Fitzpatrick
Fitzpatrick Referrals, Orthopaedic and Neurology Hospital, Halfway Lane, Eashing, Godalming GU7 2QQ, UK

B. G. Murphy, M. Y. Mok, K. D. Woolard and C. Hillman
Department Pathology, University of California, Davis, School of Veterinary Medicine, Microbiology and Immunology, Davis, CA 95618, USA

D. York, R. Rebhun, P. Dickinson and K. Skorupski
Department of Surgical and Radiological Sciences, Davis, CA 95618, USA

Index

A

Anaesthesia, 20, 24, 27-28, 30-31, 33-34, 82-84, 86, 88, 90, 126, 139-140, 191-192, 194

Appendicular Osteosarcoma, 199, 205-206

Arteriovenous Fistulas, 1

B

Bone Grafting, 133, 139, 141, 164

Bone Mineral Density, 54-55, 57-62, 144, 152

Bone Regeneration, 133-134, 136, 138-141, 149-150, 196

Bonewelding, 190-191, 195-198

C

Calcium Chloride, 74-76, 78-82

Canine Femora, 54, 60

Canine Femur, 55-56, 60, 141

Canine Osa Tissue, 199-200, 205

Canine Osa Tissue Microarrays, 205

Canine Osteosarcoma, 199, 202, 206

Canine Renal Cortical Tissue, 200, 203

Canine Spleens, 91

Canine Splenic Hemangiosarcoma, 91-92, 99-101

Canine Splenic Masses, 92

Canine Stifles, 13, 164

Cavalier King Charles Spaniel, 190-191, 193, 197

Chemical Castration, 74-75, 78, 80-82, 125

Chlorhexidine, 63-68, 82, 115, 126

Clodronate, 143-146, 148-152

Clostridium Difficile, 109, 111-113

Common Marmoset, 109, 112-113

Continuous Rate Infusion, 2

Cystadenocarcinoma, 69

D

Diaphragmatic Hernia, 19-21, 23-25

Dual-energy X-ray Absorptiometry, 54-55, 61

E

Equids, 26-27

Equine Surgery, 26, 35, 82, 107

Ethylenediaminetetraacetic Acid, 146, 151

Eublepharis Macularius, 15, 18

F

Faecal Microbiota Transplantation, 109-110, 112

G

Gelatinous Matrix, 153-154, 157, 163

German Shepherd, 5, 21, 175, 182

Green Iguana, 69-73

H

Hernioplasty, 103, 108

Hind Limb Amputation, 1-2, 13

I

Iguana Iguana, 69-70, 72-73

Immunohistochemistry, 93, 199-200, 203-205

Inflammation, 27, 33, 35, 81, 107, 115, 117-119, 123-124, 184, 195

L

Labrador Retriever, 21, 174-175, 181-182, 202

Left Displacement of Abomasum, 47, 52

Leopard Gecko, 15-16, 18

Load-sharing Classification, 38

M

Malignant Ovarian Teratoma, 69-70, 72-73

Mean Invasive Arterial Blood Pressure, 83, 86-87

Meloxicam Oral Suspension, 114-115, 118-119, 123-124

Methicillin-resistant S. Pseudintermedius, 64, 67

Metronidazole, 109-110, 112-113

Monosegmental Pedicle Instrumentation, 37-40, 42

N

Nodular Hyperplasia, 91-99

O

Oral Meloxicam, 114-115, 119, 123-124

Oscillometric Method, 83, 85-86

Ovarian Neoplasms, 69

Ovarian Tumors, 69

Ovariectomy, 71, 183-186, 188-189

Ovariohysterectomy, 21, 23-24, 35, 64, 125-126, 128-132, 183-186, 188-189

P

Pyloric Canal, 47, 49, 52

R

Reposition Surgery, 47-52

S

Septic Synovitis, 26-27

Serum Amyloid A, 26-27, 34-36

Serum Testosterone Levels, 76, 78, 80-81

Short-segment Pedicle Instrumentation, 37-40, 42-43, 45

Short-segment Pedicle Screw Instrumentation, 38

Skin Asepsis Protocols, 63-65, 67

Stereotactic Radiation Therapy, 199

Sterilisation Surgery, 125-126, 128

Surgical Castration, 74-75, 78, 81-82, 114-115, 118, 122-123, 132

Surgical Site Infections, 63-64, 66-68, 130, 132

Surgical Sterilization, 82, 132, 183-184, 186, 188

T

Tibial Tuberosity Advancement, 153-154, 163-164

Tiludronate, 143-145, 148-152

U

Ultrasonography, 20, 47-49, 51-53, 69-70, 103-106, 154, 156, 158-159, 161, 163-164

V

Veterinarians, 1, 8, 12-13, 48, 67, 115, 123, 126, 130-132, 173

Veterinary Hospital, 104, 107, 184

Veterinary Instructors, 126-127

Veterinary Medicine, 1-2, 13, 19, 25-28, 31, 35, 47, 53-55, 60-61, 63-64, 67, 69, 72-75, 82, 91, 100, 103, 107, 113, 132, 143, 151-153, 155, 163, 165, 183-184, 188, 195, 199, 205-206

Veterinary Surgeons, 127, 164-173

Titanium Mesh, 190, 193-195, 197

Traumatic Diaphragmatic Hernia, 19-20, 24-25

Traumatic Rupture, 103-104

www.ingramcontent.com/pod-product-compliance
Lightning Source LLC
Chambersburg PA
CBHW082039190326
41458CB00010B/3408